Neuropsychological Formulation

Jamie A. B. Macniven
Editor

Neuropsychological Formulation

A Clinical Casebook

Springer

Editor
Jamie A. B. Macniven
Department of Neurology
Auckland City Hospital
Auckland, New Zealand

ISBN 978-3-319-35297-8 ISBN 978-3-319-18338-1 (eBook)
DOI 10.1007/978-3-319-18338-1

Springer Cham Heidelberg New York Dordrecht London

Softcover re-print of the Hardcover 1st edition 2016

Printed on acid-free paper

Springer International Publishing AG Switzerland is part of Springer Science+Business Media (www.springer.com)

Preface

> Analysis and synthesis are thus the incessantly alternating mental activities, a stroke of the one preparing the way for a stroke of the other, much as, in walking, a man's two legs are alternately brought into use, both being indispensable for any orderly advance.
>
> William James (1890, p. 550)

Clinical neuropsychologists work across diverse cultures and clinical settings, and with an enormous range of patient presentations and health conditions. There are a number of common strands to what we do. Perhaps the three most consistent components are clinical assessment, cognitive testing, and diagnosis. There is almost always a fourth component: neuropsychological formulation. It is this core skill that perhaps sets us apart from other health professionals. It is in this process of analysis and synthesis that we draw together those disconnected facts—the history, clinical interview, and cognitive test results—and create a meaningful narrative to describe a person's experience after neurological illness or injury.

This book is an attempt to illustrate some of the complexities, themes, and diversity of neuropsychological formulation. As our profession continues to develop rapidly across the world, I believe that neuropsychological formulation will increasingly be seen as the core competency that defines our contribution to healthcare. I am enormously grateful to the chapter authors for providing such fascinating and informative insights into the process of neuropsychological formulation as practised in different clinical settings and countries, with a diverse range of referral questions and presenting problems.

Clinical psychology training typically involves a focus on formulation: A pivotal process in the assessment and therapeutic process of working with people who have mental health problems. Clinical psychologists are encouraged to utilise therapeutic frameworks such as cognitive-behavioural theory to develop hypotheses, help people understand their situation, and to plan intervention. Formulations might be diagrammatic; illustrations of a person's psychological experience. Alternatively, and perhaps more commonly, narrative formulations summarise the predisposing, precipitating, and maintaining factors that explain a person's psychological distress. The same process applies equally well to neuropsychological assessment and intervention. The added dimensions that often make this process more complex include neuropsychological data, neurological history, and neuroimaging.

In many countries, most clinical neuropsychologists are originally trained as clinical psychologists. The concept of formulation has perhaps, therefore, been intuitively integrated into the practices of many neuropsychologists. Most considered, thoughtful, neuropsychological assessments will implicitly lead to meaningful formulations. However, there is limited literature on the subject. Trainees and assistants are likely to struggle to find numerous published examples of diagrammatic or narrative formulations around which to frame their own work. This book is an attempt to add to this literature and in doing so to describe the various ideas, perspectives, techniques, and skills that make clinical neuropsychology such a valuable component of modern healthcare.

Each chapter of this book focuses on one or more cases in which an important neuropsychological process, concept, or issue is elucidated. The focus is of course always on neuropsychological formulation in its many guises. We are fortunate to have a breadth of patient ages, neurological conditions, clinical settings, and countries of practice represented across the chapters. As a UK-trained clinical psychologist and neuropsychologist now living and working in New Zealand, I am interested in the commonalities and differences in our work internationally. I believe that we can all benefit from an understanding of how neuropsychology is practised differently across cultures. This book is just a step in that direction, with an admittedly narrow focus on neuropsychology in UK, Italy, New Zealand, the USA, and Australia.

The authors of this book have my sincere gratitude for sharing their clinical and academic insights, as do the people who all kindly consented for their neuropsychological formulations to be described. Where possible, all potentially identifying client information has been altered to maintain confidentiality.

Finally, because I may never have another chance to do so, this book is dedicated to my beloved whānau: the wonderful, wilful, and always vital Georgia, Phoebe, and Rebecca.

J.A.B.M., 2015

References

James, W. (1890). *The principles of psychology*. New York: Henry Holt and Company.

Contents

Contributors

Erin D. Bigler Department of Psychology, Brigham Young University, Provo, UT, USA; Neuroscience Center, Brigham Young University, Provo, UT, USA; Magnetic Resonance Imaging Research Facility, Brigham Young University, Provo, UT, USA; Department of Psychiatry, University of Utah, Salt Lake City, UT, USA; The Brain Institute of Utah, University of Utah, Salt Lake City, UT, USA

Stephen C. Bowden Melbourne School of Psychological Sciences, University of Melbourne, Melbourne, Victoria, Australia; Neuropsychology Unit, Department of Clinical Neurosciences, St. Vincent's Hospital, Fitzroy, Victoria, Australia

Mark J. Cook Department of Medicine and Department of Clinical Neurosciences, St. Vincent's Hospital, Fitzroy, Victoria, Australia

Roberto Cubelli Department of Psychology and Cognitive Sciences, University of Trento, Corso Bettini, Rovereto, Italy

Kay L. Cunningham PO Box 152, Miramar Wellington, New Zealand

Sergio Della Sala Human Cognitive Neuroscience, University of Edinburgh, Edinburgh, 7 George Square, UK

Cathy Grant Department of Clinical Psychology and Neuropsychology, Nottingham University Hospitals NHS Trust, Nottingham, UK

Virginia M. Hogg School of Psychology and Centre for Brain Research, The University of Auckland, Auckland, New Zealand

Vicky T. Lomay Tsinajini Psychology Services, Mesa, AZ, USA

Silva Pedrizzi Rehabilitation Unit, Pierantoni Hospital, Forlì, (FC), Italy

George P. Prigatano Barrow Neurological Institute, Phoenix, AZ, USA

Ron Ruff University of California-San Francisco, San Francisco, CA, USA

Leonie C. Simpson Neuropsychology Unit, Department of Clinical Neurosciences, St. Vincent's Hospital, Fitzroy, Victoria, Australia

Martha Sorensen AT&R Unit, Middlemore Hospital, Neuropsychology and Rehabilitation, Colvin Complex, Otahuhu, Auckland, New Zealand

Arleta Starza-Smith Department of Clinical Psychology and Neuropsychology, Nottingham University Hospitals NHS Trust, Nottingham, UK

Robert D. Stephens Department of Clinical Psychology and Neuropsychology, Nottingham University Hospitals NHS Trust, Nottingham, UK

Greg Savage ARC Centre of Excellence in Cognition and Its Disorders (CCD), Department of Psychology, Macquarie University, University Avenue, Sydney, Australia

Emily Talbot Department of Clinical Psychology and Neuropsychology, Nottingham University Hospitals NHS Trust, Nottingham, UK

Lynette J. Tippett School of Psychology and Centre for Brain Research, The University of Auckland, Auckland, New Zealand

Patrick Vesey Department of Clinical Psychology and Neuropsychology, Nottingham University Hospitals NHS Trust, Nottingham, UK

Christina Weyer Jamora San Francisco General Hospital & University of California-San Francisco, San Francisco, CA, USA

Ingram Wright Department of Experimental Psychology, University of Bristol, The Priory Road Complex, Bristol, UK

Chapter 1
The Interface of Neuroimaging with Neuropsychological Findings in Traumatic Brain Injury

Erin D. Bigler

Neuropsychological assessment provides the psychometric framework to identify the neurobehavioral and neurocognitive consequences of a traumatic brain injury (TBI). Neuropsychological assessment has a long tradition as a stand-alone method to characterize the level and degree of impaired functioning from TBI. However, twenty-first century advanced neuroimaging procedures are now available, which provide anatomical and functional details about the brain, the nature of potential pathologies, and their influence over time (Bigler 2013; Chanraud et al. 2010; Jak et al. 2009), which should be routinely incorporated into the neuropsychological examination. Nevertheless, despite these improvements in neuroimaging, neuropsychological assessment techniques have made only the smallest steps in integrating neuroimaging findings into the process of neuropsychological assessment (Bilder 2011). As Jagaroo (2009) points out for neuropsychology to embrace twenty-first century technologies it needs to integrate the available neuroinformatics, the most important of which may be the information contained in neuroimaging studies.

The TBI case presented herein outlines some of the neuroimaging methods and findings that could routinely be incorporated into the neuropsychological assessment.

Case The patient was a 63-year-old truck driver involved in a head-on collision caused by another semi travelling at highway speeds that had lost control, coming from the opposite direction. As a consequence of the severity of the collision and vehicular damage an extended extrication was required. The patient was found "unconscious" by highway patrol and eyewitness accounts with obvious trauma to the head includ-

E. D. Bigler (✉)
Department of Psychology, Brigham Young University, 1001 SWKT, Provo, UT 84602, USA
Neuroscience Center, Brigham Young University, 1001 SWKT, Provo, UT 84602, USA
Magnetic Resonance Imaging Research Facility, Brigham Young University, Provo, UT, USA
Department of Psychiatry, University of Utah, Salt Lake City, UT, USA
The Brain Institute of Utah, University of Utah, Salt Lake City, UT, USA
e-mail: erin_bigler@byu.edu

J. A. B. Macniven (ed.), *Neuropsychological Formulation*,
DOI 10.1007/978-3-319-18338-1_1

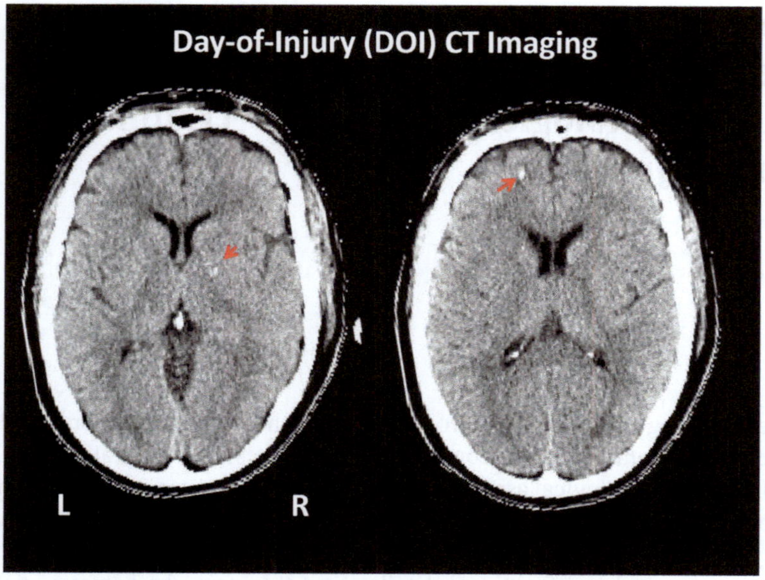

Fig. 1.1 Axial day-of-injury CT scan showing the location of two of several petechial hemorrhages *right* at the *gray–white* matter junction *(white arrow*, *right)* in the *left* frontal lobe and *right* internal capsule *(red arrow*, *left)* adjacent to the globus pallidus, common findings associated with traumatic shear lesions (Gean and Fischbein 2010)

ing extensive facial lacerations, bleeding, and multiple other injuries including an initially compromised airway. At the scene, the Glasgow Coma Scale (GCS) of the patient was rated as 7/15 by emergency medical service as the patient was being extricated, which was also the emergency department (ED) GCS score before sedation and intubation. Day-of-injury (DOI) CT imaging documented multiple intraparenchymal petechial hemorrhages, consistent with diffuse axonal injury (DAI); some of which are shown in Fig. 1.1. Several repeat scans showed stable hemorrhagic lesions with no change and no progression of the cerebral edema. No neurosurgical intervention took place although extensive surgery was needed to treat the scalp and facial lacerations; however, because of the extensive lacerations to the head with excessive blood loss and internal injuries, the patient received an ED diagnosis of hypovolemic shock. He gradually improved with conservative care over the next few days with posttraumatic amnesia persisting for about a week. He had mild motor and balance deficits likely associated in part with acute petechial hemorrhage noted in the region of the internal capsule/basal ganglia (see Fig. 1.1). The patient received limited inpatient rehabilitation, which included cognitive rehabilitation by a speech therapist.

Five Months Post-Injury

The patient was seen on two occasions for neuropsychological consultation, 5 months and 2 years post-injury. Litigation was present as the accident was caused by the other truck driver, but was settled out of court. Due to persisting memory complaints, he was evaluated approximately 5 months post-injury to assist in treatment planning. When initially seen, the patient complained of short-term memory problems and moodiness, corroborated by the spouse. From a self-report perspective, he described his problems with mood by stating "My wife thinks I have a short fuse." He characterized his memory problems as "forgetfulness." He was still receiving physical therapy for residual deficits in motor and balance function as well as cognitive rehabilitation when initially assessed. He continued to experience posttraumatic headaches on a regular basis and described a moderate headache on the day of neuropsychological assessment.

By mental status standards the patient was doing well. He was fully oriented, appropriately engaged in conversational speech without any notable impairment in fluency or prosody, and had no difficulty remembering four words on immediate recall. Although he perceived maladroitness with motor skills, they were not outwardly evident. Mental status exam was considered to be rather unremarkable.

Consistent with the rather unremarkable mental status examination the neuropsychological findings, summarized in Table 1.1, demonstrated generally average

Table 1.1 Wechsler Abbreviated Scale of Intelligence (WASI)

5 months post-injury	Standard score	Percentile
Verbal IQ	86	18
Performance IQ	96	39
Full scale	91	23
2 years post-injury		
Verbal IQ	91	27
Performance IQ	101	53
Full scale	96	40
Speed of processing—Trail making test		
5 months post-injury	Seconds	*z-score*
Trails A	77	−2.8
Trails B	149	−1.0
2 years post-injury		
Trails A	39	−0.02
Trails B	119	−0.05

California verbal learning test											
Trials											
	1	2	3	4	5	1–5	T-B	S-Free	S-Cue	L-F	L-Cue
5 Months post-injury											
Raw score	3	8	7	7	10	35	3	6	8	6	6
z-score	−2.0	0.0	−1.0	−1.0	0.00	43 (T)	−1.5	−0.5	−1.0	−1.0	−1.5
2 Years post-injury											
Raw score	5	7	9	9	9	39	4	8	11	0	9
z-score	−0.05	−0.05	0.00	−0.5	−0.5	48 (T)	−1.0	−0.5	0.5	−3.0	−0.5

scores in basic intellectual and academic abilities (Wide Range Achievement Test results were all within the average to low average range: Single Word Reading (32nd percentile), Sentence Comprehension (16th percentile), Spelling (9th percentile), and Math Computation (14th percentile)). Prior to injury, this individual had achieved a high school education with a work history of service and delivery jobs. He had no prior history of special education. Taken together these historical premorbid observations would suggest average ability prior to the head injury. As shown in Table 1.1, scores on the California Verbal Learning Test (CVLT), the worst performance was on the first trial. By the 5th CVLT trial, he performed at normative and pre-injury baseline expectations. In individuals with severe TBI, especially in the subacute timeframe, such a pattern is often reflective of initial challenges devoting attentional resources to initial processing with a slow rate of acquisition which over repeated trials normalizes (Millis and Ricker 1994; Wright and Schmitter-Edgecombe 2011). Processing speed, commonly affected in severe TBI (Kourtidou et al. 2013), was also slow, as reflected in the Trail Making Test performance (see Table 1.1). The combination of slowed processing and attentional problems can be disruptive to working memory, especially when competing stimuli are present in the natural environment.

On self-report questionnaires, including the Beck Depression Inventory, Symptom Checklist-90, and Personality Assessment Inventory, the patient reported mild to moderate levels of depression. At this point he had not been receiving any mental health intervention, including no pharmacotherapy. In light of these emotional findings, treatment recommendations including psychiatric and psychotherapy referrals were made.

Only clinical acute to subacute CT imaging had been done while hospitalized. As mentioned, a finding of petechial hemorrhage constitutes the neuroimaging marker for DAI (Scheid et al. 2003; Scheid et al. 2006). Presence of DAI implicates white matter (WM) damage, consistent with slowed processing speed and problems with working memory (Kinnunen et al. 2011; Spitz et al. 2013; Wang et al. 2011).

Two Years Post-Injury

The patient was seen at 2 years post-injury and for the most part exhibited a similar neuropsychological profile with expected improvements in processing speed noted on the Trail Making Test (see Table 1.1). However, memory complaints persisted and, in comparison to findings at 5 months post-injury, performance was reduced on several of the index scores from the Wechsler Memory Scale-Third edition (WMS-III), as shown in Table 1.2. Another notable difference was in regards to mental status where clinically the patient appeared more depressed and lethargic. Indeed, his Beck Depression Inventory which was in the moderate range (score of 20) when first assessed but had risen to severe (score of 30) at the 2 year follow-up. On the Symptom Checklist the depression subtest T-score was >80.

Table 1.2 Wechsler Memory Scale-Third edition (WMS-III)

Index score	5 months post-injury	2 years post-injury
	Standard score	*Standard score*
Auditory immediate	97	92
Visual immediate memory	88	78
Immediate memory	91	82
Auditory delayed	102	99
Visual delayed	72	81
General memory	93	88
Working memory	91	91

Physically there were no obvious stigmata of injury, except for the scars associated with the scalp lacerations. General motor abilities had returned to baseline. No motor, sensory-perceptual or language deficits were evident in the test results. Speech production and prosody appeared normal, including performance on word fluency measures. Prior to the TBI he had never accessed mental health services, but was now under the care of a psychiatrist and taking antidepressant medication. He and his wife were in marital counseling. A major source of the marital conflict was the patient's lack of drive and interest in activities which prior to the injury had been a source of mutual enjoyment. The spouse reported that her husband had diminished drive with little ambition to "do anything," including reduced interest in previous hobbies and activities that were part of his life prior to injury. Due to this, as a couple they had withdrawal from most pre-injury social activities despite his excellent physical recovery at this point in time.

Clearly by the second visit depressive symptoms and apathy dominated the clinical picture. There were no pathognomonic features to the neuropsychological findings as most test scores were within the range that could be expected, given his age, educational, and vocational background. From this perspective a reasonably good cognitive recovery from this severe TBI had occurred. With a high school educational background and vocational history of nontechnical service oriented jobs, the assumption was that premorbid abilities would have been within the broad spectrum of average, which is the same range where the majority of neuropsychological test findings were observed on both assessments. Furthermore, normative studies have shown that subjects within standardization samples have several subpar scores (Binder et al. 2009; Zakzanis and Jeffay 2011), so there was nothing distinctive about the post-severe TBI neuropsychological findings in this patient reflecting a cognitive deficit. Additionally, in the follow-up assessment below cut-score performance on some symptom validity tests occurred, likely a reflection of the severe depression and lack of test engagement that reduced test performance.

So what can be made of these neuropsychological test findings, if interpreted in isolation? Is the patient merely depressed? Is the depression independent of the TBI? Is there residual "brain damage" that affects behavioral function?

Neuropsychological Conclusions Based Solely on Neuropsychological Test Findings

If the neuropsychological test findings and the history of having sustained a severe TBI were the only information for clinical decision-making, it would be a challenge to fully understand the neurobehavioral syndrome experienced by this patient. He was administered the Delis–Kaplan Executive Function System, but on most subtests displayed scores within the average range, except distinctly slow speed on the color–word interference task, which was at the 2nd percentile. From a behavioral perspective this patient presented in a rather listless, nonengaging fashion. Eye contact was rather poor with gaze typically away from the examiner, often looking towards the floor. Mild psychomotor retardation was noted along with a depressed countenance. A separate interview with the spouse confirmed that these behavioral features were also present in the home setting and because of these behavioral changes they mostly avoided social activities. The DOI CT showed only petechial hemorrhages and no other major structural damage. With a GCS of 7/15 and a post-traumatic amnesia (PTA) in excess of a week, there can be no debate that a severe TBI had occurred, but were the emotional problems and diminished drive merely secondary to the development of a major mood disorder or something more specific to the TBI?

Added Value of Neuroimaging

Returning to the Fig. 1.1, an abnormality right at the gray–white matter junction constitutes a classic shear lesion and a marker for DAI as noted on the initial DOI CT (Gean and Fischbein 2010), but is there more to the lesion than can be shown on a DOI CT? Figures 1.2–1.6 from follow-up magnetic resonance imaging (MRI) studies, including diffusion tensor imaging (DTI) provide the answer. Figure 1.2 shows that the region where the initial small hemorrhage was detected (compare Fig. 1.1 with Fig. 1.2 and subsequent figures) in the left frontal lobe continues to display hemosiderin deposition, particularly notable on the susceptibility weighted imaging (SWI) sequence (see Fig. 1.2a). Hemosiderin is a blood by-product in TBI that reflects not only the shearing forces of the trauma to brain parenchyma but also the vasculature. Residual blood by-products indicates tissue strain-tearing at the point of hemorrhage with the implications of considerable tissue deformation, particularly involving the WM in or around where the hemosiderin is observed. In Fig. 1.2, the residual hemosiderin appears to be small, just as in the acute CT imaging in Fig. 1.1. It is also evident that the other MRI sequences were not very sensitive in detecting the hemosiderin.

Fortunately, the SWI sequence is exquisitely sensitive to hemosiderin deposition as a DAI marker and in this case, when the entire brain was viewed extensive shear pathology was evident, as shown in Fig. 1.3. This sagittally reconstructed view through the mid-left frontal lobe shows a ribbon of prior bleeding right at the gray–

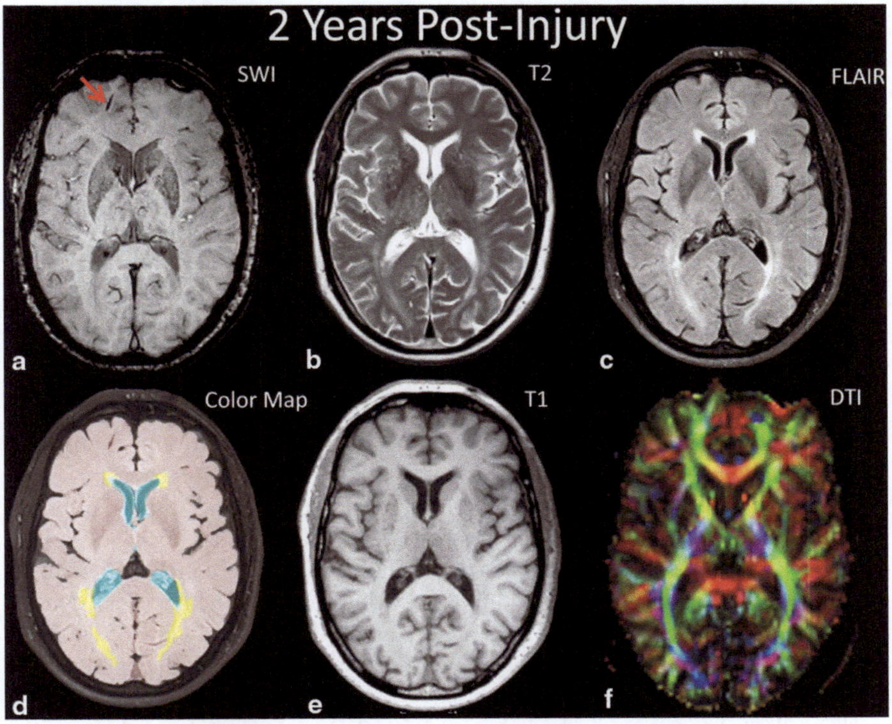

Fig. 1.2 Different Axial MRI sequences at the same level showing different sensitivities in detecting traumatic related neuropathologies. In the susceptibility-weighted imaging *(SWI)* sequence, the *red arrow* points to residual hemosiderin where the original hemorrhage was noted in the frontal lobe in the DOI CT (see Fig. 1.1). The fluid attenuated inversion recovery *(FLAIR)* sequence shows periventricular white matter hyperintensities *(WMH)* including signal changes in deeper WM regions. The color map merely colorizes the ventricular system (aquamarine) with the WMHs shown in *yellow* for easier identification. The diffusion tensor imaging *(DTI)* represents the raw color map where *green* reflects aggregate pathways that course within the anterior to posterior plane, the warm *orange-red* course laterally, or side-to-side, and the *blue* are vertically oriented pathways

Fig. 1.3 SWI cut in the sagittal plane shows multiple areas of hemosiderin deposition within the frontal lobe from the TBI

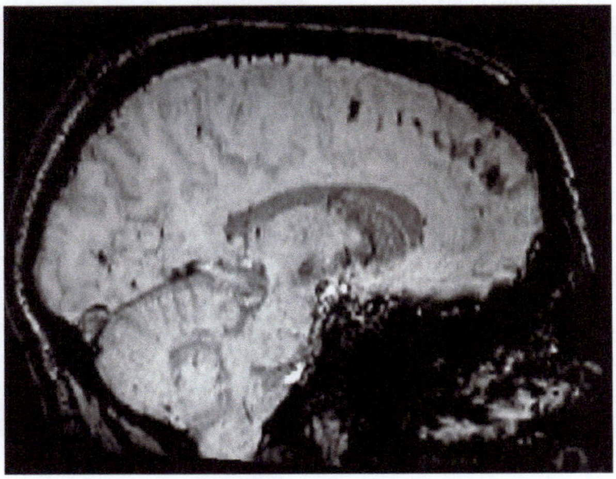

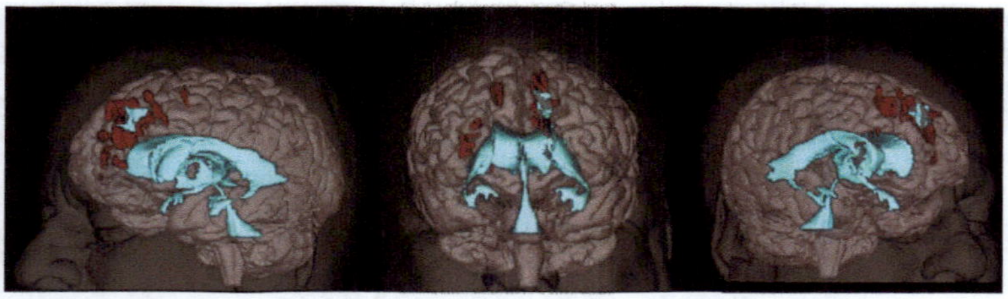

Fig. 1.4 As depicted in *red* in the various 3-D renderings of the brain of this TBI patient, the extensive hemosiderin deposition throughout both frontal lobes, but in particular the *left*. For reference, the ventricular system is shown in aquamarine. The most prominent shear lesion, originally identified in the DOI CT scan (see Fig. 1.1) left a small pocket of cerebrospinal fluid, which explains the aquamarine coloration mixed in with where the hemosiderin is frontally located

white matter junction extending from the anterior frontal region to a more posterior classic region for hemorrhagic shear lesions involving the frontal lobe.

If only viewed at a singular MRI level as in Fig. 1.2 or with only the CT information (Fig. 1.1), the extensiveness of the damage would not be appreciated. In fact, often the small petechial hemorrhages noted on the DOI CT are but a reflection of the "tip-of-the-iceberg." As shown in Fig. 1.4, the locations of hemosiderin deposition plotted in three-dimensional (3-D) space on a 3-D rendered view of the brain demonstrates the range of pathology directly related to shearing phenomena that occurred predominantly in the frontal area.

Using the tractography method also applying 3-D neuroimaging analyses of the DTI findings to extract aggregate WM tracts involving the corpus callosum, substantial tract loss had occurred at the level of the forceps minor, clearly evident in Fig. 1.5 as pointed to by the red arrow. Overall thinning of corpus callosum tracts was observed as well, so the pathology was not just restricted to the anterior aspect of the corpus callosum. Such findings would be consistent with reduced connectivity as a consequence of the TBI (Bigler 2013).

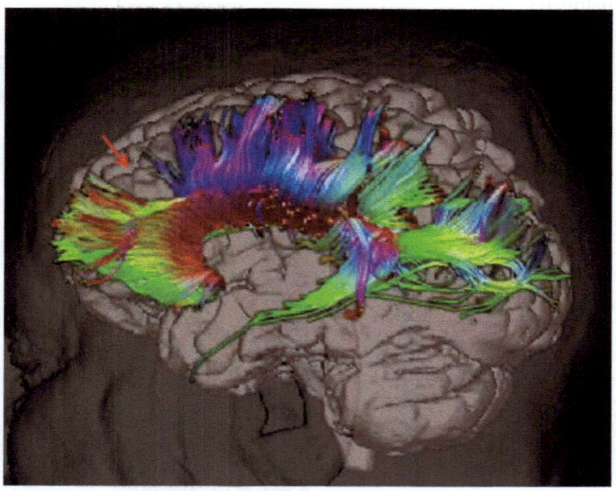

Fig. 1.5 Lateral view of the left hemisphere with tractography identified corpus callosum interhemispheric projections where a major dropout of frontal projecting tracts can be seen *(red arrow)*. See Fig. 1.3 for description of what the color maps indicate. In Figs. 1.2 and 1.6, the extent of WM pathology as reflected in FLAIR signal abnormality is depicted in *yellow*

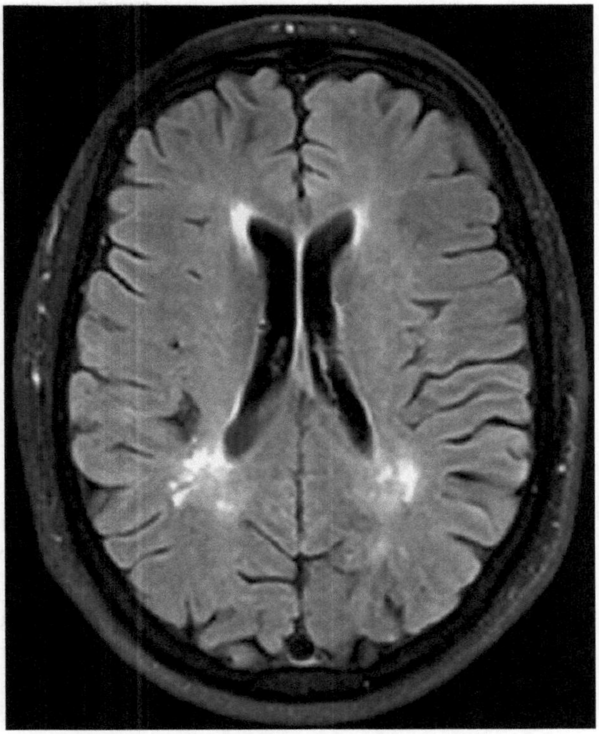

Fig. 1.6 Axial FLAIR image at the level of the centrum semiovale showing deep WM signal abnormality

Furthermore, as may be recalled from the initial description of the injury this patient experienced significant blood loss and hypovolemic shock. Presence of traumatic parenchymal injury induced edema and associated metabolic changes, intraparenchymal hemorrhage from shear injury combined with the excessive blood loss likely led to ischemic brain injury in addition to the direct trauma. In fact, extensive WM damage was evident on the FLAIR sequence (see Figs. 1.2c and 1.6) that would be consistent with ischemic injury. Hypoxic-ischemic brain injury may also be the source of microhemorrhage as well. Returning to Fig. 1.2, there is evident hyperintense signal abnormality in the deep WM of the brain, particularly in the periventricular region; however, FLAIR imaging superior to the level shown in Fig. 1.2, as seen in Fig. 1.6, demonstrates the extensiveness of the deep WM signal abnormality. This can also be plotted in 3-D as shown in yellow in Fig. 1.7. There was no density change noted on CT imaging in the central WM on the DOI scanning, indicating that the ischemic injury likely occurred as a consequence of all of the abovementioned factors associated with the TBI. This deep central WM damage would be additive to any shear injury directly from the initial trauma, as the more generalized WM damage would occur as a secondary injury.

Inspecting the sagittal view of the SWI sequence the extensiveness of the hemorrhagic lesions and the depth of the frontal pathology may be fully appreciated (see Fig. 1.3). Combining this with the corpus callosum tractography which demonstrates major disruption across the forceps minor reflecting rather exten-

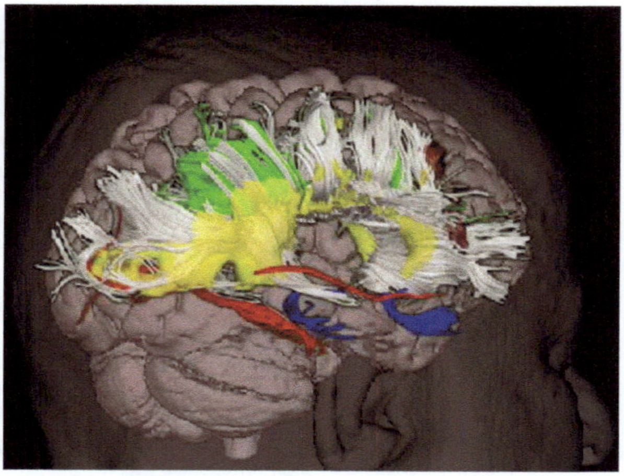

Fig. 1.7 *Right* hemisphere, posterior oblique showing different major tracts of the brain in this TBI patient as well as WM pathology *(yellow)*. *White*: corpus callosum, *green*: cingulum bundle, *blue*: Uncinate fasiculus, *red*: occipitotemporal fasciculus. *Blood red* in the front represent the locas of hemosiderin deposition in the *right* frontal lobe. Note that the occipitotemporal fasciculus on the *right* is markedly reduced in size compared to the *left*

sive disruption of frontal integration, further defines the amount of frontal pathology. Additionally, with the extensive WM pathology extending into parietofrontal connections (see Fig. 1.7) likely diminished the integrity throughout the superior longitudinal fasciculus affecting attention and default mode networks. Such pathology is likely a factor in the problems with working memory.

In examining the memory problems experienced by this patient, visual memory was consistently reduced in comparison to all other aspects of memory function on both testing occasions. Automated image analyses including volumetric assessment (Bigler et al. 2010) may be performed that provide the clinician with rather precise estimates of region of interest (ROI) volumes including the hippocam-

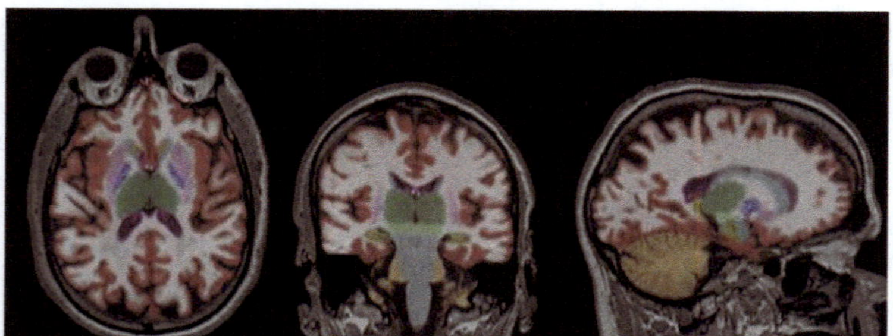

Brain Structure	Volume (cm³)	% of ICV (5–95% Normative Percentile*)	Normative Percentile*
Hippocampi	7.99	0.47 (0.43–0.59)	20.11
Lateral Ventricles	22.98	1.34 (0.31–3.38)	46.06
Inferior Lateral Ventricles	2.03	0.12 (0.07–0.25)	39.92

Fig. 1.8 NeuroQuant findings based on the color parcellation volumes from specific regions of interest: *Green*—Thalamus, *purple*—globus pallidus, *lavender*—putamen, *light blue*—caudate, *yellow*—hippocampus

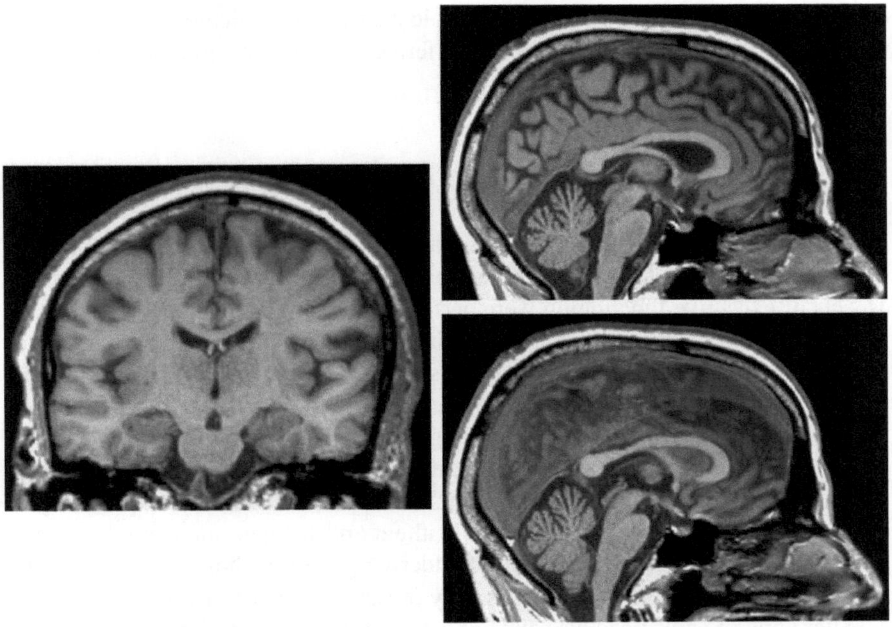

Fig. 1.9 *(Left) T1* coronal section through the level of the hippocampus. *(Top Right)* Sagittal view slightly off midline that shows generally normal appearance of the fornix without prominent atrophy of the cingulate gyrus. *(Bottom right)* Mid-sagittal view *right* at midline showing normal mammillary body size but some thinning of the posterior body of the corpus callosum

pus (Ross et al. 2012). Such analyses were performed in this case as shown in Fig. 1.8. Hippocampal volume was reduced, at the 20th percentile, but such a value is still within the lower limits of average. Furthermore, as shown in Fig. 1.9, the hippocampi are symmetric in appearance with normal size and configuration of the fornix, mammillary bodies and no prominent atrophy of the cingulate gyrus. These generally normal appearing anatomical features of Papez circuitry critical for memory suggest no obvious pathology. However, the DTI findings show not only disruption of callosal fibers but other tracts as well. For example, the occiptotemporal fasciculus in the right hemisphere was distinctly reduced in comparison to the tract on the left (see Fig. 1.7). The occipitotemporal fasciculus is involved in visual memory function (Voineskos et al. 2012). Could this be an explanation for the consistently greater deficit in visual memory impairment? Neuropathologically given the WM and DTI findings, disrupted connectivity appears to the better explanation for impaired "memory" performance, which seems to be dominated by factors associated with attention, concentration, and task engagement. Lastly, viewing the gross anatomy of the corpus callosum in Fig. 1.8, it appears generally within normal limits for an individual 63 years of age, although the posterior mid-body is thin. Viewing gross anatomy may not reveal the microstructural anatomy as depicted by DTI (see Figs. 1.5 and 1.7). Such was the case with this patient—the tractography of the corpus callosum as well as anisotropic measurements demonstrated far more widespread abnormalities that would be inferred from just the gross anatomy.

Final Case Formulation

From a cognitive perspective this individual exhibited relatively intact ability to perform neuropsychological tests, consistent with premorbid ability although some aspects of executive functioning were performed below expectation. Behaviorally, the presentation both in the assessment clinic as well as the home environment, as indicated by the spouse, suggested depressed mood which was confirmed by self-report psychometric measures. Since severe TBI is known to have a predilection for damage to frontotemporal regions and given the fact that the DOI CT scan demonstrated frontal petechial hemorrhages, it could be assumed that frontal damage from DAI had occurred in this individual, which in part would be explanatory of the findings and observations. However, without updated neuroimaging it becomes problematic to appreciate the degree of underlying brain pathology in this patient, since a major mood disorder clinically may present in this manner as well.

After applying advanced neuroimaging analyses, it became clear that the severe TBI sustained by this individual had resulted in extensive and widespread damage. Both the cognitive and neurobehavioral sequelae are likely a direct consequence of combined focal and nonspecific pathologies involving WM connectivity and network damage to limbic and frontal executive systems. As shown in the various illustrations presented in this chapter, all of this can be objectively and directly demonstrated with contemporary neuroimaging analysis methods. The mood disorder and deficits with memory, drive, and goal-directed behaviors reflected disrupted frontal lobe and integrated WM functioning as a consequence of the TBI. Post-TBI, the patient has what could be described as a "Frontal Lobe Syndrome" (see Lezak et al. 2012, pp. 91–97) characterized by both the mood and personality/behavioral changes along with a loss of drive and diminished engagement in goal-directed behaviors combined with the executive deficits in cognitive functioning.

Treatment Formulation

Continued psychiatric treatment including pharmacotherapy, individual and marital therapy were recommended. From the neuropsychological standpoint, education, and coordination with the treatment team, as well as the spouse, as to the nature of frontal lobe syndromes and WM pathology resulting from a severe TBI constituted a major role for the neuropsychologist given the type of neuropsychological test and neuroimaging information available on this patient.

Reflection/Discussion

It is now the twenty-first century and the neuropsychologist should be utilizing all technological information available in the evaluation, care, and treatment of patients with neurological and neuropsychiatric disorders. The traditional neuropsychological technique allows only inferences about neural systems. Structural neuroimaging as was done in this case provides a method for direct visualization of the brain, but the images alone possess no behavioral or cognitive information. The integration of neuropsychology with neuroimaging bring these two modalities of assessing the patient with neurological injury, disease or disorder to render a more complete and thorough clinical picture. As shown by the case used in this chapter, the clinician does not have to speculate based on just the history and neuropsychological test results that a "frontal lobe disorder" is present; confirmation comes with understanding the neuropsychological exam findings in the context of the neuroimaging where each assessment modality compliments the other.

Major advancements have been made in quantitative neuroimaging analysis and rapid image display. In my opinion, the future of neuropsychology has been outlined by Bilder (2011) where a wealth of information will be integrated algorithmically with the neuropsychological findings. Neurocognitive and neurobehavioral testing will not be examined in terms of just scores and their relation to some normative sample, but quantitatively compared to a multitude of medical and neuroimaging variables that provide information about brain anatomy, pathology as well as networks and connectivity. With the incredible sophistication of neuroimaging methods, comprehensive integration of neuroimaging findings with neuropsychological test results enhances both disciplines and provides a more complete clinical picture of the patient.

References

Bigler, E. D. (2013). Neuroimaging biomarkers in mild traumatic brain injury (mTBI). *Neuropsychology review, 23*(3), 169–209. doi:10.1007/s11065-013-9237-2.

Bigler, E. D., Abildskov, T. J., Wilde, E. A., McCauley, S. R., Li, X., Merkley, T. L., Levin, H. S., et al. (2010). Diffuse damage in pediatric traumatic brain injury: A comparison of automated versus operator-controlled quantification methods. *NeuroImage, 50*(3), 1017–1026. doi:10.1016/j.neuroimage.2010.01.003.

Bilder, R. M. (2011). Neuropsychology 3.0: evidence-based science and practice. *Journal of the International Neuropsychological Society 17*(1), 7–13. doi:10.1017/S1355617710001396.

Binder, L. M., Iverson, G. L., & Brooks, B. L. (2009). To err is human: "Abnormal" neuropsychological scores and variability are common in healthy adults. *Archives of clinical neuropsychology: The official Journal of The National Academy of Neuropsychologists, 24*(1), 31–46. doi:10.1093/arclin/acn001.

Chanraud, S., Zahr, N., Sullivan, E. V., & Pfefferbaum, A. (2010). MR diffusion tensor imaging: A window into white matter integrity of the working brain. *Neuropsychology Review, 20*(2), 209–225. doi:10.1007/s11065-010-9129-7.

Gean, A. D., & Fischbein, N. J. (2010). Head trauma. *Neuroimaging Clinics of North America, 20*(4), 527–556. doi:10.1016/j.nic.2010.08.001.
Jagaroo, V. (2009). *Neuroinformatics for neuropsychology*. New York: Springer.
Jak, A. J., Bangen, K. J., Wierenga, C. E., Delano-Wood, L., Corey-Bloom, J., & Bondi, M. W. (2009). Contributions of neuropsychology and neuroimaging to understanding clinical subtypes of mild cognitive impairment. *International Review of Neurobiology, 84,* 81–103. doi:10.1016/S0074-7742(09)00405-X.
Kinnunen, K. M., Greenwood, R., Powell, J. H., Leech, R., Hawkins, P. C., Bonnelle, V., Sharp, D. J., et al. (2011). White matter damage and cognitive impairment after traumatic brain injury. *Brain: A Journal of Neurology, 134*(Pt. 2), 449–463. doi:10.1093/brain/awq347.
Kourtidou, P., McCauley, S. R., Bigler, E. D., Traipe, E., Wu, T. C., Chu, Z. D., Wilde, E. A., et al. (2013). Centrum semiovale and corpus callosum integrity in relation to information processing speed in patients with severe traumatic brain injury. *The Journal of Head Trauma Rehabilitation, 28*(6), 433–441. doi:10.1097/HTR.0b013e3182585d06.
Lezak, M. D., Howieson, D. B., Bigler, E. D., & Tranel, D. (2012). *Neuropsychological assessment*. New York: Oxford University Press.
Millis, S. R., & Ricker, J. H. (1994). Verbal learning patterns in moderate and severe traumatic brain injury. *Journal of Clinical and Experimental Neuropsychology, 16*(4), 498–507. doi:10.1080/01688639408402661.
Ross, D. E., Ochs, A. L., Seabaugh, J., & Henshaw, T. (2012). NeuroQuant(R) revealed hippocampal atrophy in a patient with traumatic brain injury. *The Journal of Neuropsychiatry and Clinical Neurosciences, 24*(1), E33. doi:10.1176/appi.neuropsych.11020044.
Scheid, R., Preul, C., Gruber, O., Wiggins, C., & von Cramon, D. Y. (2003). Diffuse axonal injury associated with chronic traumatic brain injury: Evidence from T2*-weighted gradient-echo imaging at 3 T. *American Journal of Neuroradiology, 24*(6), 1049–1056.
Scheid, R., Walther, K., Guthke, T., Preul, C., & von Cramon, D. Y. (2006). Cognitive sequelae of diffuse axonal injury. *Archives of Neurology, 63*(3), 418–424. doi:10.1001/archneur.63.3.418.
Spitz, G., Maller, J. J., O'Sullivan, R., & Ponsford, J. L. (2013). White matter integrity following traumatic brain injury: The association with severity of injury and cognitive functioning. *Brain Topography, 26*(4), 648–660. doi:10.1007/s10548-013-0283-0.
Voineskos, A. N., Rajji, T. K., Lobaugh, N. J., Miranda, D., Shenton, M. E., Kennedy, J. L., Mulsant, B. H., et al. (2012). Age-related decline in white matter tract integrity and cognitive performance: A DTI tractography and structural equation modeling study. *Neurobiology of Aging, 33*(1), 21–34. doi:10.1016/j.neurobiolaging.2010.02.009.
Wang, J. Y., Bakhadirov, K., Abdi, H., Devous, M. D., Sr., Marquez de la Plata, C. D., Moore, C., Diaz-Arrastia, R., et al. (2011). Longitudinal changes of structural connectivity in traumatic axonal injury. *Neurology, 77*(9), 818–826. doi:10.1212/WNL.0b013e31822c61d7.
Wright, M. J., & Schmitter-Edgecombe, M. (2011). The impact of verbal memory encoding and consolidation deficits during recovery from moderate-to-severe traumatic brain injury. *The Journal of Head Trauma Rehabilitation, 26*(3), 182–191. doi:10.1097/HTR.0b013e318218dcf9.
Zakzanis, K. K., & Jeffay, E. (2011). Neurocognitive variability in high-functioning individuals: Implications for the practice of clinical neuropsychology. *Psychological Reports, 108*(1), 290–300.

Chapter 2
The Role of Cognitive Neuropsychology in Clinical Settings: The Example of a Single Case of Deep Dyslexia

Roberto Cubelli, Silva Pedrizzi and Sergio Della Sala

The Role of the Neuropsychologist

In this chapter, we first define the role of a cognitive neuropsychologist within the diagnostic team,[1] and then exemplify it by means of a case report describing the cognitive performances of a stroke patient presenting with deep dyslexia. The purpose of this chapter is to illustrate the overhauling of mere clinical labels to reach the objective of identifying the spared and impaired cognitive processes as depicted by the relevant theoretical models of mental functions. Detecting the range of spared cognitive processes is not simply a matter of completeness. Rather, it is an integral aspect of the neuropsychological diagnostic procedure. Once a deficit has been ascertained by means of reliable and standardized instruments, a hypothesis is usually formulated to account for it. To consolidate such diagnostic hypothesis requires additional supporting evidence, but a solid diagnostic confirmation comes from attempts to falsify the postulated hypothesis.

[1] The introductory text of this chapter capitalises on a previous publication by the same authors: Cubelli and Della (2011).

R. Cubelli (✉)
Department of Psychology and Cognitive Sciences, University of Trento, Corso Bettini, 31-38068 Rovereto, Trento, Italy
e-mail: roberto.cubelli@unitn.it

S. Pedrizzi
Rehabilitation Unit, Pierantoni Hospital, Via C. Forlanini 34, 47121 Forlì (FC) Italy
e-mail: s.pedrizzi@ausl.fo.it

S. Della Sala
Human Cognitive Neuroscience, University of Edinburgh, 7 George Square, Edinburgh EH8 9JZ, UK
e-mail: sergio@ed.ac.uk

J. A. B. Macniven (ed.), *Neuropsychological Formulation,*
DOI 10.1007/978-3-319-18338-1_2

The etymological meaning of term diagnosis is "to know thoroughly" (by scrutinising signs and symptoms). Diagnosing implies two consequent yet independent processes: to identify a disease and to find its cause(s). Suppose that a person with abrupt language problems seeks help from a general practitioner who acknowledges the deficits and sends her for neurological consultation. The neurologist, informed by a series of clinical and instrumental exams, confirms the presence of a deviant behaviour and formulates a possible diagnosis identifying the disease, for instance minor left hemisphere ischemia. In parallel, the language impairment needs to be identified, quantified and interpreted. The outcome of off-the-shelf psychometric assessments will assist in determining that this patient's language difficulties could be labelled as Broca's aphasia, which is a shortcut description of her impairment. The aim of a skilled neuropsychologist though is to investigate the cognitive causes of this impairment, which can be multifarious (Mohr et al. 1978; Caramazza 1984). Limiting the examination to offering a tag would only attain the scope of corroborating the problem as lamented by the patient and her carers, perhaps by labelling it more eloquently, like a doctor diagnosing a knee pain as *gonalgia*.

In sum, cognitive neuropsychologists are called to investigate the impairments of cognitive processes following brain damage and to account for the observed patterns of spared and impaired abilities "in terms of damage to one or more components of a theory or model of normal cognition" (Ellis and Young 1995, p. 4). In turn, this refined diagnosis consents to take an informed decision on whether or not to initiate a cognitive treatment and, if so, to make precise the targets and the working hypotheses of rehabilitation programmes.

Neuropsychologists use relatively simple tasks, such as reading aloud, drawing figures, recognising objects, or memorising lists of words, and are equipped with pre-packed test batteries. The apparent simplicity of the neuropsychologist's trademark instruments is deceptive. The core competence of a neuropsychologist is not solely to administer the tests (which could be presented by different professionals or by trainees), but to plan the individual assessment, to refine the testing programme, to decode the findings, and to unravel the observed pattern of performance. Central to their remit is the *interpretation* of the outcome from such tests, based on both accuracy scores and the qualitative analysis of errors. Like a radiologist who could carry out a scan, but whose main chore is to interpret it, the neuropsychologist is asked to derive hypotheses on the patient's cognitive functioning. Hence, the diagnostic process should not be merely applying gross clinical labels (i.e. Broca's aphasia, dysexecutive syndrome, unilateral neglect and episodic amnesia), but to identify the damaged component(s) of the cognitive processes in individual patients. This approach would of course require considerable time per patient asking for a different organization of the services offered. It would also entail a greater cultural and political appreciation of the relevance of the professional role of the neuropsychologists in diagnosing and managing individual issues posed by patients.

The Neuropsychological Interpretation

A single error is per se opaque. The ambiguity of single errors needs to be disentangled considering the overall pattern of spared and impaired abilities and their matching onto the relevant cognitive model.

It is paramount to distinguish between error classification and their interpretation. Take a patient who reads the word "beep" as "peep"; this error could be classed as letter substitution, but it could be interpreted by means of six different accounts. The error could be (i) perceptual (b → p), revealing a problem in coding the spatial orientation of the letter shape, which will also involve non-orthographic stimuli; (ii) orthographic (<B> → <P>), due to a deficit in processing the letter identity, specific to reading tasks; (iii) lexical semantic (beep → peep), because the stimulus and response pair include two semantically similar words; (iv) phonological (/b/→/p/), involving one distinctive feature, with a voiced stop consonant replaced by its unvoiced cognate, due to a phonetic deficit which would be apparent also in spontaneous speech; (v) attentional (beep → -eep), due to a defective coding of the beginning letter, as in neglect dyslexia; (vi) contextual (xxxP → PxxP), a sequential error called "retrograde assimilation or anticipation" (Lecours and Lhermitte 1979), due to a deficit in planning the correct phonological sequence in short-term memory. The ambiguity of single errors needs to be disentangled considering the overall pattern of spared and impaired abilities and their matching onto the relevant cognitive model.

The labelling of an error, like "letter substitution," derives from agreed mutually exclusive categories, that is, a given response could be listed under one, and one only, error category. However, this kind of errors could be interpreted by means of several different accounts. Similarly, errors which can be classed differently may derive from the same underlying problem. Consider, for instance, phonemic paraphasias (e.g. table → pable) and formal paraphasias (e.g. table → cable), whereby the response is a nonword and a word, respectively. In most cases, these two types of error reflect the same output disorder (see Blanken 1990).

Classing an error does not imply its interpretation, which instead ought to be vetted against the full assessment and nested within verified cognitive models. A naming error, e.g. tiger → lion, classed as semantic paraphasia, does not necessarily imply the impairment of semantic knowledge, rather it could be traced to a pre-semantic deficit, as in associative visual agnosia, or it could result from a post-semantic deficit, as in anomic aphasia (Caramazza and Hillis 1990a). The way to disentangle the origin of a given error is to both compare performance in different tasks and to consider the frequency of other error types. In case of semantic paraphasias in picture naming tasks, the deficit would be pre-semantic if the naming performance was within the normal limits with stimuli presented in other sensory modalities (haptic or verbal) and other errors were mainly characterised by visual paraphasias (i.e. the name of a visually similar objects; e.g. apple → ball). In contrast, the deficit would be post-semantic if the semantic errors were present in all naming tasks independently from the sensory modality of stimulus presentation and the most frequent errors were circumlocutions (e.g. camel → the animal with humps…in Egypt). Finally, the deficit could be semantic in nature. In this case, semantic errors should be coupled with “don’t know” errors and observed in all tasks requiring the access to semantic knowledge, including nonverbal tests, like drawing from memory. Only transcoding tasks, like repeating, reading or writing nonwords, should be errorless.

Psychometrics Is Not All

Good tests are furnished with norms relative to validated cut-off scores derived from a reference sample, which allow the identification of performances that deviate more than 2 standard deviations from psychometric values like the median, or fall below the 5th percentile. These arbitrary criteria can give rise to false positives or false negatives, which could be avoided by acknowledging that a poor performance does not necessarily equate to a pathological one.

To assess a given cognitive function one single test cannot suffice, as the test–function correspondence is weak. The Token Test (De Renzi and Faglioni 1978) is recognised as a good test to assess language comprehension, yet it includes only a limited number of lexical units (names of shapes, sizes and colours). It does not assess linguistic processes like inferential knowledge (“I heard a dog” conveys the information that an unknown and unseen dog is barking far from me) or the assignment of thematic roles (the role of agent is assigned to nouns occupying pre-verbal and post-verbal positions in active and passive sentences, respectively). Moreover, there are several different ways to fail the Token Test. A patient may be inaccurate, not because of aphasia, but because of colour agnosia or working memory problems in binding shapes to colours, or deficits in keeping track of the word sequence.

Moreover, the validity of a test should not be taken for granted. A test might not assess exactly what it was devised for, for instance because of faulty selection of the stimuli. The Judgement of Line Orientation Test (Benton et al. 1978), widely assumed to detect selective visuospatial deficits in right-hemisphere-damaged patients, is biased by an uneven distribution of the stimulus lines, which are easier to discriminate in the left space thus favouring left-brain-damaged patients who tend to be more accurate in processing ipsilateral information (Treccani et al. 2005).

Structure of the Neuropsychological Assessment

A sound neuropsychological assessment should entail separate but intertwined steps. After an interview aimed at gathering a targeted personal and clinical history and a screening phase, whereby a comprehensive battery of brief tests (Brazzelli et al. 1994; Dudas et al. 2005) is given, a full-blown neuropsychological examination is delivered based upon the information gleaned with the preliminary steps. Here, the neuropsychologist's tools are tests or batteries geared at investigating the presence and the severity of specific disorders (Wilson et al. 2008; Huber et al. 1984), by means of which one could attribute clinical labels. The diagnostic process should not stop at this stage, as clinical labels cover a wide range of cognitive disturbances lumped together under a syndromic umbrella. To identify the precise locus of cognitive impairment is the objective of the latter step, in which the neuropsychologist should use experimental tests, culled from the literature, or even devised ad hoc.

Case Report

BR (fictitious initials), a right-handed Italian craftman with 5 years of schooling, was 49 years old when he suffered a left middle cerebral artery stroke. A series of neuroimaging investigations disclosed a large fronto-temporo-parietal ischemia. At admission, he presented with right paresis and non-fluent aphasia.

Eight months after his stroke, he underwent a comprehensive neuropsychological assessment (see Table 2.1) which demonstrated oral and ideomotor limb apraxia (Spinnler and Tognoni 1987) but no signs of visuospatial neglect, tested by means of tasks requiring cancellation of segments (Albert 1973) or target objects (Gauthier et al. 1989; Wilson et al. 1987), drawing geometrical figures (Spinnler and Tognoni 1987) and line bisecting (Halligan and Marshall 1989). He obtained the age and education adjusted score 20/36 on the Raven's Coloured Progressive Matrices, indicating a performance within the normal range (Basso et al. 1987). The output of the Italian version of the AAT (Luzzatti et al. 1991) confirmed the diagnosis of Broca's aphasia. His language abilities were further investigated by means of the BADA (a battery for the assessment of aphasic disorders, Miceli et al. 1994; (see Table 2.2) In particular, tasks assessing language auditory input, phonemic discrimination, lexical decision and word–picture matching tasks were at, or near, ceiling. His language was non-fluent, his performance in the picture-naming task was good but characterised by some semantic errors (e.g. microfono [microphone] → voce [voice]) or agrammatic circumlocutions (e.g. serratura [lock] → buco [hole] ... chiave [key]). His reading abilities were poor and characterised by semantic

Table 2.1 BR's neuropsychological assessment. The asterisk indicates scores below age and education adjusted cut-off point corresponding to the inferential lower 5th percentile of the population

Test	Range	Cut-off	Raw score	Adjusted score
Token Test	0–36	29	13	14*
Raven's Coloured Progressive matrices	0–36	18	17	20
Copying of Geometrical Figures	0–14	7.75	10	9.5
Imitation of oral movements	0–20	16	1	0.75*
Imitation of limb movements	0–20	16	15	15.75*
Corsi spatial span	0–10	3.5	2	1.5*

Table 2.2 BR's performance on BADA, a battery for the assessment of aphasic disorders

Subtests	Correct responses (%)
Phonological discrimination	60/60 (100)
Oral repetition	
Words	17/45 (38)
Nonwords	19/36 (53)
Auditory lexical decision	76/80 (95)
Visual lexical decision	37/80 (46)
Auditory word comprehension	38/40 (95)
Visual word comprehension	34/40 (85)
Oral naming	
Objects	25/30 (83)
Actions	11/28 (39)
Reading	
Words	16/92 (17)
Nonwords	0/45 (0)

paralexias (e.g. mandorla [almond] → fiore [flower]) which are pathognomonic of deep dyslexia (Coltheart et al. 1980).

Deep dyslexia is a multi-componential syndrome resulting from heterogeneous functional deficits. Accordingly, we have further assessed BR to make precise the cognitive loci of his reading impairment. In a series of testing sessions, he was requested to read aloud a total of 1265 words and 192 nonwords. BR was unable to read nonwords and had serious difficulties in reading words (see Table 2.3).

Detailed scrutiny of subgroups of items from the list of words allowed us to further analyse the effects of relevant linguistic variables. BR read better concrete (25/92, 27 %) than abstract (1/92, 1 %) words and read better nouns (10/70, 14 %) than verbs and grammatical functors (0/140). However, his superiority in reading high-frequency words (21/138, 15 %) versus low-frequency words (13/138, 9 %) was not significant (chi-square = 0.14, ns). The presence of the lexical effect and semantic errors together with the observation of the concreteness effect and the grammatical class effect are indicative of the diagnosis of deep dyslexia (Shallice 1988, Chap. 5; Coltheart et al. 1980). The lack of a significant frequency effect is not surprising as this effect has not been consistently observed in cases of deep dyslexia, since its first description (case GR, Marshall and Newcombe 1966).

Reading errors were classified according to the categories identified by Coltheart et al. (1980, Table 6). These included semantic errors, when stimulus and response share semantic properties but differ orthographically, and visual errors which define

Table 2.3 BR's overall performance on word and nonword reading

	Words (n = 1265)	Nonwords (n = 192)
Correct responses	164 (13 %)	0
Omissions	177 (14 %)	57 (29.7 %)
Errors	924 (73 %)	135 (70.3 %)

Table 2.4 Paralexias produced by BR subdivided according to error categories

Error type	*n* (%)	Examples
Semantic	55 (5.9)	finestra [*window*]; → porta [*door*]; ieri [*yesterday*] → domani [*tomorrow*]
Visual	481 (52.1)	penna [*pen*] → pane [*bread*]; forma [*shape*] → forbici [*scissors*]
Visual and/or semantic	35 (3.8)	satellite [*satellite*] → stella [*star*]; corvo [*crow*] → cornacchia [*carrion crow*]
Visual-then-semantic	63 (6.8)	cabina → [*hut*] → fucile [*gun*] via carabina [*rifle*]; domanda [*question*] → donna [*woman*] via uomo [*man*]
Morphological	77 (8.3)	dente [*tooth*] → dentist [*dentist*]; posto [*place*] → posti [*places*]
Unclassified	213 (23.1)	senza [*without*] → sacchi [*sacks*]; genere [*gender*] → gelato [*ice cream*]

responses containing at least 50 % of the stimulus letters without sharing semantic relation with it. When responses were both visually and semantically related to the stimulus, the errors were classed as visual and/or semantic. Following the examples (sympathy → orchestra assuming the mediation of symphony) given by Marshall and Newcombe (1966), errors were classed as visual-then-semantic when a presumed, not overt, visual error preceded a semantic conversion. Reading errors were morphological when the response was characterised by a substitution of inflexional (e.g. card → cards) or derivational (e.g. teach → teacher) suffixes.

When the patient uttered more than one response for a given stimulus, the last one was considered for the error analysis. Table 2.4 details the types of word-reading errors committed by BR. The bulk of his paralexias was visual errors, corresponding to what Shallice (1988) labels as "input type," whereby the deficit involves the pre-semantic processing phase of the stimulus. With nonwords 60 % of all errors were visual; the remaining nonword paralexias included 5.2 % of visual-then-semantic and 34.8 % of unclassified errors. He never produced a nonword in response to either word or nonword stimuli; that is, he either omitted to respond or produced a wrong word.

The cognitive profile of BR was compatible with a clinical diagnosis of deep dyslexia. Within the dual-route model of reading (Coltheart et al. 2001), BR's deficits affected both the lexical and the sublexical route (nonword reading was at floor, word reading was also poor and characterised by several different error types). It was necessary though to interpret the functional loci of BR's errors, in particular his visual errors which are paramount.

Interim Formulation

BR's pattern of performance revealed a severe symptom complex due to multiple functional disorders. First of all, the sublexical procedure converting orthography to phonology appeared to be completely damaged and unavailable. BR was totally unable to read nonwords aloud; no correct responses were given. He produced only omissions ("don't know" responses) and substitutions with visually similar words; he never produced nonwords as responses.

As reading of known words was also affected, the lexical-semantic route must have been impaired. Most erroneous responses were substitutions of the stimuli with semantically and/or visually similar words. The sources of semantic errors could be various. They could result at the level of orthographic input lexicon, but if this was the case, semantic errors should be limited to reading aloud. BR produced semantic errors also in object naming; therefore, these errors should have had their origin at post-orthographic levels. If they were due to an impairment of the semantic system, tasks assessing word comprehension, like word to picture matching tasks, should have also been defective. However, as reported in Table 2.2, his performance on both auditory and written word comprehension tasks was quite normal. Finally, the source of the semantic errors could be located at the level of the phonological output lexicon. This interpretation is suggested by the presence of circumlocutions in object naming tasks, which revealed a deficit in accessing the phonological lexicon, confirmed by the very small number of errors on word comprehension.

The most frequent errors were visual paralexias, i.e., substitutions with visually similar words. Where did they come from? They cannot be attributed to the impaired grapheme-to-phoneme conversion mechanism because the patient never produced nonwords in his responses; therefore, it is highly implausible that this kind of errors could stem from the sublexical level. Visual paralexias can be phonological or orthographic in nature. However, since almost no phonemic paraphasias were observed in BR's spontaneous speech and naming tasks, these errors have to be considered orthographic and not phonological, and could be located either at the lexical or at the prelexical level.

The position of the individual letters involved in errors allows us to disentangle the origin of these errors. Indeed, errors at the lexical level should involve any letters independently of their position within the stimuli; in contrast, prelexical errors should be spatially specified and limited to a given side. As shown by the examples given in Table 2.4, the latter was the case: BR's errors often involved the endings of the words.

BR's Reading Errors: A Case of Neglect Dyslexia?

Following Hillis and Caramazza (1991), a Letter Position Effect was calculated considering a subset of 387 word whose length ranged from 4 to 7 letters (four letters $n=59$, five letters $n=170$, six letters $n=99$ and seven letters $n=59$). Figure 2.1 illustrates the outcome showing the percent correct (letter in correct position) within these words. It appears at face value that there is an order effect, whereby the beginnings of the words are better read than their endings. This asymmetrical distribution of errors is compatible with right-sided neglect dyslexia (Vallar et al. 2010).

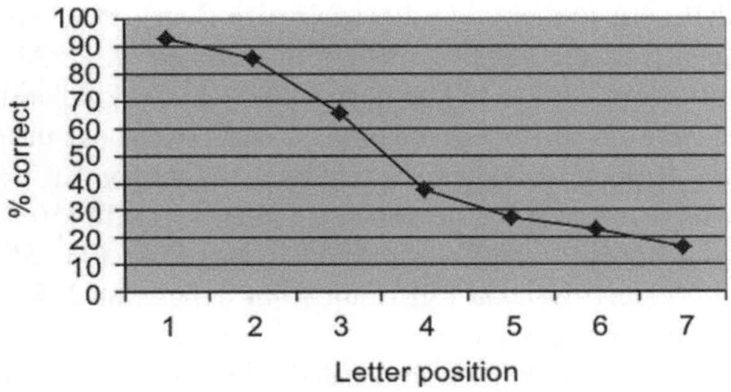

Fig. 2.1 Letter position effect in BR's single-word reading. Percent correct (letter in correct position) within 4–7 letter words is shown. An order effect emerges: the beginning of the words is better read than their ending

Indeed, several of BR's reading errors met the defining criteria of neglect paralexias set forth by Ellis et al. (1987): paralexias could be classified as right neglect errors if the target and the response were identical to the left of an identifiable neglect point and there were no letters in common to the right of this point. Neglect paralexias were identified within each error category: visual (zio [uncle] → zingara [gypsy]), visual and/or semantic (canguro [kangaroo] → cane [dog]), visual then semantic (anzi [rather] → vecchi [old] through "anziani" [elderly]), morphological (lupo [wolf] → lupa [she-wolf]) and unclassified (senso [sense] → sedia [chair]). Also errors in reading nonwords could be classified as neglect paralexias: visual (curete → cucina [kitchen]) and visual then semantic (nafò → benzina [petrol] … no! nafta [naphtha]).

Considering all BR's errors in reading words, taken from all categories with a visual component (n=869), a total of 279 errors (32 %) could be defined as right neglect paralexias according to Ellis et al. (1987). This proportion is less than that reported in cases of left neglect dyslexia due to right hemisphere damage (e.g. see Table 2.3 in Cubelli et al. 1991) and would not comply with the diagnosis of neglect dyslexia whereby neglect paralexias are the majority of observed errors. According to Ellis et al.'s criteria, none of the letters right to the neglect point should be shared between the stimulus and the response. However, in Italian almost all words end with a vowel, in particular "a, e, o." Therefore, the probability that the two words share the ending vowel simply by chance is sizeable. To overcome this confound, the less popular and looser criteria proposed by Hillis and Caramazza (1990) were adopted. These criteria assume that the diagnosis of neglect paralexia is satisfied when all the following conditions are observed: the response is identical to the target by at least two letters from the left end (beginning), there is at least one unshared letter to the right of the shared ones, and the stimulus and the response should not contain identical clusters of two or more letters to the right of the shared segment. Applying these criteria the proportion of BR's errors classifiable as right neglect paralexias rises to 61 % (n=529), which constitutes the majority of his errors and is compatible with the diagnosis of neglect dyslexia.

To tackle this hypothesis an ad hoc test was devised: the auditory–visual matching task. The patient was presented with two series of 16 trials each composed of four words characterised by having either the first three letters in common (e.g.

POLIZIA [police], POLENTA [maize flour], POLLINE [pollen] and POLMONE [lung]) or the last three letters in common (e.g. FARMACO [drug], UBRIACO [drunken], SINDACO [major] and ZODIACO [zodiac]). The four words in each trial were visually presented on flash cards one above the other; the task of the patient was to point to the word named by the examiner. BR's correct response in the trials with words sharing the same beginning was 8/16 (50 %), whereas his performance with words sharing the same ending was 15/16 (93.75 %).

Neglect dyslexia can result from deficits at different levels of representation (Hillis and Caramazza 1995): viewer-centred, stimulus-centred and word-centred. Neglect dyslexia associated with left hemisphere damage is hallmarked by the presence of word-centred neglect (Vallar et al 2010, p. 231) and may occur in the absence of unilateral spatial neglect (e.g. see case RYT by Warrington 1991). Therefore, BR should present with word-centred neglect. Should he present with an effect of spatial orientation, typical of stimulus-centred neglect sensitive to the physical features of the stimuli, the word-centred neglect hypothesis would be falsified. Word-centred representation codifies the abstract orthographic information specifying the identity and the order of the constituent letters independently of their physical appearance; hence, it should not be modulated by the spatial orientation of the stimulus. BR was assessed with a reading task in which the words were presented vertically, with individual letters one below the other. A total of 23 stimuli were used. Adopting Hillis and Caramazza's (1990) criteria, BR produced 17 (74 %) right neglect paralexias, for instance he read "mela" [apple] as "mese" [month]. This proportion of errors is akin to that observed with horizontal stimuli (i.e. 61 %).[2] The lack of spatial orientation effect suggests that BR's neglect paralexias were due to a deficit at the level of word-centred representation, which specifies the ordinal information of the letters within the word independently of their actual physical properties, such as size, font, case, spacing between letters, as well as the spatial orientation of the stimulus.

This interpretation is consistent with the performance of other patients with deep dyslexia reported in the literature. Three of them produced many errors, either visual or visual-then-semantic, that could be classified as neglect paralexias: thin → think; earl → deaf (case GR, Marshall and Newcombe 1966); bow → bowl; coward → Cowes (a place on the Isle of Wight; case KF, Shallice & Warrington 1975); revolt → revolver; charter → map (case DE, Patterson 1980). Siakaluk and Buchanan (2001) first described the case of a patient presenting with both right neglect dyslexia and deep dyslexia. Errors were semantic paralexias (e.g. ill → sick) and neglect paralexias (e.g. shown → short). Also Berndt et al. (Greenwald and Berndt 1999; Petrich et al. 2007; Berndt et al. 2005) described a series of left-brain-damaged patients who showed visual errors affecting the final letter of the stimulus words. As no visual spatial neglect and attentional disorders were detected, they stated that the positional errors were due to a selective disorder in coding orthographic ordinal information rather than being the direct consequence of neglect

[2] With Ellis et al.'s (1987) criteria the responses classified as right neglect paralexias were 35 %, again similar to the proportion identified with horizontal stimuli (i.e., 32 %).

dyslexia. Whatever the causal interpretation may be, the deficit ought to be located at the prelexical stage, at the level of the abstract orthographic representation where information about letter position is specified. The asymmetric performance may be spatial in nature (as assumed in word-centred neglect dyslexia, by Hillis and Caramazza 1995) or be the consequence of a defective activation of individual letters, as hypothesized by Petrich et al. 2007). Both impairments depend on positional information and involve the ending letters of all orthographic stimuli (the right part of normally oriented stimuli).

If BR's visual errors reflected prelexical impairment, it would be possible to account for the visual-then-semantic errors which characterise deep dyslexia: these errors have to be interpreted as the effect of two independent and consecutive errors occurring in response to a single item.

Diagnosis of BR's Reading Impairments—Reformulation

BR is affected by three independent deficits (see Fig. 2.2), which can be observed separately: impaired sublexical route in phonological dyslexia, defective access to phonological lexicon in anomic aphasia, and asymmetrical orthographic representation in neglect dyslexia or positional dyslexia.

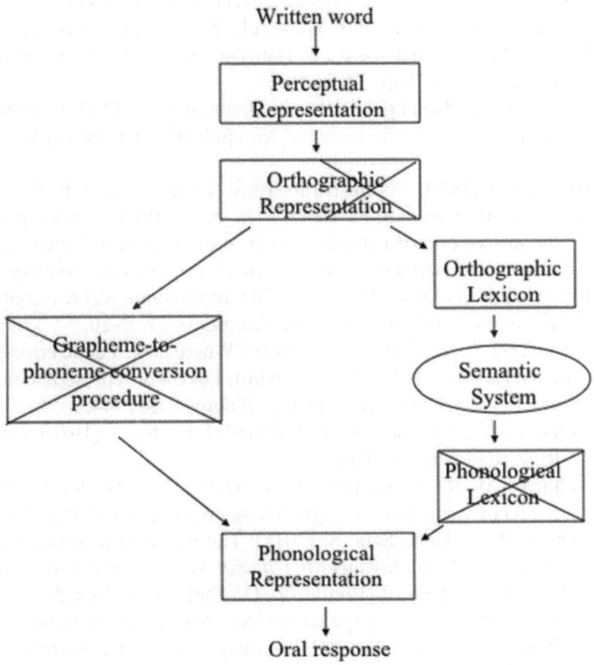

Fig. 2.2 BR's reading deficits superimposed to and interpreted according to Coltheart's dual-route cognitive model of reading. BR is affected by three separate deficits: phonological dyslexia shown by the impaired sublexical route, anomic aphasia expressed by the defective access to phonological lexicon, and neglect dyslexia illustrated by the asymmetrical orthographic representation

Conclusions

Neuropsychological formulation is a complex endeavour geared at investigating human cognition, not a second tier approach for ascertaining possible abnormalities in brain functions. Scores achieved in any neuropsychological test are not per se indicative of brain damage, as a test can be failed for several and different reasons; nor should their aim simply be that of grossly indicating the possible lesion localization, as conceived in the pre-neuroimaging era.

Knowledge advances stepwise by identifying, isolating and fractionating phenomena. The aim of formulating a thorough clinical diagnosis is the same. Within cognitive neuropsychology, scientific investigation and clinical analysis converge both in scope and procedures. In clinical settings patients present with a constellation of symptoms and signs; their cognitive profile is rarely straightforward and seldom reflects textbook descriptions. Clinical assessment should mirror the methods of a scientific investigation within the frame of a single case analysis, as the case of BR demonstrates. Similarly, researchers should make precise the clinical diagnosis of potential candidate cases to test predictions derived from established cognitive models.

References

Albert, M. (1973). A simple test of visual neglect. *Neurology, 23*(6), 658–664.

Basso, A., Capitani, E., & Laiacona, M. (1987). Raven's coloured progressive matrices: Normative values on 305 adult normal controls. *Functional Neurology, 2,* 189–194.

Benton, A. L., Varney, N. R., & Hamsher, K. (1978). Visuospatial judgement: A clinical test. *Archives of Neurology, 35,* 364–367.

Berndt, R. S., Haendiges, A. H., & Mitchum, C. C. (2005). Orthographic effects in the word substitutions of aphasic patients: An epidemic of right neglect dyslexia? *Brain and Language, 93*(1), 55–63.

Blanken, G. (1990). Formal paraphasias: A single case study. *Brain and Language, 38*(4), 534–554.

Brazzelli, M., Capitani, E., Della, S. S., et al. (1994). A neuropsychological instrument adding to the description of patients with suspected cortical dementia: The milan overall dementia assessment. *Journal of Neurology, Neurosurgery, and Psychiatry, 57,* 1510–1517.

Caramazza, A. (1984). The logic of neuropsychological research and the problem of patient classification in aphasia. *Brain and Language, 21,* 9–20.

Caramazza, A., & Hillis, A. E. (1990a). Where do semantic errors come from? *Cortex, 26,* 95–122.

Caramazza, A., & Hillis, A. E. (1990b). Levels of representation, co-ordinate frames, and unilateral neglect. *Cognitive Neuropsychology, 7,* 391–445.

Coltheart, M., Patterson, K., & Marshall, J. C. (Eds.). (1980). *Deep dyslexia*. Henley-on-Thames: Routledge & Kegan Paul.

Coltheart, M., Rastle, K., Perry, C., Langdon, R., & Ziegler, J. (2001). DRC: A dual route cascaded model of visual word recognition and reading aloud. *Psychological Review, 108,* 204–256.

Cubelli, R., & Della Sala, S. (2011). The purposes of neuropsychological assessment and how to achieve them. *Advances in Clinical Neuroscience & Rehabilitation (ACNR), 11*(1), 36–37.

Cubelli, R., Nichelli, P., Bonito, V., De Tanti, A., & Inzaghi, M. G. (1991). Different patterns of dissociation in lateral spatial neglect. *Brain and Cognition, 15,* 139–159.

De Renzi, E., & Faglioni, P. (1978). Development of a shortened version of the token test. *Cortex, 14,* 41–49.

Dudas, R. B., Berrios, G. E., & Hodges, J. R. (2005). The Addenbrooke's Cognitive Examination (ACE) in the differential diagnosis of early dementias versus affective disorders. *The American Journal of Geriatric Psychiatry, 13,* 218–226.

Gauthier, L., Dehaut, F., & Joanette, Y. (1989). The bells test: A quantitative and qualitative test for visual neglect. *International Journal of Clinicle Neuropsychology, 11,* 49–54.

Greenwald, M., & Berndt, R. (1999). Impaired encoding of abstract letter order: Severe alexia in a mildly aphasic patient. *Cognitive Neuropsychology, 16,* 513–556.

Ellis, A. W., & Young, A. W. (1995). *Human cognitive neuropsychology. A textbook with readings.* Hove: Psychology Press.

Ellis, A. W., Flude. B. M., & Young, A. W. (1987). "Neglect dyslexia" and the early visual processing of letters in words and non words. *Cognitive Neuropsychology, 4,* 439–464.

Halligan, P. W., & Marshall, J. C. (1989). Line bisection in visuo-spatial neglect: Disproof of a conjecture. *Cortex, 25,* 517–521.

Hillis, A. E., & Caramazza, A. (1990). The effects of attentional deficits on reading and spelling. In A. Caramazza (Ed.), *Cognitive neuropsychology and neurolinguistics: Advances in models of cognitive function and impairment* (pp. 211–275). Hillsdale: Lawrence Erlbaum Associates.

Hillis, A. E., & Caramazza, A. (1991). Deficit to stimulus-centered, letter shape representations in a case of "unilateral neglect". *Neuropsychologia, 29,* 1223–1240.

Hillis, A. E., & Caramazza, A. (1995). A framework for interpreting distinct patterns of hemispatial neglect. *Neurocase, 1,* 189–207.

Huber, W., Poeck, K., & Willmes, K. (1984). The Aachen Aphasia test. *Advances in Neurology, 42,* 291–303.

Lecours, A. R., & Lhermitte, F. (1979). *L'aphasie.* Paris: Flammarion.

Luzzatti, C., Willmes, W., & De Bleser, R. (1991). *Aachener Aphasia Test (AAT): Versione Italiana.* Florence: Organizzazioni Speciali.

Marshall, J. C., & Newcombe, F. (1966). Syntactic and semantic errors in paralexia. *Neuropsychologia, 4,* 169–176.

Miceli, G., Laudanna, A., Burani, C., & Capasso, R. (1994). *B.A.D.A. Batteria per l'analisi dei deficit afasici [A Battery for the assessment of aphasic disorders].* Rome: CEPSAG.

Mohr, J. P., Pessin, M. S., Finkelstein, S., et al. (1978). Broca aphasia: Pathologic and clinical. *Neurology, 28*(4), 311–324.

Petrich, J. A., Greenwald, M. L., & Berndt, R. S. (2007). An investigation of attentional contributions to visual errors in right "neglect dyslexia". *Cortex, 43*(8), 1036–1046.

Patterson, K. E. (1980). Derivational errors. (1980). In M. Coltheart, K. Patterson, & J. C. Marshall (Eds.), *Deep Dyslexia* (pp. 286–306). Henley-on-Thames: Routledge & Kegan Paul.

Shallice, T. (1988). *From neuropsychology to mental structure.* Cambridge: Cambridge University Press.

Shallice, T., & Warrington, E. K. (1975). Word recognition in a phonemic dyslexic patient. *Quarterly Journal of Experimental Psychology, 27,* 187–199.

Siakaluk, P. D., & Buchanan, L. (2001). Stimulus-specific neglect in a deep dyslexic patient. *Brain and Cognition, 46*(1–2) 268–271.

Spinnler, H., & Tognoni, G. (1987). Standardizzazione e taratura italiana di Test Neuropsicologici. *The Italian Journal of Neurological Sciences, 6*(Suppl. 8), 1–120.

Treccani, B., Torri, T., & Cubelli, R. (2005). Is judgement of line orientation selectively impaired in right brain damaged patients? *Neuropsychologia, 43,* 598–608.

Vallar, G., Burani, C., & Arduino, L. S. (2010). Neglect dyslexia: A review of the neuropsychological literature. *Experimental Brain Research, 206,* 219–235.

Warrington, E. K. (1991). Right neglect dyslexia: A single case study. *Cognitive Neuropsychology, 8,* 193–212.

Wilson, B. A., Cockburn, J., & Halligan, P. W. (1987). *Behavioural inattention test.* Titchfield: Thames Valley Test Company Ltd.

Wilson, B., Greenfield, E., Clare, L., et al. (2008). *Rivermead Behavioural Memory Test–Third Edition (RBMT–3).* Toronto: Pearson.

Chapter 3
A Case of Traumatic Brain Injury in Adolescence, Complicated by a History of Premorbid Learning Difficulties and Significant Social Concerns

Emily Talbot

Introduction

Cases referred to paediatric neuropsychology tend to be complex (Anderson et al. 2011). Few cases are straightforward, and each child is different. Complexity is increased by complications post-injury, but also by a host of premorbid factors which are essential to account for in the formulation process, both to isolate the difficulties related to the brain injury and to place the brain injury within the context of premorbid factors. For example, for the purposes of rehabilitation when specific specialist neuropsychology assessment environments allow for only limited time for each child to be seen, the formulation process has to be particularly focused and undeterred, reserving most of the allocated clinical time for the administration, processing and interpretation of neuropsychological test data in order to inform the referral question. Careful formulation is required to allow for simplicity of interpretation. To illustrate a formulation approach for a very complex case within a time-restricted assessment clinic in the NHS, the case of a child with premorbid social care and subsequent severe brain injury has been selected.

To highlight the complexities of such cases, and the need to simplify the remit towards an effective formulation, this chapter focuses on a systemic approach adopted within the context of the neurological event and sequelae. Such focus will ensure a stepwise formulation to arrive at a simplified explanation of the problem.

Services for children and adolescents within the social care system in the UK have greatly improved in recent years with dedicated clinical nurse specialists for looked-after children (children in the care of a local authority in the UK; Royal

The author would like to acknowledge Dr. Daniel Smith, Lincoln College, Oxford, for his invaluable assistance in the proofreading of this chapter.

E. Talbot (✉)
Department of Clinical Psychology and Neuropsychology, Nottingham University Hospitals NHS Trust, QMC Campus, Derby Road, Nottingham NG7 2UH, UK
e-mail: Emilytalbot@nhs.net

J. A. B. Macniven (ed.), *Neuropsychological Formulation*,
DOI 10.1007/978-3-319-18338-1_3

College of Nursing and the Royal College of Paediatrics and Child Health 2015; Department for Education and Department for Health (2015). NICE and the Social Care Institute for Excellence (SCIE) 2010). Child and Adolescent Mental Health Services (CAMHS) teams also employ clinical nurse specialists (Department for Children, Schools and Families 2009). However, the complexities of these young peoples' social care histories, including previous trauma, abuse and learning difficulties can make formulation more challenging if a child in care sustains an acquired brain injury (ABI). In addition, the ability to gather accurate information regarding prior medical, health, school and social backgrounds can at times be problematic due to children relocating, or moving across the country into adoptive families, or returning to birth families. Such moves create specific challenges both for the formulation and for subsequent targeted recommendations.

Background

This chapter introduces the case of Megan who sustained an ABI at 14 years old and who was seen for neuropsychological assessment on two occasions. She was initially seen soon after her discharge from hospital and again for reassessment 18 months later. Megan had been referred by the Consultant Neurologist. She sustained a significant traumatic brain injury (TBI) after being involved in a road traffic accident (RTA) when she was a pedestrian at the age of 14 years. A computerised tomography (CT) scan at the time of her admission to hospital had identified bilateral frontal contusions with an acute subdural haematoma, and she was admitted to the Paediatric Intensive Care Unit (PICU). Following her accident Megan underwent neurosurgery for evacuation of the haematoma.

The referral question was to assess Megan's cognitive function and memory following her ABI to identify ways to best support her within the home and educational environment. Megan was originally seen for an early baseline neuropsychological assessment only three months following the ABI in order to inform her return to school. A further reassessment was conducted as a routine follow-up 18 months after the original assessment.

This chapter will consider Megan's background information and history, the original assessment, formulation and intervention, and further reformulation following the second assessment. The outcome and issues raised will also be discussed.

Clinical Interview

Medical and Family

Megan sustained a significant ABI after being involved in an RTA. Megan was admitted to hospital and was found to have bilateral frontal contusions and an acute subdural haematoma. She spent 10 days in the PICU before being transferred to a children's neurosciences ward. During her stay in PICU she underwent surgery to evacuate the left frontal haematoma and had a partial frontal lobectomy to resect the contused frontal lobe. She was reported to show good progress during her stay in hospital although during the first 10 days she was observed to be agitated, at times aggressive, and to have poor speech. During her time in hospital, she greatly improved and at the time of her discharge was reported to be settled and having normal conversations demonstrating logical thinking. She was discharged two months after her admission to hospital.

Megan was reported to be short-sighted and wore glasses. There were no reported prior head injuries, though accurate early information was lacking due to her foster carers having limited amounts of detail regarding her background history and her new social worker also being unsure of very specific details. She was on no medication at the time of the original neuropsychological assessment and the foster carer was not aware of any significant major early childhood illnesses or periods of time in hospital.

Family

Megan had been in foster care since before she sustained the TBI. She had been placed in social care at eight years old, having been neglected by her birth parents. At the time of the accident and the original assessment, Megan was living with foster carers, with whom she had been for approximately 18 months. Her half-brother, Ben, aged 10, was also staying with them. Prior to this she had been placed with two other foster families, always with her brother. Each of these foster placements had been short term. This had resulted in Megan needing to change schools and therefore her relationships and friendships had been affected throughout her childhood.

Education

At the time of the original assessment Megan was in her third year of a state secondary school. Reports indicated that she required additional special educational needs support at school and had identified learning difficulties, contributed to by her early neglect and limited early education. It was reported that as a young child she had not been sent to school and her education had been disrupted through school changes due to her foster care placements changing. Due to her early childhood experiences and disrupted education, she was having difficulties in developing friendships, often coming across as overbearing and controlling with her peers. This was also evident in her relationship with her brother where she took on a mothering role, a characteristic that she had already adopted when living with her birth family.

At the time of the original assessment, however, Megan had not yet returned to school and therefore details of her presentation and abilities were as yet unclear. She had received support from the hospital school that recognised her difficulties with learning but were unsure how much of this related to premorbid difficulties and how much was related to the ABI and any acquired cognitive/neuropsychological impairments.

Assessment

Observations During Assessment and Assessment Conducted

During the assessments, Megan was observed to engage well and was happy to answer questions when asked. She often became distracted but could be directed back to the task with encouragement.

Neuropsychological Assessment

Megan was assessed using the Wechsler Intelligence Scale for Children-Fourth UK Edition (WISC-IV^{UK}), Children's Memory Scale (CMS), Behaviour Rating Inventory of Executive Function (BRIEF) and Delis–Kaplan Executive Function System (D–KEFS).

Wechsler Intelligence Scale for Children-Fourth UK Edition (WISC-IV^{UK})

Megan was assessed using the WISC-IV^{UK} to provide an overall profile of her cognitive strengths and weaknesses. As can be seen from Tables 3.1 and 3.2, Megan's performance placed her within the Borderline to Extremely Low range of functioning across all domains of the assessment. She demonstrated lower performance on the verbally mediated tasks of the Verbal Comprehension and Working Memory indices. Her performance was slightly higher on the visual tasks of the Perceptual Reasoning and Processing Speed indices, although these remained below the 10th percentile and within the Borderline range of ability (Tables 3.1 and 3.2).

Table 3.1 Composite index scores

Scale	Composite score	Percentile rank	Qualitative description
Verbal Comprehension (VCI)	67	1	Extremely Low
Perceptual Reasoning (PRI)	73	4	Borderline
Working Memory (WMI)	65	1	Extremely Low
Processing Speed (PSI)	78	7	Borderline
Full Scale (FSIQ)	64	1	Extremely Low

Table 3.2 Subtest scores

Index	Subtest	Subtest scaled score
Verbal Comprehension	Similarities	5
	Vocabulary	3
	Comprehension	5
	(Information)	(4)
	(Word Reasoning)	(4)
Perceptual Reasoning	Block Design	5
	Picture Concepts	4
	Matrix Reasoning	8
	(Picture Completion)	(5)
Working Memory	Digit Span	2
	Letter–Number Sequencing	6
	(Arithmetic)	(5)
Processing Speed	Coding	6
	Symbol Search	6
	(Cancellation)	(9)

() = supplementary subtests

Children's Memory Scale (CMS)

Megan was also assessed using the CMS to get a detailed profile of her memory abilities. Her scores on the CMS indicated that she has significant difficulties with her memory. Her overall performance gave her a General Memory Index score of 52, which was at the 0.1st percentile, and fell within the Extremely Low range of ability. Megan performed within the Extremely Low to Borderline range across all indices of the assessment with particularly low scores on the verbal memory tasks compared to the visual tasks (Tables 3.3 and 3.4).

Table 3.3 Composite index scores

Index	Index score	Percentile rank	Qualitative description
Visual Immediate	72	3	Borderline
Visual Delayed	69	2	Extremely Low
Verbal Immediate	60	0.4	Extremely Low
Verbal Delayed	60	0.4	Extremely Low
General Memory	52	0.1	Extremely Low
Attention/Concentration	78	7	Borderline
Learning	82	12	Low Average
Delayed Recognition	57	0.2	Extremely Low

Table 3.4 Subtest scores

Subtest	Subtest scaled score	Percentile rank
Dot Locations		
Learning	9	37
Total Score	6	9
Long Delay	6	9
Stories		
Immediate	3	1
Delayed	4	2
Delayed Recognition	4	2
Faces		
Immediate	5	5
Delayed	4	2
Word Pairs		
Learning	5	5
Total Score	4	2
Long Delay	3	1
Delayed Recognition	2	<1
Numbers		
Total Score	6	9
Sequences		
Total Score	7	16

Delis–Kaplan Executive Function System (D–KEFS)

Megan performed well on two subtests of the D–KEFS executive function assessment. It is important to note that executive function can be difficult to measure, particularly in children and teenagers where skills are still emerging or are yet to emerge (Anderson 2001). This can lead to patients with dysexecutive difficulties doing well on standardised assessments whilst being observed to experience significant difficulties in everyday life (Table 3.5).

Behaviour Rating Inventory of Executive Function (BRIEF)

Megan's foster carers completed this questionnaire in relation to Megan. She was scored below the clinical cut-off *T*-score of 65 on all of the domains of this questionnaire, indicating no clinically significant difficulties in executive function. During the course of this original assessment, she was not yet attending school again and therefore it was not possible to get a teacher report version, which would have been particularly advantageous in this case. When considering her presentation during assessment, her foster carers' responses on the BRIEF appeared to be an underestimate of her difficulties (Table 3.6).

Table 3.5 Subtest scores

Subtest	Subtest scaled score
Verbal Fluency	
Letter Fluency	9
Category Fluency	10
Category Switching (total correct responses)	10
Category Switching (total switching accuracy)	12
20 questions	
Initial Abstraction score	10
Total Questions asked	9
Total Achievement Weighting score	10

Table 3.6 Composite and subscale scores

	T-score	Percentile
Behavioural Regulation Index	58	83
Inhibit	60	86
Shift	52	65
Emotional Control	59	81
Metacognition Index	53	70
Initiate	50	59
Working Memory	60	84
Plan/Organize	60	83
Organisation of Materials	35	10
Monitor	58	81
General Executive Composite	56	76

Formulation

Megan's case required formulation from a number of approaches. Although it was important to consider the specific neuropsychological models and theories of cognition and early child and adolescent brain development, in this case it was also increasingly important to consider the systems around her and the impact they had on the neuropsychological aspects of her history and presentation. To demonstrate this I will focus on her neuropsychological presentation within a systemic formulation of her difficulties and use this to offer recommendations of how best to intervene to support her at home and school. We must also consider the impact of the severe frontal brain injury on her ongoing cognition and social functioning. These would be likely to evolve over time as the frontal lobes of the brain continue to develop (Fig. 3.1).

At this stage the remit of the formulation is about better understanding Megan, starting from the outer circles of the formulation diagram to gather information and build up a picture and impression of Megan together with direct contact with her.

Society This section of the formulation relates to how UK society views children in the social care system and young people with ABI. Intervention at this level may be

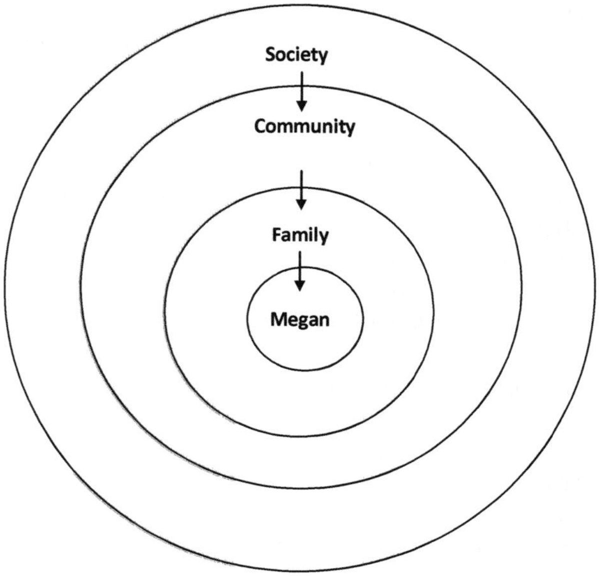

Fig. 3.1 Formulation diagram

focused towards increasing general understanding of these issues through the media and literature, including charities and the work that they do.

Community This level of the formulation considers how Megan's closer community such as her school, social care system, friendships and health-care teams relate to her functioning. For her, understanding within her local community was quite limited, particularly when living in the foster placement where she was at the time of her accident and hospital stay. Changes in behaviour were attributed to her premorbid personality, despite school reports that indicated significant differences post-injury.

Family For Megan, this includes consideration of her foster carers, previous foster carers and their families, plus her birth family. Furthermore, many complexities arose from ongoing contact with her family and extended family. In particular, her relationship with her younger brother was important to contemplate as they were fostered together. For Megan, this level also encompassed key people from her social care team, such as her social worker, especially those that had been consistent and present for her for many years. Megan had encountered a large number of social workers and therefore lacked a key adult with whom she had developed a particularly close relationship.

Early in Megan's rehabilitation, Megan and her family and part of the community section would be most prominent with regards to intervention. As time goes on, more work with the wider circles becomes increasingly important to consider as Megan moves out into wider society. Later rehabilitation will thus become broader in remit.

Megan At this level, issues specific and personal to Megan need to be addressed, such as premorbid personality, acquired cognitive and behavioural difficulties, psychological and emotional impact of life in social care, history of neglect, separation from birth parents and lack of early schooling.

Intervention/Feedback/Reformulation

Feedback following assessment was provided initially to the original school which Megan attended after discharge from hospital. Regrettably, in the first instance direct feedback could not be provided to the foster carer or Megan as they were unable to be contacted. This was an example of one of the complexities of interacting with the social care system. Eventually, made contact with social services who then informed that Megan had since moved into an adoptive placement and therefore feedback was provided to her new parents. Information was also provided to the referrer and general practitioner (GP) in the form of a full neuropsychological report.

Reassessment

Megan was referred for a further assessment 18 months following the original assessment in order to monitor her neuropsychological functioning and development.

Wechsler Intelligence Scale for Children-Fourth UK Edition (WISC-IV^{UK})

Tables 3.7 and 3.8 show that Megan's performance on the WISC-IV^{UK} revealed a similar pattern of performance and areas of strength and difficulty as her previous assessment.

Children's Memory Scale (CMS)

Tables 3.9 and 3.10 describe Megan's performance on the CMS.

Table 3.7 WISC-IV^{UK} composite index scores

Scale	Composite score	Percentile rank	95 % confidence interval	Qualitative description
Verbal Comprehension (VCI)	63	1	58–72	Extremely Low
Perceptual Reasoning (PRI)	79	8	73–88	Borderline
Working Memory (WMI)	68	2	63–78	Extremely Low
Processing Speed (PSI)	70	2	65–83	Borderline
Full Scale (FSIQ)	63	1	59–69	Extremely Low

Table 3.8 WISC-IV^{UK} subtest scores

Index	Subtest	Subtest scaled score
Verbal Comprehension	Similarities	5
	Vocabulary	2
	Comprehension	4
	(Information)	(2)
	(Word Reasoning)	(6)
Perceptual Reasoning	Block Design	4
	Picture Concepts	9
	Matrix Reasoning	7
	(Picture Completion)	(5)
Working Memory	Digit Span	4
	Letter–Number Sequencing	5
	(Arithmetic)	(3)
Processing Speed	Coding	3
	Symbol Search	6
	(Cancellation)	(11)

Table 3.9 CMS results

Index	Index score	Percentile rank	Qualitative description
Visual Immediate	66	1	Extremely Low
Visual Delayed	73	3	Borderline
Verbal Immediate	60	0.4	Extremely Low
Verbal Delayed	69	2	Extremely Low
General Memory	54	0.1	Extremely Low
Attention/Concentration	57	0.2	Extremely Low
Learning	72	3	Borderline
Delayed Recognition	50	<0.1	Extremely Low

Table 3.10 CMS subtest scores

Subtest	Subtest scaled score	Percentile rank
Dot Locations		
Learning	8	25
Total Score	5	5
Long Delay	3	1
Stories		
Immediate	4	2
Delayed	2	<1
Delayed Recognition	2	<1
Faces		
Immediate	4	2
Delayed	8	25
Word Pairs		
Learning	3	1
Total Score	3	1
Long Delay	8	25
Delayed Recognition	1	<1
Numbers		
Total Score	3	1
Sequences		
Total Score	3	1

Wechsler Individual Achievement Test-Second UK Edition (WIAT-II^{UK})

Due to Megan's reported difficulties with academic attainment such as reading and spelling, she was assessed using the Word Reading, Pseudoword Decoding and Spelling subtests of this assessment, which assesses achievement of children aged 4 to 16 years old on a number of domains such as reading and written language.

Megan achieved a standard score of 43 (<0.1st percentile) on the Word Reading subtest, 67 (1st percentile) on the Pseudoword Decoding and 47 (<0.1st percentile) on the Spelling subtest, all falling within the Extremely Low range for her age. These scores are below what would be expected based on Megan's Full Scale IQ (FSIQ) and this may well be the consequence of disrupted and lacking early education when building the foundations of reading, writing and spelling and/or pre-existing specific learning difficulties.

Table 3.11 Delis–Kaplan Executive Function System (D–KEFS)

Subtest	Subtest scaled score
Verbal Fluency	
Letter Fluency	7
Category Fluency	6
Category Switching (total correct responses)	6
Category Switching (total switching accuracy)	3
20 questions	
Initial Abstraction score	5
Total Questions asked	13
Total Achievement Weighting score	9

Delis–Kaplan Executive Function System (D–KEFS)

Megan was assessed using two subtests of the D–KEFS; the Verbal Fluency Test and 20 Questions Test, the results of which are shown in Table 3.11.

On the Verbal Fluency Test, Megan completed the Letter Fluency Test, in which she was required to name words beginning with a particular letter; the Category Fluency Test, in which she had to name words within a semantic category; and the Category Switching Test, which required her to switch between semantic categories. Megan scored in the Low Average range on the Letter and Number Fluency trials and the Category Switching Total Correct responses. She scored below average on the Category Switching (Total Switching Accuracy) Test.

On the 20 Questions Test, Megan was required to identify a target picture chosen by the examiner from an array of pictures by asking the fewest number of yes/no questions as possible. On this test Megan performed in the Average range for her age for Total Questions Asked and Total Weighted Achievement scores. However, although Megan developed a more effective style of questioning as each trial continued, initially she demonstrated an inefficient strategy of questioning for her first question which eliminated only a small number of possible pictures (Table 3.12).

Behaviour Rating Inventory of Executive Function (BRIEF)

Megan's adoptive parents completed the BRIEF questionnaire in relation to Megan (see Table 3.12). Megan scored above the clinical cut-off *T*-score of 65 on all of the domains of this questionnaire, indicating clinically significant difficulties in executive function, including behavioural regulation and metacognition, such

Table 3.12 BRIEF scores

	T-score	Percentile
Behavioural Regulation Index	76	96
Inhibit	76	97
Shift	70	94
Emotional Control	73	96
Metacognition Index	76	97
Initiate	69	95
Working Memory	69	95
Plan/Organize	80	98
Organisation of Materials	64	92
Monitor	79	99
General Executive Composite	78	98

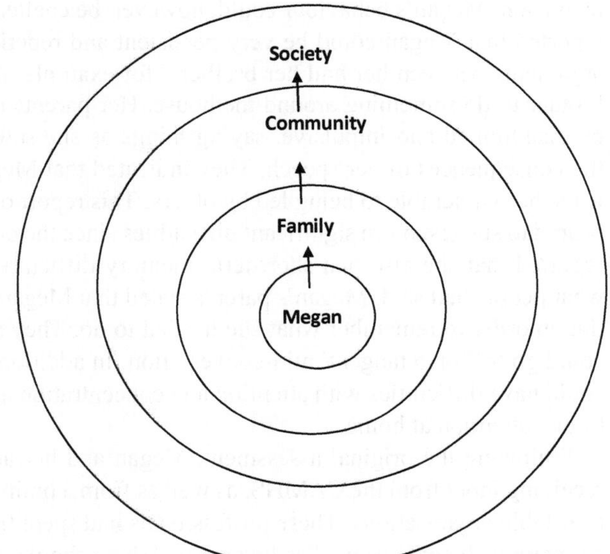

Fig. 3.2 Reformulation diagram

as inhibition, working memory, planning and organising, and initiation. This score identifies significant problems compared with the previous scores obtained by the foster carers.

Reformulation

At this stage of the formulation, Megan is known better and therefore the reformulation starts from Megan and moves towards the outer circles (Fig. 3.2). Information is gathered to build upon the original formulation and intervene and influence Megan's environment at various levels of her needs, personality and strengths. At this stage, the neuropsychologist becomes a true advocate for Megan. This formulation provides a two-step approach for the paediatric neuropsychologist in a time-limited specific assessment setting.

Megan Since the original assessment Megan and her younger half-brother, Ben, now aged 12, were living in an adoptive placement. Megan reported that she enjoyed living with her new parents and felt well supported by them. Both parents had an understanding of Megan's additional learning needs. Since living with her new family, Megan had had no direct contact with her birth family. At clinical interview Megan's parents provided detailed information regarding their understanding and observations of Megan and her presentation, demonstrating their insight into Megan's needs.

At home, Megan's parents reported that Megan could be very helpful and assisted in carrying out household tasks. She enjoyed listening to music and watching television. Megan's behaviour could, however, be challenging at times. Her parents reported that Megan could be very persistent and repetitive, and this could create arguments between her and her brother—for example, if Megan was ordering her brother to do something around the house. Her parents reported that Megan could be disinhibited and impulsive, saying things as she saw them before considering the consequences of her speech. They indicated that Megan's impulsiveness could leave her vulnerable to being led by others. This report of executive difficulties appeared to suggest more significant difficulties since the original assessment. Parents reported that she also had short-term memory difficulties, for example forgetting what people had said. Megan's parents stated that Megan needed structure and routine in order to remember what she needed to do. They also described that Megan could go 'off on a tangent' mid-conversation. In addition they reported that Megan could have difficulties with attention and concentration and also sought lots of one-to-one attention at home.

Following the original assessment, Megan and her adoptive parents were now receiving input from the CAMHS, as well as from a brain injury support worker and charitable organisations. These professionals had spent time supporting Megan and her parents directly, as well as liaising with her school and social care team.

At the time of the reassessment she had just entered her fifth year of secondary school. Megan's placement at her previous school had broken down since the first assessment due to her difficulties with behavioural regulation and interaction with her peers. Importantly though, Megan's original school had indicated a noticeable difference in Megan's memory and learning following her brain injury. They reported that she had always presented with learning difficulties, including reading and numeracy, but that she had demonstrated more difficulties with learning and behaviour since the accident.

At her new school Megan was supported by a dedicated special education needs centre and a statutory assessment of special educational needs had been requested. Prior to Megan's school move, her academic work and reading was reported to be improving. She was in a nurture group at her previous school for the majority of her lessons.

Premorbid personality, acquired cognitive and behavioural difficulties, psychological and emotional impact of life in social care, history of neglect and lack of early schooling are all contributing factors to Megan's formulation. Megan demonstrated a very similar neuropsychological profile to her original assessment, though her results on testing of executive function were more impaired at the time of reassessment. This may reflect a more considered report from her parents compared with her foster carers during the previous assessment and the emerging deficits as a result of her acquired frontal brain injury as she has developed through her adolescent years.

Family For Megan this includes consideration of her adoptive parents, previous foster carers and their family, as well as her birth family and all the complexities that come with her ongoing contact with her family and extended family. This may also include key people from her social care team, such as her social worker if they have been consistent and present for her for many years. Megan had developed a close relationship with her new adoptive parents which was providing a great deal of support. She had, however, experienced losses such as no longer having contact with her birth parents and moving on from her previous foster carers. However, she continued to live with her brother.

Community The focus at this level includes how Megan's closer community such as school, social care system, friendships and health-care teams relate to her functioning. Megan's new school did not know her medical background: although this gave her a new start, her difficulties could have been overlooked or misinterpreted. She experienced difficulties settling in and developing friendships. However, the new setting also meant professionals could liaise with staff and pupils to inform and educate them regarding Megan's difficulties and how best to aid her learning. Having CAMHS and a brain injury support worker supporting Megan and her family greatly improved information sharing across services and helped the family.

Society As detailed in the formulation section, this level of the formulation relates to how UK society views children in the social care system and young people with ABI. Intervention at this level would include how we can increase general understanding of these issues through the media and literature, including charities and the work that they do. As can occur with children with nonaccidental brain injuries who enter the care system, accidental brain injury cases such as Megan's may get lost to regular neuropsychological and neurological follow-up within the NHS. Children may move to different care placements and schools across the country and the brain injury and its consequences may get lost in the lists of other factors and reports concerning the child and their needs.

Outcome

At the time of reassessment Megan was living in an adoptive placement. This created changes and losses for Megan that needed to be included in the reformulation. Changes included living a long distance from her existing school and losing the community in which she used to live. However, this also included positive changes amongst a new community setting which appeared to be more supportive and understanding of her difficulties. In terms of intervention there was a new hospital service with a brain injury coordinator which led to joint working with the neuropsychologist to provide training for staff at the new school. Health-care professionals' regular attendance at CAMHS consultations and contact with the parents was important. Also, work was done with school peers to help them understand why Megan behaved the way that she did for them to have more understanding and be more accommodating of her difficulties.

Summary and Discussion

Megan was a young person living in the social care system who sustained a significant head injury at the age of 14. She had pre-existing learning difficulties and disrupted early education, as well as a disrupted domestic environment due to changes in foster carers and social work support. Serial neuropsychological assessment on two occasions revealed that Megan continued to experience significant difficulties across a range of cognitive domains including verbal comprehension, perceptual reasoning, working memory, processing speed, visual and verbal memory, and executive function. It was difficult to ascertain Megan's premorbid abilities before the accident due to the challenges in accurately estimating this in children and also her disrupted education and lack of family report. Within the limitations of the NHS assessment process, it was possible to obtain further information about Megan through detailed neuropsychological testing. At the second assessment, further details were obtained about the changes in her life and schooling, and it was now possible to corroborate her difficulties with a repeat neuropsychological assessment.

Recommendations were made regarding the support Megan recieved at home and school. Megan's pre-existing learning difficulties meant that it was problematic to ascertain precisely how much of her impairment results from her significant head injury and how much derives from a pre-existing learning disability. However, observations of behaviour change and performance at school were noted post-accident and these changes would be unsurprising given the significance of the head injury that Megan sustained.

It would be imperative for Megan's learning and development that she continue to receive additional support at home and school as she was a vulnerable young person as a result of her social background, disrupted education, pre-existing learning difficulties and ABI. The importance of consistency and understanding of the severity of her brain injury was of paramount importance as much of her behaviour could be attributed to her previous life experiences.

It is important in the context of brain injury to have details of premorbid ability to distinguish what was accident related and what was premorbid ability. Assessing this is always more difficult in children where most of the information to determine premorbid ability is provided by parents/carers and education. There may be little family background, developmental and medical history available about a child living in local authority care. For example, this is the case if a child comes to an appointment with a foster carer who has limited background information. These challenges raise the importance of health and education professionals talking to and liaising with other social care professionals such as social workers to gain the most information possible should a child sustain a brain injury while living in local authority care.

The means of intervening for a child with an executive deficit may differ from the intervention used with a child with a history of abuse or neglect. Joint intervention with experts in social care thus becomes essential. Additional executive function difficulties together with additional needs (as the result of early abuse and/or neglect) may increase vulnerability of these young people and increase the possible breakdown of foster and potential adoptive placements. Joint multi-agency collaboration would be aimed at working pro-actively to reduce risk for children like Megan within the social care system with ABI's accidental, nonaccidental or acquired through infections. Future cases should consider all the levels, the impact on the child or adolescent and the importance of intervening at each level to ensure the understanding of all parties who are making decisions about this child. This consideration will be of paramount importance when considering placements, decisions about schooling, decisions about adoption or foster placements or returning to birth parents/families. This is the case for accidental and nonaccidental injuries where the head injury may get lost or be underestimated when a child is being moved from placement to placement.

Learning points in this case include the need for greater liaison with the local community during the first assessment as having more information led to a more positive outcome in the second assessment phase. The value of formulation and reformulation in this case lies in the many complexities and missing pieces of information that needed to be pulled together. A formulation such as this can be difficult to pull together when working within an acute hospital trust where access to community and social service records may be more limited. However, the importance of liaison with other health and social care professionals is identified in this case and those similar cases where children may have moved home a number of times and moved through different medical professionals, schools and families. This is particularly pertinent if they have moved across different counties or regions of the country where information may get lost.

References

Anderson, V. (2001). Assessing executive functions in children: Biological, psychological, and developmental considerations. *Pediatric Rehabilitation, 4*(3), 119–136.

Anderson, V., Spencer-Smith, M., & Wood, A. (2011). Do children really recover better? Neurobehavioural plasticity after early brain insult. *Brain, 134*, 2197–2221.

Department for Children, Schools and Families. (2009). *Statutory guidance on promoting the health and well-being of looked after children*. Nottingham: Department for Children, Schools and Families.

Department for Education and Department for Health. (2015). Promoting the health and well-being of looked-after children. Department for Education and Department for Health. http://www.rcpch.ac.uk/system/files/protected/page/DH_Promoting_the_health_and_well-being_of_looked-after_children.pdf. Accessed 26 May 2015.

NICE and the Social Care Institute for Excellence (SCIE). (2010). *Looked-after babies, children and young people*. https://www.nice.org.uk/guidance/ph28. Accessed 7 Nov 2014.

Royal College of Nursing and the Royal College of Paediatrics and Child Health. (2015). *Looked after children: Knowledge, skills and competences of health care staff*. London: Royal College of Nursing and the Royal College of Paediatrics and Child Health. http://www.rcpch.ac.uk/system/files/protected/page/Looked%20After%20Children%202015_0.pdf. Accessed 26 May 2015.

Chapter 4
All in the Family: Huntington's Disease, Variability and Challenges for Clinical Neuropsychology

Lynette J. Tippett and Virginia M. Hogg

Some clinical neuropsychologists work in settings, or communities, in which clients with Huntington's disease (HD) are relatively frequent, but many clinicians may be asked to assess an individual with the HD gene just a few times in their careers, if at all. Although HD, a progressive neurodegenerative disorder, is caused by a single autosomal dominant gene, there is surprising variability in the symptoms and problems that result from its action, and from the interactions between the neural effects of the gene and the characteristics of the person and their environment. Whilst variability is commonplace amongst many neurological conditions and diseases, most clinicians develop the ability to produce skilled formulations of the complex presentations of patient groups as a result of experience and exposure to multiple clients with the same neurological condition. Producing valid and useful formulations of low frequency client groups, however, is more challenging. This chapter will provide a brief background to HD, before outlining and illustrating some of the challenges and issues related to generating useful neuropsychological formulations in clients with the HD gene. We illustrate some of these issues, particularly related to variability, in the presentation of the cases of two brothers carrying the HD gene.

HD is inherited through an autosomal-dominant gene. Each child of an affected parent, therefore, has a 50:50 chance of inheriting the gene and developing the disease. In 1993, the Huntington's Disease Collaborative Research Group identified the gene defective in HD on the short arm of chromosome 4 (The Huntington's Disease Collaborative Research Group 1993). The HD gene (IT15) has a CAG trinucleotide repeat that is expanded to 36 repeats or more. This produces an expanded polyglutamine sequence in the derived protein (huntingtin), which results in neurodegeneration in the basal ganglia and cerebral cortex of the forebrain (Vonsattel

L. J. Tippett (✉) · V. M. Hogg
School of Psychology and Centre for Brain Research, The University of Auckland, Room 660, Level 6, Main Office, Human Sciences Building, 10 Symonds Street, Auckland, New Zealand
e-mail: l.tippett@auckland.ac.nz

V. M. Hogg
e-mail: vhogg@adhb.govt.nz

J. A. B. Macniven (ed.), *Neuropsychological Formulation*,
DOI 10.1007/978-3-319-18338-1_4

et al. 1997). Since 1993, it has been possible in many countries for individuals aged 18 years or over to undergo a test to determine their genetic status, usually following completion of a predictive testing process in keeping with the current international guidelines (MacLeod et al. 2013). Uptake of presymptomatic genetic testing varies amongst nationalities, but, however, is generally low, ranging from 3 to 4% in Germany, to 24% in The Netherlands, with the United Kingdom and Canada at 18% (Tibben 2007).

Perhaps surprisingly, it is still relatively common that individuals at risk of inheriting the gene are unaware of their risk. Family members may not disclose the at-risk status to an individual for a variety of reasons; unease, shame, prejudice, denial, lack of knowledge, adoption, or because families have lost contact with one another by geographical or social separation. In addition, at-risk status may be obscured because a similarly at-risk parent or sibling died prior to the emergence of symptoms of the disease, or because their CAG repeat length fell within the reduced penetrance range (CAG repeat length 36–39), or intermediate range (27–35) (Langbehn et al. 2004). A CAG length in the intermediate range (sometimes called mutably normal range) means that person will not develop clinical HD, but their offspring may be at risk of developing the disease due to expansion of the CAG repeat length into the disease range during meiosis (Imarisio et al. 2008).

The clinical course of HD is characterised by a triad of impairments: movement disorder, impaired cognition and mood/psychiatric disturbance (Vonsattel and DiFiglia 1998). It is mostly known for the presence of involuntary choreiform movements, but motor problems also involve alterations in eye movements, coordination, impaired gait, motor impersistence, dystonia, loss of balance and impaired swallowing (Biglan et al. 2009; Marshall 2004; Young et al. 1986). Cognitive changes include slowed processing speed, attentional and executive difficulties (poor concentration, difficulty multitasking, loss of mental flexibility, poor planning, working memory and initiation) and problems with recognition of emotions and with some aspects of visuospatial processing (Brandt and Butters 1986; Paulson 2011; Stout et al. 2011; Wahlin et.al 2007). Mood and psychiatric disturbance commonly includes anxiety, irritability and depression, but can also include aggressive outbursts, psychotic disturbance and suicide (Duff et al 2007; Julien et al 2007; Rosenblatt 2007; van Duijn et al. 2007). Whilst the high incidence of depression in HD is likely to be partially a natural consequence of reactive stress, it appears also to reflect neural changes occurring with the disease (Du et al. 2013; Julien et al. 2007; Thu et al. 2010). As the disease progresses weight loss occurs, and sleep disorders are common. Clinical progression is also accompanied by functional changes that gradually erode the individual's level of independence; they are unable to maintain employment at the level prior to symptom onset, eventually are no longer safe to drive, and develop difficulty in completing domestic tasks such as cooking, cleaning and managing finances. Ultimately, some individuals, although certainly not all, require full hospital care (Novak and Tabrizi 2011).

Diagnosis of clinical onset of HD (commonly in the 30 or 40s, but reported range from 2 to 80 years) is currently provided by neurologists. It is defined only by the development of unequivocal HD motor signs, even though it is generally accepted that there may be cognitive, psychological and perhaps psychiatric symptoms for some years prior to this (Kieburtz et al. 1996; Biglan et al. 2013). The onset of clinical symptoms in individuals is roughly negatively correlated with the number of CAG repeats in the HD gene, although this accounts for only approximately 50 % of the variance. Of the remaining variance, 60 % is thought to be due to environmental factors (Ross and Tabrizi 2011; Wexler et al. 2004). In transgenic mouse models of HD, environmental enrichment significantly delays the onset and slows the progression of disease (Hockly et al. 2002; van Dellen et al. 2000). Trembath et al. (2010) also found that a passive lifestyle contributed to the earlier onset of symptoms in a sample of 154 individuals symptomatic for HD.

The familial effects of HD extend beyond inheritance of the autosomal-dominant HD gene. The clinical onset of HD in early-to mid-adult years commonly leads to many sources of stress within the family of origin: financial (reduced capacity to work over a normal lifespan for individual and carer), shame and embarrassment for children (parents who are perceived as drunk or mentally unstable), children who have to take on adult roles (cook/cleaner/carer for their parent), children, spouses and relations coping with severe behavioural disturbances in the HD-affected individual, and at worst, coping with childhoods of abuse and neglect. Within any given family, there may be multiple generations as well as multiple siblings who are symptomatic for the disease at one time. Others watch and wonder, with varying degrees of certainty, if this is also their future. Understanding the broader familial impacts of HD for gene-positive and gene-negative family members is crucial when interviewing family members.

Clinical Formulation in Huntington's Disease

The role of a clinical neuropsychologist and neuropsychological assessment and formulation in HD will depend upon the stage of clinical HD in the client, and the particular circumstances that led to the referral. Sometimes the neuropsychologist may be asked to contribute to the diagnosis of clinical onset of HD, although the current general practice is to base diagnosis of clinical onset only on the presence of motor features that are unambiguously Huntington's related. Nevertheless, the referring clinician and/or client may ask whether there is any sign of disease-related cognitive decline in neuropsychological performance. This is a difficult question to respond to as it requires having: (i) a valid estimate of "normal" or pre-disease level of functioning for that person; (ii) a well-selected neuropsychological battery that is likely to be sensitive to the earliest cognitive changes that occur in HD and (iii) the ability to gain optimal performance from a client who may have a number of mood issues that could be reactive or part of the HD disease process.

Just as in other domains of clinical neuropsychology, delineation of behavioural strengths and weaknesses often provides the most useful type of formulation. This can contribute to the client's and family's understandings of functional difficulties (and how these relate or are a consequence of the neural changes associated with HD), and of HD progression and severity (or to the contrary, normalise behaviours that are being misattributed to HD). This may also be useful for understanding family interactions, have implications for work and other roles with responsibility (e.g. childcare) and other functional questions. Some clients may want the neuropsychologist to provide predictions for their future/s, which, as in the case of most neurodegenerative conditions, is a request that cannot be well answered. Nevertheless, it may be possible to identify specific areas of strength, which may assist with managing areas of weakness. This may include generating recommendations on coping with environmental demands in the face of particular behavioural deficits, providing input into the individual's ability to manage themselves and behave adaptively in society, and into possible forensic issues.

Challenges to Useful Formulations in HD

When working with HD clients (either presymptomatic or symptomatic), there are a number of challenges to providing valid and useful formulations, particularly for clinicians without a broad understanding of HD. Many of these challenges are particularly marked in assessment of individuals who are approaching, or in the very early stages of symptom onset, when the presence of clinical problems may be subtle.

First, the selection of an appropriate test battery requires selection of measures sensitive to the cognitive problems associated with various disease stages (Ho et al. 2003; Paulsen 2011; Stout et al. 2011). The neuropsychologist must also consider possible variability in types of cognitive difficulties experienced from person to person, possibly due to variability in patterns of cortical degeneration, although evidence for this is very preliminary (Rosas et al. 2008, Scahill et al. 2013; Thu et al. 2010).

Second, the selection and interpretation of performance on neuropsychological measures must take account of the extent of any motor problems (typically bilateral) present. The presence of involuntary movements, such as chorea, will affect speed of response, exactness of response, and may make tasks requiring fine motor movements and coordination extremely difficult. Even when chorea is not present or not marked, there may be subtle changes in voluntary movements (fine motor coordination, motor impersistence and bradykinesia) that influence performance on tasks requiring a motor response, particularly a speeded response.

A third challenge to the development of valid formulations is the presence of clinical variability in the disease. Not only does age of symptom onset vary in HD, but the symptoms present at onset vary from person to person and the extent of functional difficulties resulting from particular symptom-domains may continue to vary across the span of clinical disease. Some individuals experience mainly motor symptomatology at clinical onset and minimal dysfunction of either mood or cognition. Others show mainly mood and/or cognitive changes, with minimal movement dysfunction until later stages of the disease. Others experience concomitant motor, mood and cognitive symptoms at onset and throughout the course of the disease (Folstein 1989; Claes et al. 1995; Loy and McCusker, 2013; Tippett et al. 2007; Zappacosta et al. 1996). This issue is often misunderstood because of the single-gene aetiology of HD, but even in the case of monozygotic twins there are descriptions of variable clinical phenotypes (e.g. Georgiou et al. 1999; Gomez-Esteban, et al. 2007; Panas et al. 2008). Loy and McCusker (2013) provide a depiction of the dimensions along which this variability may be present in HD. There is no clear correlation between the variable symptom profile and CAG repeat number.

The variability of the presence of mood disturbance poses particular challenges. Anxiety, depression and irritability may be present early in the disease course and may influence neuropsychological performance in this population in a number of ways (Berrios et al. 2002; Duff et al. 2007; Rosenblatt 2007; Thompson et al. 2012). We have found in our extensive longitudinal research that mood difficulties may not always be reported in the clinical interview by individuals (either presymptomatic or symptomatic), yet their responses to formal mood scales may indicate marked levels of mood disturbance, particularly anxiety and irritability. Apathy is also common in both presymptomatic and symptomatic HD (van Duijn et al. 2007), but may have multiple origins. It is important to select mood scales that have removed items that have a strong focus on somatic or motor symptoms to avoid inflated estimates of mood disturbance due to motor symptoms.

If the client has undertaken predictive gene testing, it is important to consider the timing of the assessment in relation to when the person received their results of predictive gene testing. Tibben (2007) reported that individuals identified as gene positive for HD experienced increased distress for a number of weeks, but returned to baseline psychological functioning within 1 year of testing, despite the knowledge that they will develop this devastating disorder at some point in their futures. Non-carriers also experience distress after initial feelings of relief, with most distress 6 months after receiving the result.

Integrating mood disturbance appropriately into a clinical formulation is particularly difficult, as determining whether mood symptoms are direct results of the disease process, secondary responses to current difficulties, or pre-existing traits is complex. When mood disturbance is only present at a low level, it is difficult to ascertain to what extent this has impacted performance on the neuropsychological measures.

Another challenge to clinical formulation (although one that is not unique to HD) is that individuals who are symptomatic frequently do not accurately report symptoms and issues they face. Cognitive deterioration may mean the client will lack insight, or they will have difficulty in articulating their concerns. Indeed, it is not uncommon for symptomatic individuals to present as if in total denial of any HD symptoms at all. In these cases, and more generally, a separate clinical interview with a significant other is important to gain useful insight into current functioning and problems.

A final important point is the modulating effects of situational and social factors in the expression of the clinical symptoms of HD. As described earlier, many HD families will have a history that includes chaos and uncertainty resulting from the altered/reduced functioning of an HD-affected parent. Situational factors can modulate the nature and extent of these disturbances, and possibly also the rate of progression of the symptoms in the HD individual (particularly given recent findings that social factors modulate the progression of mild cognitive decline in older adults; Marioni et al. 2012). The presence of a stable and supportive partner/family can sometimes help to reduce stress and the extent of pressure experienced by the person with HD. This in turn reduces the severity of symptoms, particularly, behavioural disturbances.

To illustrate some of these issues, particularly of the variability in HD presentation and development, we present the cases of two brothers carrying the HD gene. Our knowledge of these two men has come from direct observations, clinical and neuropsychological assessments, as well as significant input from family members. We report neuropsychological data collected at two time points approximately 2 years apart, with follow-up information some years later. These assessments were carried out as a part of a longitudinal observational study that included an extensive, tailored, neuropsychological assessment with reports provided to participants. The brothers have been visited at their homes on a biennial basis over a 12-year period by one of the researchers (VH). During the first 10 years, neither of these men took any HD-related medication, nor did they have any HD-related medical oversight by specialists (e.g. neurologist or psychiatrist).

A Tale of Two Brothers and HD

Common Background The two brothers, George and Bob, inherited the HD gene from their father, testing positive for the gene presymptomatically. George's expanded CAG repeat length was 42, Bob's was 41. (A difference of one in CAG repeat length falls within the margin of error associated with the genetic test; Benjamin et al. 1994.) It is plausible to presume that these two brothers would have a similar age of onset and experience of the disease. This, however, was not the case.

The brothers grew up unaware of the existence of HD in their family. Their father's HD symptoms were always attributed to his serious tractor accident. By chance one of the brother's wives read an article in a magazine and from this she determined that her father-in-law actually had HD. He was finally diagnosed just prior to his death around the age of 72. Three of his six siblings had also inherited the gene, two were gene negative and one had died as a young child. The existence of HD in the family had been known by a few, but kept from those at risk. By the time the brothers became aware they were adults, each with two children. The brothers' children and grandchildren, who are at risk of inheriting the gene, have thus far elected not to know their genetic status.

George and Bob grew up on a farm in rural New Zealand. All four siblings in their family of origin inherited the HD gene. Their two elder sisters both died from HD, the eldest aged 55 years, the next aged 73 years. George and Bob share not only their family of origin and childhood experiences but many aspects of their adult lives. Both men married women who had grown up in the same local area; both the marriages have spanned more than 40 years and both wives remain very supportive of their husbands.

George and Bob both left school at 16 years of age to assist their father on the family farm. They both demonstrated high average academic ability (performing at a high average to superior level in their school exams at 15 years of age). They both have long careers as dairy farmers and are passionate about their work and lifestyle. Both of them own their own farms, which are situated in the rural area of their birth. Whilst for much of their careers they have been involved in the hands-on activities of farming, for example milking cows, rearing animals, cropping, property maintenance, they have also been responsible for the overall productivity and viability of the farm and to this extent they are very much managers of their own businesses. They train and employ and manage staff, and make the economic and financial decisions for a business of significant value. Both the brothers enjoy the intellectual, as well as the practical, aspects of farming.

The strong similarities in the lives of these two brothers make their very different experiences of HD particularly striking.

Bob Assessment 1

Bob, aged 61, was first seen 5 years after he had received his HD test results. At this time neither Bob nor his wife Wendy considered there were any issues causing concern, nor any definite signs of HD. The only reported probable prodromal symptom was mild motor restlessness in his feet when seated. Bob thought his short-term memory was not as good as it had been, but felt he was not significantly worse than his peers.

In addition to farming life, Bob enjoyed boating and fly fishing and travelling abroad. He was an avid reader, reading up to five books (generally non-fiction) a week. His wife described him as "intelligent," "a deep thinker" and "a hard worker." Bob highly valued his family and his farming lifestyle. Bob had told his children and some close friends of his genetic test result. He presented as a considered, private, thoughtful man.

Bob had no significant health concerns, no history of cigarette use or abuse of alcohol or drugs, no known head injuries or other neurological disorders. He was taking medication for a heart arrhythmia and joint pain. Bob stated that when under stress he tended to "go quiet" and "take things out on himself." Throughout his life Bob had been prone to days when he would "get down to it." He had never been on any mood altering or antidepressant medication and had never been formally diagnosed with depression. His most recent and persistent period of low mood occurred for approximately 6 months following his HD test results (aged

55). Since this time, however, Bob felt he had experienced fewer episodes of low mood and that he was better able to manage any such incident. He has a place on the farm where he goes if feeling low, and uses self-statements to calm himself, to reassure himself of his relative fortune, and to remind himself to accept things as they come. At the time of his first assessment, Bob's scores of "0" on the depression component and "3" on the anxiety component of the Hospital Anxiety and Depression Scale (HADS) were in the normal range, as was his score of "2" on the Snaith Outward Irritability scale. During neuropsychological testing, however, Bob did exhibit noticeable anxiety, which was particularly evident during verbal fluency: difficulty on the first letter led to considerable observable distress when he tried the next letter.

Neuropsychological Assessment Overall Bob's pattern of performance on the neuropsychological assessment (see Table 4.1) revealed a number of areas of clear strength and a number of areas of mild concern. Verbal skills were an area of strength with his performance on tasks of word knowledge, confrontation-naming abilities and abstract reasoning, within or above his estimated level of premorbid ability (high average). Overall his performance on tasks involving visual perceptual and visuospatial processing also fell consistently in the expected range, with the exception of Block Design, on which his score fell just below the mean. Processing speed (particularly psychomotor speed) is frequently one of the first domains in which HD-related neuropsychological impairment may emerge. Given this, Bob's relatively poor performance on Symbol Digit Modalities and Stroop Colour suggested early HD-related neuropsychological changes may be emerging. Notably, however, his performance on other measures of psychomotor and processing speed was relatively good (SCOLP Comprehension, Trails A, Stroop Word), as was his performance on motor speed measures (finger tapping and Purdue pegboard). Executive functioning (including mental flexibility, problem solving and strategy generation and working memory) and complex attention (set-shifting) are influenced by frontostriatal dysfunction and are considered to be key indicators of an HD-related cognitive decline. Bob's performance raised mild concerns in the domain of executive functioning. Catastrophic performance on oral word fluency was striking, with relatively poor performance also on Stroop interference, which involves inhibition of a prepotent or automatic response. However, the performance on other relevant measures did not indicate difficulties (category fluency, Trails B and working memory). Finally as noted by Bob, his performance on memory measures involving new learning and recall was mildly, but not significantly, lower than predicted. This is not, however, a domain typically affected in the earliest stages of HD.

Summary Bob's performance revealed two areas of concern for the onset of HD symptoms: psychomotor processing speed, and aspects of executive functioning. His performance was noted to have been negatively affected by anxiety at some points, which in itself could have been part of another early HD symptom, namely HD-related mood disturbance. In our formulation, we opted at this point to be cautious in our interpretation. Bob had a long-standing struggle with mild depression,

Table 4.1 Neuropsychological performance of two brothers with HD gene overa 2-year interval

	Bob		George	
	T1: 61 years	T2: 63 years	T1: 57 years	T2: 59 years
Mini-Mental Status (/30)	25	27	29	28
Boston Naming (short version)/30	30	28	27	27
z-score	*1.79*	*0.55*	*0.43*	*0.43*
WAIS-R Similarities (scaled score)	15	13	13	12
z-score	*1.67*	*1.0*	*1.0*	*0.67*
Fluency: Phonemic (COWA)	10	31	30	27
z-score	*−2.05*	*−0.37*	*−0.98*	*−1.26*
Category (animals)	15	12	17	16
z-score	*−0.33*	*−1.02*	*−0.67*	*−0.90*
SCOLP Spot The Word (scaled score)	12	12	11	12
z-score	*0.67*	*0.67*	*0.33*	*0.67*
Speed of Comprehension (scaled score)	13	10	10	10
z-score	*1.0*	*0*	*0*	*0*
Symbol Digit Modalities	39	47	35	29
z-score	*−0.47*	*0.52*	*−0.97*	*−1.62*
Trail Making Test: Trails A (secs)	34	35	58	35
z-score	*0.09*	*0.20*	*2.09*	*−0.01*
Trails B (seconds)	69	97	95	106
z-score	*−0.28*	*1.15*	*0.85*	*1.42*
Trails: B–A	35	62	37	71
z-score	*−0.21*	*1.43*	*−0.22*	*1.53*

Table 4.1 (continued)

	Bob		George	
	T1: 61 years	T2: 63 years	T1: 57 years	T2: 59 years
Stroop (UHDRS) Colour	65	64	40	49
z-score	*− 1.28*	*− 1.36*	*− 3.19*	*− 2.50*
Word	94	80	67	68
z-score	*− 0.18*	*− 1.28*	*− 2.31*	*− 2.23*
Interference	31	33	22	23
z-score	*− 1.42*	*− 1.24*	*− 2.25*	*− 2.16*
Attention Set Shifting:				
Perseveration Condition				
Intra-dimensional shift (errors)	N/A	4	1	1
z-score		*0.36*	*− 0.42*	*− 0.42*
Extra-dimensional shift (errors)	N/A	3	29 (discont.)	22
z-score		*− 0.54*	*>3.12*	*2.14*
Learned Irrelevance Condition				
Intra-dimensional shift (errors)	N/A	4	22 (discont.)	3
z-score		*0.31*	*>5.6*	*0.01*
Extra-dimensional shift (errors)	N/A	2	–	18
z-score		*− 0.18*		*7.82*
WAIS-R Digit Span (scaled score)	11	11	10	11
z-score	*0.33*	*0.33*	*0*	*0.33*
Maximum Forwards	6	6	7	7
Maximum Back	5	6	4	4

Table 4.1 (continued)

	Bob		George	
	T1: 61 years	T2: 63 years	T1: 57 years	T2: 59 years
WMS-R Spatial Span				
Maximum Forwards	6	6	7	8
Maximum Back	5	5	6	6
VOSP:				
Position Discrimination (/20)	20	20	17	16
z-score	*0.44*	*0.44*	*− 2.89*	*− 4.0*
Number Location (/10)	10	10	9	8
z-score	*0.55*	*0.55*	*–0.36*	*− 1.27*
BORB:				
Unusual Views (/50)	50	50	N/A	50
z-score	*2.22*	*2.22*		*2.22*
Object Decision (/32)	26	29	N/A	27
z-score	*–0.45*	*0.91*		*0*
WAIS-R Block Design (scaled score)	9	14	10	11
z-score	*–0.33*	*1.33*	*0*	*0.33*
Rey Complex Figure (RCF) Copy	31	N/A	25	N/A
z-score	*0.05*		*− 1.68*	
RCF Recall (30 mins)	21	N/A	15.5	N/A
z-score	*0.91*		*0.09*	
Hopkins Verbal Learning Test				
Total Recall	23	13	14	14
z-score	*− 0.82*	*− 3.06*	*− 3.33*	*− 3.33*
Delayed Recall	8	5	5	3
z-score	*− 0.78*	*− 2.34*	*− 2.74*	*− 3.83*

Table 4.1 (continued)

	Bob		George	
	T1: 61 years	T2: 63 years	T1: 57 years	T2: 59 years
Hopkins Verbal Learning Test (cont.)				
Percentage Recall	100	83.33	100	50
z-score	*0.70*	*−0.53*	*0.47*	*−3.49*
Recognition True Positives	11	11	10	6
z-score	*−0.47*	*−0.47*	*−1.74*	*−6.24*
Recognition False Positive	1	2	4	3
z-score	*0.35*	*1.48*	*3.63*	*2.53*
Finger Tapping Test: Preferred Hand	50	49.8	N/A due to difficulty using finger	N/A due to difficulty using finger
z-score	*1.45*	*1.45*		
Non-Preferred Hand	43	36.4	N/A	N/A
z-score	*0.60*	*−0.48*		
Purdue Pegboard				
Right Hand	16	14	9	7
z-score	*1.38*	*0.23*	*−2.51*	*−3.44*
Left Hand	13	13	9	8
z-score	*−0.06*	*−0.06*	*−2.24*	*−2.69*
Both Hands	9	12	6	6
z-score	*−1.30*	*0.75*	*−2.66*	*−2.66*

WAIS-R Wechsler Adult Intelligence Scale-Revised, *SCOLP* The Speed and Capacity of Language-Processing Test *UHDRS* Unified Huntington's Disease Rating Scale, *WMS-R* Wechsler Memory Scale-Revised, *VOSP* The Visual Object and Space Perception Battery *BORB* Birmingham Object Recognition Battery which may have included features of anxiety. Importantly there was no suggestion from his wife, that he had any significant deterioration or exaggeration of his mood. In short, there was no evidence to suggest this testing-related anxiety was an HD-related symptom. Whilst there were a small number of measures on which Bob performed relatively poor, these may have been affected by the anxiety within the testing context, which was a context in which Bob felt uncomfortable. In his day-to-day life, all available evidence indicated he was competently running his farm. So again there was a lack of converging evidence to support the possibility that the lowered test scores reflected early HD. Our summary formulation, based upon the clinical interview with Bob, input from his wife and the neuropsychological assessment, was that there was no evidence that Bob was showing early symptoms of clinical HD.

Bob Assessment 2

Neuropsychological Assessment and Summary Second Testing Bob was now 63 years of age and continued to work without difficulty or concerns about his performance. He continued to feel anxious in the testing environment. Nevertheless Bob's scores on this second occasion supported our earlier formulation that he was showing no evidence of HD-related clinical difficulties. On many measures improvements were evident, at times dramatically bringing previously low scores into expected ranges (e.g. oral word fluency, Symbol Digit Modalities and Block Design), and Bob continued to show strengths in verbal functioning, as well as visual processing. He did perform more poorly on one measure of complex working memory and attentional shifting (Trails B), but there were no other clear indications of problems in this domain, including normal performance on measures of set-shifting involving perseveration and learned irrelevance. Memory performance on the Hopkins Verbal Learning Test (HVLT) had declined, but there were no functional difficulties that indicated memory functioning was causing any problem in daily life or was of clinical significance. Despite the anxiety evident during testing, there continued to be no mood issues evident in Bob's daily life. At this point, we had much more certainly in interpreting Bob's neuropsychological and clinical presentation as presymptomatic for HD.

George Assessment 1

George, 4 years younger than his brother, was 57 years old when first assessed. He was a socially outgoing man, said to have a "wide circle of friends" with whom he was completely open about his illness. Like his brother, George was hard working and enjoyed fishing and boating. He loved "a challenge," such as backpacking around the world, loved to party, and generally had a very positive outlook, enjoying things "150 %." George did not smoke cigarettes or take drugs. He enjoyed alcohol, occasionally to excess, at social events.

George's wife Mandy believed that he first started to show subtle signs of HD when 47 years of age. These were motor in nature, with involuntary feet movements that were particularly noticeable in bed and a non-specific change in gait. At the age of 57, when we first met, George was experiencing some difficulties with fine motor movements, such as tying shoelaces and writing, and he had become increasingly accident prone. His gait had a widened base and chorea was peripheral at this stage, which he often masked when sitting by crossing his hands under his arms. He had noticed that he had reduced tolerance to alcohol.

George had no history of depression, anxiety, or significant irritability. Since age 55, however, he had begun to throw what the family termed "burkes." These verbal outbursts were totally out of character, at times associated with stress, and sometimes seemingly out of the blue. George said he could feel these coming on; in the past, he would have been able to control it and communicate reasonably, but now he felt unable to shut off the words. When under stress he would usually go for a walk or take time out alone.

At the time George was first tested, he was under a considerable amount of pressure on the farm, including the added demands of a new farm, training new personnel and financial pressures. In addition, he was dealing with a recent family tragedy. His score of 5 on the depression component of the HADS was in the normal range, as was his score of 2 on the SNAITH outward irritability scale. On the anxiety component of the HADS, however, his score of 15 fell in the abnormal range.

Neuropsychological Assessment George had completed the National Adult Reading Test in a previous research study, from which his full scale, verbal and performance IQs were estimated to fall in the high average range. This was consistent with his educational and occupation achievements. Overall George's pattern of performance on the neuropsychological assessment (see Table 4.1) revealed a number of areas of concern. His performance on measures of verbal skills (including measures of word knowledge, abstract reasoning and confrontation naming) indicated this was a relative strength. In the domain of perceptual and visuospatial processing, George's performance was mixed. On constructional tasks his scores were lowered, but not significantly so (Block Design, copy of the Rey Figure), but he did have difficulty on measures of spatial judgements.

In the key domain of processing speed, George's performance fell consistently more than 1 standard deviation below the mean (with the exception of the SCOLP comprehension subtest which fell on the mean), suggesting impairment in this domain. Executive functioning and complex attention (set-shifting), also considered key when monitoring for HD-related cognitive decline, raised mild concerns. George's performance on measures of mental flexibility (Trails B) and strategy generation (both fluency tasks) were lowered but within 1 standard deviation of the mean. Although his performance on Stroop interference was poor, it was not differentially lower than the speeded control conditions. Working memory was mildly lowered for verbal material (Digits Back) but not for visual material (Span Back). Of most concern in this domain was his performance on the set-shifting task. On the perseveration condition, George failed to make the extra-dimensional shift to a new stimulus dimension, whilst on the learned irrelevance condition he failed when required to make an intra-dimensional shift (to a new exemplar within a dimension).

George struggled on both the visual (Rey Figure Recall) and verbal (HVLT) memory measures. On the HVLT George's total recall and delayed recall were significantly lowered, and he made a high number of false-positive responses on the recognition condition. Finally, George was unable to complete the finger tapping task, as he was unable to use his finger to make the taps. His performance on the Purdue pegboard was significantly lowered.

Summary George's neuropsychological performance raised multiple areas of concern related to the onset of HD symptoms reduced basic motor speed, psychomotor processing speed, verbal working memory, set-shifting, spatial processing and additionally, new learning, recall and recognition. His self-rating on the HADS indicated high levels of anxiety, which may have negatively influenced his performance, although this anxiety was not visibly evident during the session. The presence of anxiety and the verbal outbursts of irritation in his daily life that were noted as out of character may be indicators of early HD-related mood symptoms, although the presence of significant stressors in George's life made it difficult to interpret mood and behavioural changes with confidence at this timepoint. Our formulation was that George's pattern of neuropsychological difficulties was consistent with early-stage cognitive change attributable to early clinical HD. The presence of significant anxiety, however, was something that may have negatively influenced his performance and thus there was a need to be cautious at this point in our interpretation. His visible chorea and poor motor speed performance indicated the early stages of motor impairments linked with clinical HD symptoms. In summary, George's clinical and neuropsychological assessment revealed reduced or altered functioning in two domains classically affected by HD, namely motor and cognitive functioning, suggesting he was no longer presymptomatic. Even so, in his day-to-day life George continued to cope with the high-level management and running of his farm in the presence of major stressors.

George Assessment 2

Neuropsychological Assessment and Summary Second Testing George, now 59 years of age, continued to experience high levels of stress. His score of 9 on the anxiety component of the HADS, although lower than at the first assessment, fell in the borderline range. George's out-of-character outbursts still occurred, he felt more easily fatigued, found it increasingly difficult to focus on more than one thing at a time (e.g. he could no longer have the radio on whilst working on the tractor), and he had become slower and more cautious, for example when driving. Socially George had begun to feel less confident, and at times could be somewhat disinhibited with his comments. He continued, however, to work more than full time on his farm.

George's scores showed a similar pattern to that of 2 years earlier, with no marked improvements and, in general, a mild decline. His performance on measures of verbal skills was comparable and remained a relative strength. In the key domain of processing speed, George's performance on Symbol Digit Modalities had declined to more than 2 standard deviations below the mean. Whilst other measures in this domain showed some improvement, George scored more than 1.5 standard deviations below the mean on all bar the SCOLP Comprehension and Trails A subtests (on which he scored close to the mean). Performance on most measures of executive functioning and complex attention (set-shifting) showed mild deterioration with George mostly scoring between 1 and 1.5 standard deviations below the mean. On the attention set-shifting task, George failed to make the extra-dimensional shift to a new stimulus dimension in both the perseverative and learned irrelevance conditions. Finally, George's performance on the HVLT continued to indicate marked impairment. His total recall and delayed recall remained significantly lowered, and his recognition performance had deteriorated. He was still unable to complete the finger tapping tasks, and his performance on the Purdue pegboard had slightly declined. In summary, George's clinical and neuropsychological assessment continued to show reduced or altered functioning in all three domains classically affected by HD, namely motor, mood and cognition, with little improvement and mild decline in some domains. George's management and running of his farm was less effective, suggesting the emergence of functional decline, although George was still experiencing major stressors which may have contributed. Overall the second assessment reinforced the earlier formulation that George was showing HD-related clinical difficulties in the motor and cognitive domains, with a mild disturbance to mood that may have been HD-related.

Longer Term Follow-Up of the Two Brothers

We continued to be involved with these two brothers over a 10-year period. During this time, the course of the development of symptoms of these two men, who shared so much in terms of genetic, family and environment, continued to diverge.

Bob, as can be seen in Table 4.2, showed little evidence of significant decline on an abbreviated test battery. By 69 years of age there was evidence of mild slowing on Digit Symbol and Stroop, particularly the control conditions (colour and word). His memory performance remained poor, although there were still no functional memory problems in day-to-day life. At the age of 70, Bob continued to farm (with the help of workers, much as he had throughout most of his farming career), read widely, travelled overseas, and reported no significant change or deterioration in any of his activities of daily life, although he noted approaching things more quietly and circumspectly, pulling back in times of stress. His wife commented "I wish he would just slow down and have more holidays." His moods

Table 4.2 Neuropsychological performance on abbreviated battery of two brothers with HD gene during long-term follow-up

	Bob		George	
	65 years	69 years	62 years	64 years
Mini-mental status (/30)	28	N/A	27	–
Fluency: Phonemic (COWA)	26	Abandoned	31	25
z-score	*− 0.77*	(Stress)	*− 0.37*	*− 0.85*
Symbol Digit Modalities	44	30	26	22
z-score	*0.15*	*− 1.58*	*− 2.08*	*− 2.57*
Stroop (UHDRS) Colour	65	53	33	29
z-score	*− 1.28*	*− 2.20*	*− 3.73*	*− 4.03*
Word	86	77	53	50
z-score	− 0.81	− 1.52	− 3.41	− 3.64
Interference	32	32	14	17
z-score	− 1.33	− 1.33	− 2.98	− 2.71
Hopkins Verbal Learning Test				
Total Recall	18	16	12	13
z-score	*− 1.93*	*− 2.39*	*− 3.28*	*− 3.06*
Delayed Recall	6	5	2	3
z-score	*− 1.82*	*− 2.34*	*− 3.91*	*− 3.39*
Percentage Recall	85.71	71.4	40	100
z-score	*− 0.36*	*− 1.41*	*− 3.72*	*0.70*
Recognition True Positives	7	8	9	N/A
z-score	*− 4.47*	*− 3.47*	*− 2.74*	
Recognition False Positive	0	0	6	
z-score	*− 0.86*	*− 0.86*	*6.37*	

UHDRS Unified Huntington's Disease Rating Scale

remained generally even, as they had been over the 10-year period. Moderate chorea was, however, evident even to a lay observer, in his trunk, head, arms and legs when he was relaxed, sitting or standing. His writing was legible, his speech clear, requiring no repetitions. There had been no concerns regarding weight loss, sleep, swallowing, choking or driving. Overall he remained highly functional in his working, social, family and personal contexts. When last visited, Bob, aged 73, showed little functional change. Wendy reported that under stress Bob was mildly irritable, and had some sleep disturbance. There was some progression of motor symptoms. Involuntary motor problems, chorea and dystonia, were evident in the mild to moderate range, with minimal ocular changes. There was a slight widening of gait, and slowing on voluntary fine motor tasks, but speech remained clear. He remained generally in good health and was able to enjoy activities that were important to him. Bob felt very privileged that his experience of HD to date had been more benign, with a later onset and slower progression than other members of his family.

George, in contrast, had more difficulties and a more rapid progression of HD symptoms. Table 4.2 shows his increasing psychomotor slowing, and very poor memory functioning. By the age of 64, he was experiencing significant functional impairments in daily life. He continued to work, although at times made errors (e.g. fertilising the same paddock three times, bringing in the wrong herd of cows). Efforts were made to reduce both his hours at work and the complexity of the tasks he undertook. There were concerns over his perseverative thinking, driving and weight loss. Swallowing and choking problems had led to the avoidance of some foods. Overseas travel required more forward planning, to avoid excess stress. Chorea was noticeable to outsiders and to George himself. By the age of 68, a typical day for George involved a slow walk, reading, playing computer games and minimal domestic tasks. At this point, his chorea was continuous and of moderate amplitude.

Over the 12 years, George experienced difficulties that are common in HD. First, although he was often able to describe his feelings, there were occasions when he could not. One example of this was when Mandy and George were planning a trip to the USA. Although they were both excited when discussing plans, George often became distressed but was unable to articulate his distress or what was causing it. Although initially puzzled, Mandy noticed the distress appeared to be associated with discussion of the New York leg of the trip. George had been unable to express his anxiety about being in a big city like New York. It was not until Mandy asked him directly that he was able to voice his concerns. Alternate plans were then made for George whilst Mandy was to visit New York. After that he happily continued to plan, and later enjoy, the trip.

Mood issues emerged intermittently over the years. In addition to verbal outbursts George developed social anxiety (he felt people were looking at him), whereas he had previously been a very able socialiser, someone "who worked a room" with ease. Additionally, he would occasionally appear very anxious, distressed, frustrated and irritable. These periods were generally intermittent and adeptly dealt with by his wife for a number of years. Mandy found that not arguing back, allowing George space to recover his composure, reducing levels of stress and pressure and increasing the frequency of nutritious snacks helped to reduce and manage the levels of mood disturbance.

This approach did not work, however, when significant behavioural disturbance accompanied an undetected health issue. Frequently, HD persons may have health issues such as urinary tract or ear infections, or tooth decay, or they may just be hungry, and be either unaware of or unable to give accurate details of their symptoms. Instead the patient may present with irritability, anxiety, frustration and sleep disturbances. In this example, George began having sleep problems; he would get up repeatedly during the night, would pace restlessly, take off and put on his clothes and bed coverings. Sleep medication alone gave him fewer than 4 h undisturbed sleep. When asked about his sleep he responded that he felt "panicked." During the day there were no behavioural problems. Months later George was diagnosed with severe urinary retention, and surgery was scheduled. George had not previously been able to report the severe discomfort that is associated with this condition. Physical health checks are an important and useful prerequisite before deciding whether out of character behavioural changes are related to physical health or a mood-related issue that needs to be addressed.

General Summary and Overview

After 12 years the contrast between the two brothers, who inherited the same HD gene and shared many lifestyle and environmental factors, was striking. Bob (age 73) conversed normally whilst making coffee, continuing farming life, driving and travelling abroad. George (age 69) was unable to work, travel or undertake more than simple domestic tasks. His ability to participate fully in conversation was markedly reduced.

Onset of earliest HD symptoms of these brothers, with CAG's of 41 and 42, differed by approximately 15 years. Despite Bob struggling with premorbid mood issues, these reduced over the previous 12 years. Meanwhile George who, had no premorbid mood issues and was socially gregarious, had experienced both out of character irritable outbursts and heightened anxiety in social situations.

Just as with other clients, an important part of the recommendations of a neuropsychologist's report of an HD client is identification of strategies, which will enable them to manage more effectively in their workplace, in their daily lives, and with their families. Naturally, these strategies will be tailored to each individual, his or her strengths and situation, but there are some general points about HD that may be useful to practitioners.

Cognitive changes in HD that cause the most distress are those related to executive dysfunction, and impaired functioning in social and interpersonal contexts (likely reflecting changes in social cognition, apathy and/or mood disturbance). Difficulties are magnified with stress, even at very early stages. Identifying ways to reduce stress is very important, which, as difficulties progress, might mean reducing hours of work, or ensuring that others undertake the more complex tasks.

Development of practical strategies with the family and/or individual to reduce the effects of executive dysfunction will be very helpful. For example, (i) identifying ways to reduce the demands of everyday multitasking (e.g. turning the radio off if reading or doing complex tasks, asking questions of the individual only when they are free to concentrate and not engaged in other activity); (ii) developing external structure for the days via the use of technology such as programming smart phones (if the client is already using one), otherwise via visibly displayed white boards, diaries and planners (iii) developing routines. Slowed cognitive processes mean extra time needs to be allowed for the completion of tasks. However, it is important to set time limits (with a timer) for tasks, work or exercise so that concentration remains and perseverative excesses are avoided.

Social occasions can be a source of difficulty for reasons ranging from social anxiety, to impaired social cognition and impulsiveness. Modifications that may help include selecting social functions with smaller numbers of people, reducing sources of extra stress, such as food preparations, reducing alcohol intake, and being honest and open with respect to their HD condition. Apathy is a very real symptom of HD as are the frustrations that are almost inevitably associated with advanced motor symptoms (speech and movement). These issues need to be acknowledged in planning.

The nutritional needs of individuals with clinical HD are a high priority. Developing ways to ensure that food intake is regular and often, and they are getting required amounts of nutrition (which, as the disease progresses, far exceeds that of normal adult consumption) is important. Swallowing issues may mean clients need to have smaller amounts of food more often, for example, before bed and between meal snacks. Choking issues may mean that certain foods, such as dry or chewy foods, need to be avoided and replaced with something more easily swallowed.

Routine is important in all areas of daily living for those with HD, ensuring that appropriate eating, sleep, exercise and task routines are established early and maintained or adapted as needs change. When change to a routine is required, the person with HD needs to be forewarned.

Difficulties of insight, communication or perception may lead to difficulty in reporting pain, illness, temperature changes and/or emotional distress. These domains should always be investigated carefully when an individual presents with an abrupt change in behaviour. As the clinical disease emerges and progresses, often individuals will require the assistance of specialist neurologists and/or psychiatrists for medical management of the disease. There is currently no cure for HD, however medication can improve motor symptoms, and mood and psychiatric disturbance. At different points in the disease course, referrals to other health-care professionals, (e.g. social workers, care agencies who provide home help, speech and language therapists, dieticians, physiotherapists) may also be useful to manage symptoms which can otherwise lead to behavioural distress. Families and support services can be incredibly resourceful in devising strategies to support and assist those with HD to manage as best as can be possible.

Finally, it is crucial to remember always that this is a disease which impacts on the family; many individuals who are assisting with care could be at risk of inheriting the disease or have relatives that are at risk of having the disease.

The Value of Neuropsychological Formulation

HD, like other neurodegenerative conditions, has for many years fallen predominantly in the domain of neurologists, with input from psychiatrists and occasionally specialist neuropsychiatrists. These roles have typically been limited to diagnosis by neurological evaluation of motor signs, or management of psychiatric phenomenon or disruptive behaviours (predominantly via medications). As illustrated throughout this chapter, HD is clinically complex with variable changes in neuropsychological functioning, mood and motor functioning contributing to the clinical picture of each individual, with progression over time. A sound neuropsychological formulation involves not only interpreting and integrating information obtained during neuropsychological assessment, but evaluating and integrating functioning across multiple domains, including familial, work and social contexts in which the individual participates. Thus, it has the potential to capture the clinical complexity of HD at the same time as providing crucial information regarding the cognitive strengths and weakness of the individual, and documenting change across time.

The potential value of such a formulation for coping with and managing HD is multifactorial. For example, one important outcome of the richness of a skilled and informed neuropsychological formulation in individuals with the HD gene is that it can contribute meaningfully to the client's and family's understandings of functional difficulties being experienced. Understanding how these functional issues relate to, or are a likely consequence of, the neural changes associated with HD and with disease progression, can have a substantial and positive influence on family interactions and relationships generally. Similarly, being able to normalise behaviours that are being misattributed to HD can have a profound impact.

Another example relates more specifically to changes in neuropsychological functioning that frequently develop with HD, which can have a significant impact on the person's behaviour and ability to function in multiple situations, including work and other roles with responsibility (e.g. childcare), interpersonal relations, and accomplishing the complex activities of daily living. Thus, an accurate formulation that includes the cognitive strengths and weakness of the individual will facilitate the generation of useful recommendations for managing areas of weakness, for decision-making related to occupational and other life roles, for coping with environmental demands in the face of particular behavioural deficits, and for the individual's ability to manage themselves and behave adaptively in society.

Few of these benefits are truly unique to HD. Most neurodegenerative conditions are associated with clinical variability and complexity and deterioration over time. Thus, many of the lessons learned when developing proficiency in neuropsychological formulations of individuals with HD can be applied to a range of neurodegenerative conditions.

References

Benjamin, C. M., Adam, S., Wiggins, S., Theilmann, J. L., Copley, T. T., Bloch, M., et al. (1994). Proceed with care: Direct predictive testing for Huntington disease. *American Journal of Human Genetics, 55,* 606–617.

Berrios, G. E., Wagle, A. C., Markova, I. S., Wagle, S. A., Rosser, A., & Hodges, J. R. (2002). Psychiatric symptoms in neurologically asymptomatic Huntington's disease gene carriers: A comparison with gene negative at risk subjects. *Acta Psychiatrica Scandinavica, 105,* 224–230.

Biglan, K. M., Ross, C. A., Langbehn, D. R., Aylward, E. H., Stout, J. C., Queller, S., Carlozzi, N. E., Duff, K., Beglinger, L. J., & Paulsen, J. S. (2009). Motor abnormalities in premanifest persons with Huntington's disease: The PREDICT-HD study. *Movement Disorders, 24*(12), 1763–1772.

Biglan, K. M., Zhang, Y., Long, J. D., Geschwind, M., Kang, G. A., Killoran, A., et al. (2013). Refining the diagnosis of Huntington disease: The PREDICT-HD study. *Frontiers in Aging Neuroscience, 5,* (Article 12). doi:10.3389/fnagi.2013.00012.

Brandt, J., & Butters, N. (1986). The neuropsychology of Huntington's disease. *Trends in Neuroscience, 9,* 118–20

Claes, S., Van Zand, K., Legius, E., Dom, R., Malfroid, M., Baro, F., et al. (1995). Correlations between triplet repeat expansion and clinical features in Huntington's disease. *Archives of Neurology, 52,* 749–53.

Du, X., Pang, T. Y. C., & Hannan, A. J. (2013). A tale of two maladies? Pathogenesis of depression with and without the Huntington's disease gene mutation. *Frontiers in Neurology, 4,* (Article 8). doi:10.3389/fneur.2013.00081

Duff, K., Paulsen, J. S., Beglinger, L. J., Langbehn, D. R., Stout, J. C., & Predict-HD Investigators of the Huntington Study Group. (2007). Psychiatric symptoms in Huntington's disease before diagnosis: The Predict-HD study. *Biological Psychiatry, 62*(12), 1341–1346.

Folstein, S. E. (1989). *Huntington's disease: A disorder of families*. Baltimore: Johns Hopkins University Press.

Georgiou, N., Bradshaw, J. L., Chiu, E., Tudor, A., O'Gorman, L., & Phillips, J. G. (1999). Differential clinical and motor control function in a pair of monozygotic twins with Huntington's disease. *Movement Disorders, 14*(2), 320–325.

Gómez-Esteban, J. C., Lezcano, E., Zarranz, J. J., Velasco, F., Garamendi, I., Pérez, T., et al. (2007). Monozygotic twins suffering from Huntington's disease show different cognitive and behavioural Symptoms. *European Neurology, 57,* 26–30.

Ho, A. K., Sahakian, B. J., Brown, R. G., Barker, R. A., Hodges, J. R., Ané, M. N., et al. (2003). Profile of cognitive progression in early Huntington's disease. *Neurology, 61,* 1702–1706.

Hockly, E., Cordery, P. M., Woodman, B., Maha, A., van Dellen, A., Blakemore, C., et al. (2002). Environmental enrichment slows progression in R6/2 Huntington's disease mice. *Annals of Neurology, 51,* 235–242.

Huntington's Disease Collaborative Research Group. (1993). A novel gene containing a trinucleotide repeat that is unstable in Huntington's disease chromosomes. *Cell, 72,* 971–983.

Imarisio, S., Carmichael, J., Korolchuk, V., Chen, C. W., Saiki, S., Rose, C., et al. (2008). Huntington's disease: From pathology and genetics to potential therapies. *Biochemical Journal, 412,* 191–209.

Julien, C. L., Thompson, J. C., Wild, S., Yardumian, P., Snowden, J. S., Turner, G., et al. (2007). Psychiatric disorders in preclinical Huntington's disease. *Journal of Neurology, Neurosurgery and Psychiatry, 78,* 939–943.

Kieburtz, K., Penney, J. B., Como, P., Ranen, N., Shoulson, I., Feigin, A., et al. (1996). Unified Huntington's disease rating scale: Reliability and consistency. *Movement Disorders, 11*(2), 136–142.

Langbehn, D. R., Brinkman, R. R., Falush, D., Paulsen, J. S., & Hayden, M. R. (2004). A new model for prediction of the age of onset and penetrance for Huntington's disease based on CAG length. *Clinical Genetics, 65,* 267–277.

Loy, C. T., & McCusker, E. A. (2013). Is a motor criterion essential for the diagnosis of clinical Huntington Disease? *PLoS Currents*. doi:10.1371/currents.hd.f4c66bd51e8db11f55e1701af937a419.

MacLeod, R., Tibben, A., Frontali, M., Evers-Kiebooms, G., Jones, A., Martinez-Descales, A., Roos, R. A., & Editorial Committee and Working Group. (2013). Genetic testing counselling' of the European Huntington disease network: Recommendations for the predictive genetic test in Huntington's disease. *Clinical Genetics, 83*(3), 221–231. doi:10.1111/j.1399-0004.2012.01900.x.

Marioni, R. E., Valenzuela, M. J., van der Hout, A., Brayne, C., Mathhews, F. E., & MCR Cognitive Function and Ageing Study. (2012). Active cognitive lifestyle is associated with positive cognitive health transitions and compression of morbidity from age sixty-five. *PLoS ONE, 7*(12), e50940. doi:10.1371/journal.pone.0050940.

Marshall, F. J. (2004). Clinical features and treatment of Huntington's disease In R. L. Watts & W. C. Koller (Eds.), *Movement disorders: Neurological principles and practice* (2nd ed.). New York: McGraw Hill.

Novak, M. J., & Tabrizi, S. J. (2011). Huntington's disease: Clinical presentation and treatment. *International Review of Neurobiology, 98,* 297–323. doi:10.1016/b978-0-12-381328-200013-4.

Panas, M., Karadima, G., Markianos, M., Kalfakis, N., & Vassilopoulos, D. (2008). Phenotypic discordance in a pair of monozygotic twins with Huntington's disease. *Clinical Genetics, 74,* 291–292.

Paulsen, J. S. (2011). Cognitive impairment in Huntington disease: Diagnosis and treatment. *Current Neurology And Neuroscience Reports, 11*(5), 474–483.

Rosas, H. D., Salat, D. H., Lee, S. Y., Zaleta, A. K., Pappu, V., Fischl, B., et al. (2008). Cerebral cortex and the clinical expression of Huntington's disease: Complexity and heterogeneity. *Brain, 131,* 1057–1068.

Rosenblatt, A. (2007). Neuropsychiatry of Huntington's disease. *Dialogues in Clinical Neuroscience, 9*(2), 191–197.

Ross, C. A., & Tabrizi, S. J. (2011). Huntington's disease: From molecular pathogenesis to clinical treatment. *Lancet Neurol, 10*(1), 83–98. doi:10.1016/s1474-4422(10)70245-3.

Scahill, R. I., Hobbs, N. Z., Say, M. J., Bechtel, N., Henley, S. M. D., Hyare, H., et al. (2013). Clinical impairment in premanifest and early Huntington's disease is associated with regionally specific atrophy. *Human Brain Mapping, 34,* 519–529.

Stout, J. C., Paulsen, J., Queller, S., Solomon, A. C., Whitlock, K. B., Campbell, J. C., et al. (2011). Neurocognitive signs in prodromal Huntington disease. *Neuropsychology, 25,* 1–14.

Thompson, J. C., Harris, J., Sollom, A. C., Stopford, C. L., Howard, E., Snowden, J. S., & Craufurd, D. (2012). Longitudinal evaluation of neuropsychiatric symptoms in Huntington's disease. *The Journal of Neuropsychiatry and Clinical Neurosciences, 24,* 53–60.

Thu, D. C., Oorschot, D. E., Tippett, L. J., Nana, A. L., Hogg, V. M., Synek, B. J., & Faull, R. L. (2010). Cell loss in the motor and cingulate cortex correlates with symptomatology in Huntington's disease. *Brain, 133*(Pt 4), 1094–1110. doi:10.1093/brain/awq047.

Tibben, A. (2007). Predictive testing for Huntington's disease. *Brain Research Bulletin, 72,* 165–171.

Tippett, L. J., Waldvogel, H. J., Thomas, S. J., Hogg, V. M., van Roon-Mom, W., Synek, B. J., et al. (2007). Striosomes and mood dysfunction in Huntington's disease. *Brain, 130,* 206–21.

Trembath, M. K., Horton, Z. A., Tippett, L., Hogg, V., Collins, V. R., Churchyard, A., et al. (2010). A retrospective study of the impact of lifestyle on age at onset of Huntington disease. *Movement Disorders, 25*(10), 1444–1450.

van Dellen, A., Blakemore, C., Deacon, R., York, D., & Hannan, A. J. (2000). Delaying the onset of Huntington's in mice. *Nature, 404,* 721–722.

van Duijn, E., Kingma, E. M., & van der Mast, R. C. (2007). Psychopathology in verified Huntington's disease gene carriers. *Journal of Neuropsychiatry & Clinical Neurosciences, 19*(4), 441–448. doi:http://dx.doi.org/10.1176/appi.neuropsych.19.4.441

Vonsattel, J. P., & DiFiglia, M. (1998). Huntington disease. *Journal of Neuropathology and Experimental Neurology, 57*(5), 369–84.

Vonsattel, J. P. G., Ge, P., & Kelly, L. (1997). Huntington's disease. In M. M. Esiri & J. H. Morris (Eds.), *The neuropathology of dementia* (pp. 219–233). Cambridge: Cambridge University Press.

Wahlin, T. B. R., Lundin, A., & Dear, K. (2007). Early cognitive deficits in Swedish gene carriers of Huntington's disease. *Neuropsychology, 21*(1), 31–44. doi:10.1037/0894-4105.21.1.31

Wexler, N. S., Lorimer, J., Porter, J., Gomez, F., Moskowitz, C., Shackell, E., et al. (2004). Venezuelan kindreds reveal that genetic and environmental factors modulate Huntington's disease age of onset. Proceedings of the National Academy of Sciences of the United States of America. *101*(10), 3498–3503.

Young, A. B., Shoulson, I., Penney, J. B., Starosta-Rubinstein, S., Gomez, F., Travers, H., & Wexler, N. S. (1986). Huntington's disease in Venezuela: Neurologic features and functional decline. *Neurology, 36*(2), 244–244.

Zappacosta, B., Monza, D., Meoni, C., Austoni, L., Soliveri, P., Gellera, C., et al. (1996). Psychiatric symptoms do not correlate with cognitive decline, motor symptoms, or CAG repeat length in Huntington's disease. *Archives of Neurology, 53,* 493–7.

Chapter 5
Neuropsychological Aspects of Temporal-Lobe Epilepsy: Seeking Evidence-Based Practice

Stephen C. Bowden, Leonie C. Simpson and Mark J. Cook

Literature Review The study of seizure disorders has occupied a prominent position in the history of neuropsychology (Baxendale and Thompson 2010), and many clinical research groups have contributed in understanding the role of neuropsychology in the care of patients with seizure disorders (Lee 2010). Despite the attention accorded to the neuropsychological understanding of patients with seizure disorders, many aspects of the cognitive and psychosocial status of this diverse patient group remain to be understood (Lee 2010; Loughman et al. 2014). Assessment of patients undergoing surgical treatment for temporal-lobe epilepsy (TLE) is one of the facets of seizure disorders most commonly studied by neuropsychologists (Bell et al. (2011). Because TLE is often resistant to control with medication, unilateral anterior-temporal lobectomy (surgical resection of the epileptogenic focus) is a treatment of choice (Lee 2010; Wiebe et al. 2001). Foremost questions in neuropsychological research include how to provide optimal assessment of presurgical candidates and how to predict the likelihood of postoperative memory and other cognitive disabilities together with effective mental health care.

S. C. Bowden (✉)
Melbourne School of Psychological Sciences, University of Melbourne, Redmond Barry Building, Melbourne, Victoria 3010, Australia
e-mail: sbowden@unimelb.edu.au

S. C. Bowden · L. C. Simpson
Neuropsychology Unit, Department of Clinical Neurosciences, St. Vincent's Hospital, Fitzroy, Victoria 3065, Australia

L. C. Simpson
e-mail: leonie.simpson2@svma.org.au

M. J. Cook
Department of Medicine and Department of Clinical Neurosciences, St. Vincent's Hospital, Fitzroy, Victoria 3065, Australia
e-mail: mark@neurology.net.au

J. A. B. Macniven (ed.), *Neuropsychological Formulation,*
DOI 10.1007/978-3-319-18338-1_5

In the earliest published surgical series, some patients were significantly disabled by memory impairment after unilateral temporal lobectomy (Lee 2010). Extensive research effort has been devoted to identifying the risk of postoperative memory disability in patients with TLE. A wide variety of presurgical assessment techniques have been advocated to pinpoint those most at risk. Perhaps, the best known of these is the sodium-amatyl ablation or 'Wada' technique designed to simulate the effects of unilateral medial temporal resection with a transient period of a few minutes of ipsilateral anaesthesia (see Lee 2010). However, due to the uncertainty regarding the validity of the Wada test, combined with developments in structural and functional imaging to identify the focus of seizure activity (the so-called epileptogenic focus), popularity of the Wada test has waned over the last couple of decades (Kanner 2008). Instead, many research studies have targeted neuroimaging variables, together with better measurement of the cognitive and other psychological variables that may influence cognitive and psychosocial status after anterior-temporal lobectomy.

Several reviews have appeared recently that highlight current understanding of presurgical assessment. These reviews show that the risk of memory disability has changed dramatically with improvements in identifying the epileptogenic focus in patients with temporal-lobe epilepsy. In an excellent review, Bell et al. (2011) illustrate the complexity of issues in understanding the neuropsychological status of patients with TLE and the number of questions that remain unresolved regarding prediction of postsurgical effects. Bell and colleagues show that despite dramatic improvements in methods of clinical neurology and neuroimaging, 30–60 % of patients undergoing left (dominant) anterior-temporal lobectomy show a decline in verbal memory postsurgically. A smaller proportion of patients with right-sided anterior-temporal lobectomy show reduced memory postsurgically, although most visuospatial memory assessments do not use tests of allocentric (extra-personal) space which appear to be most sensitive to nondominant hippocampal disease (Bowden and McCarter 1993; Hocking et al. 2013). Unfortunately, there do not appear to be any standardised tests of allocentric memory with quality norms for clinical purpose.

Bell et al. (2011) also review a variety of cognitive as well as structural and functional imaging studies, showing that cognitive function in TLE is a result of diffuse cortical and subcortical network disruption rather than specific damage to one or other specific brain structure (Dulay and Busch 2012, see their Table 5.1). The diffuse, multisystem nature of brain changes associated with TLE illustrate the importance of taking a comprehensive approach to the neuropsychological evaluation of cognition in patients with TLE, rather than focusing on the assessment of a limited number of abilities hypothesised to have localizing value.

With regard to specific predictors of postsurgical cognitive status, Bell et al. (2011) summarise some of the factors that have been investigated particularly with respect to memory decline. They include (1) hippocampal integrity preoperatively (greater hippocampal sclerosis (HS) is associated with a better memory outcome, e.g. Rausch and Babb 1993), (2) preoperative memory ability (presumably

Table 5.1 WAIS-III—index scores. (Wechsler Adult Intelligence scale, Third edition)

	Preoperative	Postoperative	Change
	Index score (95% CI)	*Index score (95% CI)*	
Verbal comprehension	100 (94–106)	100 (94–106)	n/s
Working memory	102 (95–109)	108 (101–114)	n/s
Perceptual organisation	128 (119–133)	128 (119–133)	n/s
Processing speed	93 (85–103)	114 (103–121)	Increase[a]

CI confidence interval, *VC* verbal comprehension, *WM* working memory, *PO* perceptual organisation, *PS* processing speed

[a] Change between preoperative and postoperative assessments was statistically significant at the 95% level, allowing for regression to the mean and test reliability

n/s change between preoperative and postoperative assessments did not reach statistical significance

a consequence of hippocampal integrity, better preoperative memory is associated with a greater memory decline postoperatively, e.g. Baxendale and Thompson 2010), (3) age at onset of recurrent seizures (reflecting the increased incidence of HS with a younger onset of seizures, e.g. Saykin et al. 1989), (4) language lateralisation measures on fMRI and Wada (more left lateralisation is associated with worse memory outcome in left-sided surgery, e.g. Binder et al. 2010) and (5) Wada memory testing asymmetry, for example, poor recall when the left hemisphere is anaesthetised is associated with a poor outcome with left-sided anterior lobectomy.

Impairments in naming skills are also common following dominant hemisphere temporal lobectomy with around 34% of people experiencing a decline, although improvements in fluency are more common than decline (27% vs. 10%; Sherman et al. 2011). Absence of HS and to a lesser extent age at the onset of epilepsy are predictors of postoperative decline (Ives-Deliperi and Butler 2012).

Gargaro et al. (2013) found that 'atypical' cognitive profiles (not matching the expected material-specific memory profile or verbal memory impairment with left hippocampal focus, or visual memory impairment with right focus) were in fact common, present in about 75% of their sample. In Gargaro and colleagues' series, only patients with normal range memory scores, and contralateral profile (for example, better verbal and poorer visual memory and left HS) experienced any decline in memory. Bilateral memory impairment (poor verbal and visual memory) was associated with decline in naming. Right-sided surgery was associated with a stable profile with some groups experiencing an improvement.

There have been various attempts to combine these predictors of postsurgical cognitive function into multivariate models of postoperative memory risk prediction in people with TLE. However, Bell et al. (2011) note that, to date, the published predictive models appear to have promise as research tools but rely on local implementations of neuropsychological assessment and imaging techniques (particularly in functional imaging paradigms). So, Bell and colleagues conclude that the reviewed multivariate predictive models are in need of independent replication and may not generalise to other clinical centres. Nevertheless, all of the recent reviews argue that neuropsychological evaluations provide one of the 'non-redundant' sources of information to predict memory and other cognitive outcome after seizure surgery.

In view of the large number of epilepsy surgery centres and large number of neuropsychologists involved in epilepsy care worldwide, it is surprising that there is no stronger consensus regarding guidelines on the neuropsychological contributions to management of presurgical candidates, notwithstanding the various efforts to develop predictive models, as described in the preceding paragraph. Baxendale and Thompson (2010) describe the traditional role of neuropsychology in: (1) presurgical evaluation, seeking to predict side of seizure focus, noting that this is a task now more effectively achieved by structural and functional imaging and (2) predicting postsurgical risk of cognitive disability. They suggest that the best use of neuropsychological evaluations in the current era should be the comprehensive assessment of cognitive and psychological wellbeing. Assessment should be based on providing presurgical or baseline cognitive assessment to facilitate accurate and effective management of any concerns regarding cognitive function postsurgery, together with careful evaluation of psychological wellbeing prior to surgery, to identify any psychological adjustment issues that may require treatment prior to surgery and special care after surgery (Baxendale and Thompson 2010).

In view of the high prevalence of psychological adjustment issues in patients with seizure disorders (Busch et al. 2011; Foran et al. 2013; Seidenberg et al. 1998), care of psychological wellbeing remains one of the most important and often neglected aspects of patients with seizure disorders (Lee 2010). Many diagnosis-specific formulations of psychopathology have been advanced to account for the high prevalence of psychological distress in patients with seizure disorders. However, diagnosis-specific psychopathology formulations risk confusing nosology and diminish the opportunities to offer treatment, whether pharmacological or psychotherapeutic. If it is thought that the symptoms of psychopathology in a patient with a seizure disorder are attributable to the effects of the seizure disorder rather than being symptoms of common forms of psychopathology (such as depression and anxiety which occur with high frequency in any patient population with significant or chronic disability), then treatment opportunities may be missed (Busch et al. 2011; Foran et al. 2013; Reilly et al. 2006; Seidenberg et al. 1998). Direct evaluation of the evidence suggests that symptoms of psychopathology in patients with seizure disorders should be treated as evidence of common treatable forms of psychopathology rather than evidence for seizure-disorder-specific variants (Foran et al. 2013; Reilly et al. 2006).

The current case is designed to illustrate some of the challenges in providing effective care for a patient undergoing anterior-temporal lobectomy.

Case Description: Julia

Setting Julia was a 21-year-old woman with a diagnosis of temporal-lobe epilepsy since the age of 3. She decided to undergo a temporal lobectomy to attempt to alleviate her seizures and as part of the routine presurgical workup, she was referred for a neuropsychological assessment. The assessments reported here were conducted 1 month before and 13 months after Julia's left temporal lobectomy.

History Julia's seizures started at the age of 3. Since that time, she had experienced persistent seizures, initially up to 2–3 per week, but in the years leading up to surgery she had been experiencing approximately 2–4 seizures per day. Julia's seizures typically involved an aura of gastric discomfort. During a seizure, Julia was described as staring blankly, making unformed vocalisations and occasionally collapsing. Post-ictally, she had no memory of the seizure, and was typically quite fatigued.

Approximately 2 months prior to the presurgical neuropsychological assessment, she was admitted to the Victorian Epilepsy Centre at St. Vincent's Hospital, Melbourne for a period of video monitoring that confirmed the diagnosis of TLE comprising mostly of absence seizures with infrequent complex partial seizures. HS is the most common pathological cause of TLE. In Julia's case, a structural MRI showed a smaller left hippocampus with increased T2 signal which was interpreted as being left-sided HS (see Fig. 5.1). Volumetric measurement of the hippocampi

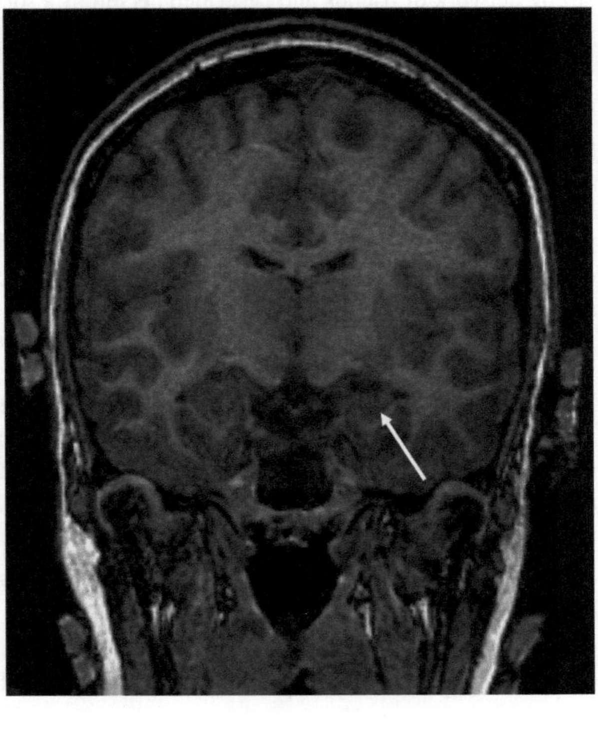

Fig. 5.1 Coronal MRI showing left-sided hippocampal sclerosis *(HS)* with reduced left hippocampus volume *(at white arrow head)* compared to *right* (*left* and *right* reversed in line with radiological convention)

revealed a significant left–right asymmetry with smaller left volume. A single-photon emission computerized tomography (SPECT) study comparing an ictal (injection of the radiotracer during a seizure) with an interictal (injection of a radiotracer not during a seizure) scan suggested a focus in the inferior and lateral margins of the rostral left temporal lobe.

Julia was undertaking 8–16 h of voluntary work per week and contemplating tertiary study in fashion design. Her seizures had also interfered with her school performance and she completed high school education part-time as a mature age student. Prior to surgery, she described her memory as her most concerning cognitive symptom with frequent lapses in everyday memory, for example, struggling to remember school work, forgetting family events and forgetting the plotline in favourite television shows.

Julia had been managed on a variety of medications over the years and was taking phenytoin, tiagabine and clobazam at the time of the surgery. Apart from her epilepsy, Julia's medical history was unremarkable. She was a nonsmoker and drank alcohol occasionally on a social basis, with no known history of substance abuse. There was no significant family history of epilepsy or any other relevant medical condition. As a child, Julia reportedly attained all major developmental milestones appropriately. She is right handed.

By way of psychosocial background, Julia had one brother, 2 years younger than her, and they both lived with their parents. Julia described having difficulty 'fitting in' at school because of her epilepsy and having only one or two other good friendships at secondary school. However, since leaving school she had established a strong network of friends and described herself as a sociable person.

Presurgical Cognitive Assessment Removal of the well-lateralised HS could be predicted to be associated with a lower risk of postoperative cognitive disability (Bell et al. 2011; Cook et al. 1992; Lee 2010). Therefore, the purpose of the presurgical assessment was primarily to provide a baseline for comparison purposes postoperatively. The presurgical assessment results were also analysed in terms of possible predictors of postoperative cognitive impairment as reviewed above. The presurgical assessment was conducted with Julia during an out-patient visit under optimal medication regimen, rather than during an admission for video monitoring, because of the greater risk of disruption of the cognitive assessment due to lowered seizure control and sleep deprivation during the telemetry visit (Lee 2010). The tests administered were chosen to provide optimum coverage of cognitive domains, according to the CHC model of cognition, along with optimum reliability. Of note, 'executive functions' are covered in the CHC model by measures of fluid intelligence, working memory and processing speed (Bowden 2013; Jewsbury et al. 2015; Larrabee 2000). Tests administered included:

- Wechsler Adult Intelligence Scale, Third Edition (WAIS-III)
- Wechsler Memory Scale, Third Edition (WMS-III)
- Boston Naming Test
- Controlled Oral Word Association Test (COWAT or FAS)

- Animal Fluency
- Beck Depression Inventory II (BDI-II)
- State-Trait Anxiety Inventory (STAI)

Summary of Results Julia was not known to have had a seizure in the 24 h preceding the assessment and she was not observed to have any seizures during the assessment. All normative data were obtained from the relevant test manuals, except for the Boston Naming Test and verbal fluency tasks. Naming and verbal fluency were scored from norms provided by Spreen and Strauss (1998) and Tombaugh et al. (1999) and adjusted for age and education. As seen in Table 5.1, at the time of the presurgical neuropsychological assessment (1 month before surgery), Julia's overall intellectual capacity was in the 'average' to 'high average' range. Significant base rate discrepancies between the four factors measured by the WAIS-III were observed. Perceptual Organisation (PO) scored higher than the other three: indexes of Verbal Comprehension (VC), Working Memory (WM) and Processing Speed (PS). The base rates of a difference like this between visuospatial reasoning PO and the other index scores were all below 5.8 %, that is, uncommon. Acquired knowledge VC, WM and mental speed fell close to the average for her age group. There were no significant base rate discrepancies between subtest scaled scores that contributed to the respective WAIS-III index scores. Therefore, her cognitive abilities are best summarised in terms of the four WAIS-III ability factors and not in terms of separate subtest scores (Bowden 2013; Kaufman and Lichtenberger 1999).

Anterograde memory function was slightly lower than general intellectual function. Although, she performed poorly on immediate (16th percentile) and delayed (1st percentile) recall of verbally presented short stories (WMS-III Logical memory I and II, see Table 5.2, 5.3), there was no clinically significant difference in terms of base rates (Wechsler 1997a) between verbal and visual memory at immediate or delayed recall (Table 5.3). The base rate of pairwise discrepancies between indexes (verbal or visual, immediate or delayed) were all above 5 %. The one exception was the difference between verbal immediate and verbal delayed index (Table 5.3).

Table 5.2 WMS-III—Scores on subtests. (Wechsler Memory Scale, Third edition)

	Preoperative		Postoperative	
	Raw	*SS (age)*	*Raw*	*SS (age)*
Logical memory I—recall	32	7	23	5
Faces I—recognition	41	11	45	15
Verbal paired associates I—recall	24	11	23	10
Family pictures I—recall	52	11	53	11
Letter-number sequencing	13	12	14	13
Spatial span	19	12	20	12
Logical memory II—recall	10	3	6	2
Faces II—recognition	41	10	39	10
Verbal paired associates II—recall	4	6	8	12
Family pictures II—recall	48	9	59	14

Table 5.3 WMS-III—index scores. (Wechsler Memory Scale, Third edition)

	Preoperative	Postoperative	Change
	Index Score (95% CI)	*Index Score (95% CI)*	
Auditory immediate	94 (87–101)	86 (80–94)	n/s
Visual immediate	106 (95–115)	118 (105–125)	n/s
Immediate memory	100 (92–108)	102 (94–110)	n/s
Auditory delayed	67 (62–81)	83 (76–94)	n/s
Visual delayed	97 (87–108)	112 (100–120)	n/s
General (delayed) memory	81 (75–91)	92 (85–101)	n/s
Auditory recognition delayed	90 (82–104)	85 (78–100)	n/s
Working memory	111 (100–119)	115 (104–122)	n/s

CI confidence interval
n/s change between preoperative and postoperative assessments did not reach statistical significance, allowing for regression to the mean and test reliability

However, the best estimate of verbal and visual memory is likely to be the average of the respective immediate and delayed index scores. This was demonstrated in the latent variable analysis of the WAIS-III, and Wechsler Memory Scales (WMS), in representative seizure disorder and other clinical and community samples (Bowden et al. 2008a; Bowden et al. 2008b; Tulsky et al. 1997). As a result, our interpretation is that there was no clinically meaningful explanation for the verbal immediate versus verbal delayed index discrepancy, other than situational factors, for example, a lapse in concentration, idiopathic increased rate of forgetting or perhaps the effects of an undetected seizure. The average of the WMS-III immediate and delayed auditory-verbal indexes was 81, and the average of the immediate and delayed visual memory indexes was 102. Although no convenient normative WMS-III data provide a basis for statistical comparison (but now available for the WMS-IV), the difference between these averages conforms to the common observation of lower verbal memory prior to surgery in patients with dominant hemisphere HS (Lee 2010).

Confrontation naming, measured by the Boston Naming Test, and fluency or lexical retrieval was impaired relative to her general cognitive abilities and also relative to age and education matched norms, see Table 5.4 (Spreen and Strauss 1998; Tombaugh et al. 1999). As discussed above, lowered language function and lexical retrieval are also a common preoperative finding in patients with dominant hemisphere TLE (Lee 2010).

Table 5.4 Miscellaneous other test scores

	Preoperative	Postoperative
Beck Depression Inventory-II (BDI-II)	5	5
State-Trait Anxiety Inventory (STAI)		
State	26 (17th percentile)	26 (17th percentile)
Trait	27 (18th percentile)	28 (22nd percentile)
Boston naming test	48 (< 10th percentile)	44 (< 10th percentile)
Controlled Oral Word Association Test: Total words (FAS)	27 (10th percentile)	27 (10th percentile)
Animal Fluency	13 (< 10th percentile)	18 (25th percentile)

Mood and risk of self-harm was screened at an initial face-to-face interview and also with the Beck Depression Inventory-II (BDI-II; Beck et al. 1996), on which she reported minimal symptoms of depression, and the State-Trait Anxiety Inventory (STAI; Spielberger 1989), on which she reported low levels of anxiety.

The conclusion of the presurgical neuropsychological assessment was that for this young woman with well-characterised HS on structural MRI, there was no clearly lateralizing memory deficit in terms of base rate discrepancies. Significant weakness in specific language skills was observed, no obvious psychosocial needs and therefore, no contraindications to left ATL.

Surgical Treatment and Medical Outcome Julia underwent a left temporal lobectomy and her postoperative recovery was unremarkable. Histology on sections of the resected brain tissue showed normal lateral neocortex and amygdala but severe HS with virtually total loss of neurons and gliosis in sector CA1, a common finding in TLE (Lee 2010). Julia reported being more alert postoperatively. She continued on Dilantin, Gabatril and Frisium, but had also participated in a trial of Levetiracetam (Keppra). She reported a significant reduction in frequency of seizures, from approximately 2 per day before surgery to around 3 per month after surgery. In terms of standard seizure outcome she would be rated as Engel Scale II—rare disabling seizures.

Postsurgical Cognitive Assessment The purpose of the postoperative assessment was to measure any changes in cognition that may have occurred following surgery. Because Julia did not express any concerns postoperatively to her neurologist regarding changes in cognitive function, postsurgical neuropsychological assessment was undertaken when postoperative course was thought to have thoroughly stabilised (Lee 2010). The same tests used preoperatively were readministered postoperatively including the WAIS-III for the most direct comparison with postoperative assessment, despite the WAIS-IV (Wechsler 2008) becoming available in the interim. Postoperative assessment also included further evaluation of psychopathology symptoms. Change in test scores was evaluated using a reliable change index (RCI) method which involves calculating a predicted true score (PTS) from the preoperative assessment scores and constructing a 95 % confidence interval using test reliability and standard deviation (Hinton-Bayre 2010; Nunnally and Bernstein 1994). Tests administered included:

- Wechsler Adult Intelligence Scale, Third Edition (WAIS-III)
- Wechsler Memory Scale, Third Edition (WMS-III)
- Beck Depression Inventory-II (BDI-II)
- Controlled Oral Word Association Test (COWAT, FAS)
- Animal Fluency
- State-Trait Anxiety Inventory (STAI)
- Boston Naming Test
- Minnesota Multiphasic Personality Inventory Restructured Form (MMPI-2-RF)

Summary of Results Again, all tests were scored and interpreted in relation to normative data. Assessment 13 months after left-sided anterior-temporal lobectomy found Julia's postoperative cognitive abilities to be mostly consistent with her preoperative levels. As shown in Table 5.1, the VC, PO and WM indexes of the WAIS-III were all unchanged as defined by the RCI. There was a significant improvement on PS from the low average to average range to the average to high average range.

At her preoperative assessment, Julia's verbal memory was relatively weak. However, as was the case preoperatively, this would not be described as a lateralising memory impairment (not clinically significant) as differences like this between visual and verbal memory occur in 6.8 % of the normative sample for the WMS-III (Wechsler 1997b). On this occasion her verbal memory scores were more consistently in the low average to average range (i.e. at both immediate and delayed recall) and importantly the RCI analysis showed that her scores had not changed significantly when compared to her preoperative scores (see Table 5.3). Julia's visual memory scores were also unchanged after the surgery.

Julia's scores on specific language tasks (verbal fluency and naming) were again a weakness in her overall cognitive profile, but they did not significantly change postsurgery (Sawrie et al. 1996).

Julia's responses on the BDI-II and STAI questionnaires did not indicate significant depression or anxiety or any change in her level of mood symptoms after the surgery. In view of the high frequency of psychological distress in patients with seizure disorders (Busch et al. 2011; Foran et al. 2013), the more detailed MMPI-2-RF was also administered at the postoperative assessment. Results of selected MMPI-2-RF scores are shown in Table 5.5 and were interpreted with the aid of the computerised interpretive report. Julia did not indicate any tendency to over- or under-reporting in the context of consistent responding and an otherwise valid profile. In the responses to the clinical scales, Julia reported experiencing poor health and feeling tired, lacking energy, and reported nonspecific neurological symptoms and multiple somatic symptoms, likely to be worsened in times of stress (MLS, COG and NUC Scales in Table 5.5). She is likely to be stress-reactive and engage in ruminative worry (ACT Scale in Table 5.5) and reports unusual ideation that may be related to seizure events or other idiosyncratic thinking styles. Finally, her responses reflect heightened excitation and energy levels that may emerge as episodes of elevated mood (RC8 Scales in Table 5.5). There was no evidence of interpersonal difficulties.

Neuropsychologist's Recommendations for Postoperative Management Julia was planning to return to study part time. Her verbal memory function, though unchanged from presurgical assessment, was nevertheless likely to affect her ability to recall new information, such as class content and reading material. Her language skills were also likely to require some support particularly regarding written work required for her course of study. It was felt that these cognitive aspects would be likely to influence her ability to perform to the best of her capabilities during her studies, particularly in examinations. A letter of support was written to her tertiary institution requesting special consideration and assistance with study skills, for example, suggesting that written examinations should be replaced with take-home exams or written assignments, and that Julia be allowed extra time on such

Table 5.5 MMPI-2-RF Scores at postoperative assessment

MMPI-2-RF—Validity scales														
	VRIN-r	**TRIN-r**	**F-r**	**Fp-r**	**Fs**	**FBS-r**	**RBS**	**L-r**	**K-r**					
T	58	50	65	42	66	64	65	62	48					
MMPI-2-RF—Higher order (HO) and restructured clinical (RC) scales														
	Higher order			**Restructured clinical**										
	EID	**THD**	**BXD**	**RCd**	**RC1**	**RC2**	**RC3**	**RC4**	**RC6**	**RC7**	**RC8**	**RC9**		
T	54	63	40	57	61	61	49	39	61	53	70	48		
MMPI-2-RF—Somatic/cognitive and internalizing scales														
	Somatic/cognitive					**Internalizing**								
	MLS	**GIC**	**HPC**	**NUC**	**COG**	**SUI**	**HLP**	**SFD**	**NFC**	**STW**	**AXY**	**ANP**	**BRF**	**MSF**
T	75	64	53	76	84	45	52	52	64	65	44	47	63	51
MMPI-2-RF—Externalizing, interpersonal and interest scales														
	Externalizing				**Interpersonal**					**Interest**				
	JCP	**SUB**	**AGG**	**ACT**	**FML**	**IPP**	**SAV**	**SHY**	**DSF**	**AES**	**MEC**			
T	40	41	37	75	49	52	47	52	44	45	47			
MMPI-2-RF—PSY-5 scales														
	AGGR-r		**PSYC-r**		**DISC-r**		**NEGE-r**		**INTR-r**					
T	43		63		44		56		47					

tasks. In discussing the results with Julia, she was encouraged to use a variety of memory strategies, such as utilising her stronger visual memory abilities, recording her lectures, reducing the amount of material to be remembered in one go and simplifying and logically structuring information she needed to remember. Julia was also referred to a specialised rehabilitation service and the neuropsychologist liaised with the rehabilitation service which became involved with assisting Julia's return to study.

This MMPI-2-RF interpretation was discussed with Julia in a collaborative assessment context (Finn and Kamphuis 2006). Julia's responses confirmed these impressions derived from objective assessment. The importance of maintaining good mental wellbeing was also discussed with Julia as was the desirability of seeking counselling or psychotherapeutic support in future if she wished to address mood or anxiety concerns.

Discussion

Presurgical Assessment In line with the practice of neuropsychologists in most epilepsy centres, we sought to provide a comprehensive assessment of cognitive abilities addressing general cognitive aptitudes, risk for postoperative disability and psychopathology screening. On the cognitive assessment front, we were guided by the CHC model of cognitive function which is perhaps the best researched model of cognition in healthy and clinical populations (Jewsbury et al. 2015; Larrabee 2000; McGrew 2009). In addition, the CHC model accommodates major neuropsychological constructs including 'executive' function and provides a rational basis for test selection and interpretation (Jewsbury et al. 2015; Loughman et al. 2014). Importantly, many of the most widely used cognitive ability tests now refer to the CHC model for theoretical interpretation (Bowden 2013; Kaufman 2013). In addition, the CHC model, as implemented in recent editions of the Wechsler Intelligence and Memory Scales, displays measurement invariance across diverse populations including representative community controls, participants with learning difficulties, neurosciences populations and representative samples of patients with seizure disorders (Bowden et al. 1999; Bowden et al. 2008a; Bowden et al. 2008b; Bowden et al. 2006). The observation of measurement invariance provides the strongest available statistical test of the precise generalisation of the construct validity of a model of cognition, in this case a variant of the CHC model, across diverse community and clinical populations (Bowden et al. 1999, 2006, 2008a, b; Jewsbury et al. 2015).

In line with common practices (Baxendale and Thompson 2010; Lee 2010), Julia was administered a standardised ability battery that addressed the core aspects of cognition including acquired knowledge (Gc in the CHC model or the VC index on the WAIS-III), fluid intelligence and visual processing (Gf/Gv or the PO index), working memory (Gsm or the WM index), processing speed (Gs or PS on the WAIS-III) and long-term retrieval (Glr or the immediate and delayed memory indexes on the WMS-III). This last ability of long-term retrieval measured by the WMS-III can of course be further divided into auditory-verbal and visuospatial long-term memory when the difference between indexes (or subtests) merits rejection of the null hypothesis of a single memory factor, that is, when the base rate of the difference between the verbal and visual memory indexes is small (Bowden et al. 2006; Kaufman and Lichtenberger 1999; Tulsky et al. 1997).

One of the reasons a comprehensive assessment of cognition is routinely administered in our epilepsy surgery program is that assessment of cognitive function prior to surgery often reveals unexpected findings in terms of the profile of factor scores including, occasionally, unexpected diagnostic issues such as intellectual disability. Without a comprehensive baseline assessment, unrecognised individual needs will be missed and patients will not receive an appropriate standard of care. In addition, in view of the frequent 'atypical' findings in terms of individual cognitive profiles (e.g. Gargaro et al. 2013 as discussed above), effective postsurgical assessment relies on individual baseline data. This strategy of individualised assessment reflects the practice of other clinicians also (Baxendale and Thompson 2010; Gargaro et al. 2013; Lee 2010).

In Julia's case, at the preoperative assessment, differences between certain of her WMS-III indexes approached significance in terms of base rates reported in the interpretative software, although, only one exceeded the 5 % (i.e., less than 5 %) base rate criterion that we routinely employ, namely the auditory-immediate versus auditory-delayed discrepancy. Although this 5 % base rate criterion provides a moderate degree of control over false-positive rate, the multiple comparisons possible between the various Wechsler Intelligence and Memory Scale indexes mean it would be reasonable to apply a more stringent criterion of base rate infrequency (i.e. less than 5 % base rate in the normative population), to control for false-positive findings (Kaufman and Lichtenberger 2005; Lichtenberger and Kaufman 2012).

Of course the Wechsler Memory indexes are also administered for reasons of practical utility as the best researched measures of the long-term retrieval or anterograde memory constructs known to be affected by resection of medial temporal lobe structures (Baxendale and Thompson 2010; Lee 2010). At the presurgical assessment there was a trend toward a weaker auditory-verbal versus visuospatial memory discrepancy (Table 5.3), but the differences did not exceed the 5 % base rate criterion. The poorer score on the auditory-verbal delayed memory index at this assessment was attributed to be situational as opposed to neurobiological factors, perhaps a lapse in concentration, test-related anxiety or an unrecognised seizure event during recall of the verbal-delayed subtests. Julia also displayed lower scores on the VC index of the WAIS-III, compared to her other cognitive ability indexes at this presurgical assessment, possibly explained by disrupted learning opportunities due to the frequent nature of her seizures.

Mood screening at the presurgical assessment with the BDI-II and STAI revealed no elevated scores indicating unusual levels of depression or anxiety and together with a semi-structured interview conducted by the examining neuropsychologist and consultation with the epilepsy service psychiatrist, no issues in the realm of psychopathology were identified at this time.

Overall, in terms of her neuropsychological profile at her presurgical assessment, there were no contraindications to successful anterior-temporal lobectomy. In view of the well-lateralised HS identified on structural MRI, consistent with other neurological investigations, Julia proceeded to have the surgery.

Postsurgical Assessment As seen in Table 5.1, Julia's postsurgical scores on the WAIS-III showed very similar scores on the VC, PO and WM indexes, but PS showed a significant increase, compared to her presurgical assessment. There were no clinically significant base rate discrepancies between subtests contributing to her respective index scores, so the postsurgical indexes were interpreted as trait-homogeneous measures of the respective latent factors, that is, the subtests are all measuring the same basic cognitive skill (Kaufman and Lichtenberger 1999; Tulsky et al. 1997). The common observation of improved processing speed (PS: Table 5.1) after anterior-temporal lobectomy is usually attributed to reduction in seizure frequency, reduction in medications or improved wellbeing (Baxendale and Thompson 2010; Lee 2010). Julia continued to have seizures after surgery, albeit at a greatly reduced frequency, and she therefore had not had a dramatic reduction in her medications. In her case, the improved processing speed may be attributed to the reduction in seizure frequency, although in any individual case, the interpretation is inevitably speculative (Lee 2010).

In contrast to her presurgical scores, postsurgical WMS-III Memory indexes (Table 5.4) displayed markedly less divergence, all falling within the below-average to average range, with no differences approaching significant (5 %) base rate discrepancies, and no significant within-index discrepancies. Importantly, there was no evidence of postoperative reduction in memory function, of the sort reported for a proportion of patients undergoing anterior-temporal lobectomy (Bell et al. 2011; Lee 2010). Language function as assessed by lexical-retrieval tests such as the fluency tests and object naming (Table 5.4) also showed no significant change from preoperative scores. Again, change in these scores was interpreted in terms of 95 % confidence intervals centred on the predicted true scores derived from the first (presurgical) assessment. These results suggest that in line with extensive research evidence language function is affected by dominant-hemisphere seizure focus, including a focus in the hippocampus, and that resection of diseased tissue will not necessarily lead to reductions in language function, although, transient or lasting postoperative reductions in language function are a common observation (Bell et al. 2011; Lee 2010).

We aim to routinely administer the MMPI-2 and now the MMPI-2-RF (Ben-Porath and Tellegen 2008) to every patient at presurgical assessment, because it is usually helpful to understand the patient's broader wellbeing and often informs interpretation of cognitive assessment issues (Foran et al. 2013). In this case, the routine screening of Julia with established brief tests (BDI-II and STAI) at presurgical assessment revealed no elevated scores and the issue of psychological distress could easily have been interpreted as unimportant. At postoperative assessment, these test scores were unchanged in terms of 95 % CI's and indicated no elevated psychological distress. However, as a comprehensive care strategy, the MMPI-2-RF was administered at postsurgical assessment and, as noted above, identified some mild issues in psychological function that might benefit from therapeutic support. It is notable that the MMPI-2-RF interpretation contrasts with the asymptomatic self-report, BDI-II and STAI scores at presurgical and initial postsurgical assessment, both of which have very high face validity. Face-to-face interview, and the BDI-II and STAI are readily susceptible to response-sets and contain no validity indicators, potentially leading to misinterpretation of the observed scores or self-report. The MMPI-2-RF provides better construct validity for the assessment of psychopathology including measurement of response-sets which may distort the clinical (diagnostic) scales (Sellbom et al. 2006). The model of construct validity has been replicated in our seizure disorder population, that is, the same basic psychopathological symptom validity characteristics that were identified in the normative population were identified in our epilepsy patients (Bowden et al. 2014). Lee (2010) emphasises the importance of assessment of quality of life in people with seizure disorders. Although, the MMPI-2-RF is not a conventional quality of life measure, much of the variance in quality of life measures is explained by current mood, so the MMPI-2 provides an important mechanism by which to gauge some of the critical underpinnings of quality of life.

We can consider whether these results of essentially unchanged memory and mood postoperatively are consistent with the literature. The overall quoted rate of cognitive decline postoperatively can be turned around to show that 40–70 % of people, who have anterior-temporal lobectomy, do not experience any change in their cognition (Bell et al. 2011). This can be easily forgotten when statistical significance is used to evaluate outcomes of the groups as a whole (a mean change in test scores can be assumed to be the result for every patient) rather than focusing on base rates, which allow us to consider how many people got the result and extrapolate to how likely it is that our individual patient will get the same result. From this point of view Julia's cognitive outcome is typical of the majority of people who undergo dominant anterior-temporal lobectomy in our program. In terms of some of the specific factors, Julia certainly had HS identifiable preoperatively (with the assistance of volumetric hippocampal measurements) and onset of her seizures was at a young age, both of which predict a lower likelihood of memory decline postoperatively. Her memory would be best described as mildly impaired overall when compared to her other cognitive skills preoperatively (most studies of people with 'normal' memory preoperatively categorise this as above 25th percentile). Her lack of memory change postoperatively is quite consistent with the literature and our practice. She had left-sided surgery which is associated with a greater chance of language impairment postoperatively, but again more people have stable naming skills than experience a decline, as was the case for Julia.

These results illustrate that anterior-temporal lobectomy can be offered to patients with the expectation of a reduction seizure activity and also that cognition in general and memory in particular may not be adversely affected if the advice is based on modern neurological and neuroimaging methods including, as in Julia's case, the use of quantitative MRI (Cook et al. 1992).

References

Baxendale, S., & Thompson, P. (2010). Beyond localization: The role of traditional neuropsychological tests in an age of imaging. *Epilepsia, 51,* 2225–2230.

Beck, A. T., Steer, R. A., & Brown, G. K. (1996). *Beck depression inventory* (2nd ed.). San Antonio: The Psychological Corporation.

Bell, B., Lin, J. J., Seidenberg, M., & Hermann, B. (2011). The neurobiology of cognitive disorders in temporal lobe epilepsy. *Nature Reviews Neurology, 7,* 154–164.

Ben-Porath, Y., & Tellegen, A. (2008). *Minnesota multiphasic personality inventory-2 restructured form: Manual for administration, scoring, and interpretation*. Minneapolis: University of Minnesota Press.

Binder, J. R., Swanson, S. J., Sabsevitz, D. S., Hammeke, T. A., Raghavan, M., & Mueller, W. M. (2010). A comparison of two fMRI methods for predicting verbal memory decline after left temporal lobectomy: Language lateralization versus hippocampal activation asymmetry. *Epilepsia, 51,* 618–626.

Bowden, S. C. (2013). Theoretical convergence in assessment of cognition. *Journal of Psychoeducational Assessment, 31,* 148–156.

Bowden, S. C., & McCarter, R. M. (1993). Spatial memory in alcohol-dependent subjects: Using a push-button maze to test the principle of equiavailability. *Brain and Cognition, 22,* 51–62.

Bowden, S. C., Carstairs, J. R., & Shores, E. A. (1999). Confirmatory factor analysis of combined Wechsler adult Intelligence scale—revised and Wechsler memory scale—revised scores in a healthy community sample. *Psychological Assessment, 11,* 339.

Bowden, S. C., Weiss, L. G., Holdnack, J. A., & Lloyd, D. (2006). Age-related invariance of abilities measured with the Wechsler Adult Intelligence Scale-III. *Psychological Assessment, 18,* 334.

Bowden, S. C., Gregg, N., Bandalos, D., Davis, M., Coleman, C., Holdnack, J. A., & Weiss, L. G. (2008a). Latent mean and covariance differences with measurement equivalence in college students with developmental difficulties versus the Wechsler adult intelligence scale–III/Wechsler memory scale–III normative sample. *Educational and Psychological Measurement, 68,* 621–642.

Bowden, S. C., Weiss, L. G., Holdnack, J. A., Bardenhagen, F. J., & Cook, M. J. (2008b). Equivalence of a measurement model of cognitive abilities in U.S. standardization and Australian neuroscience samples. *Assessment, 15,* 132–144.

Bowden, S. C., White, J., Simpson, L., & Ben-Porath, Y. (2014). Elevation discrepancies between MMPI-2 clinical and MMPI-2-RF restructured clinical (RC) scales in people with seizure disorders. *Epilepsy & Behavior, 34,* 92–98.

Busch, R. M., Dulay, M. F., Kim, K. H., Chapin, J. S., Jehi, L., Kalman, C. C., Najm, I. M. (2011). Pre-surgical mood predicts memory decline after anterior temporal lobe resection for epilepsy. *Archives of Clinical Neuropsychology, 26,* 739–745. (acr067).

Cook, M. J., Fish, D. R., Shorvon, S. D., Straughan, K., & Stevens, J. M. (1992). Hippocampal volumetric and morphometric studies in frontal and temporal lobe epilepsy. *Brain, 115,* 1001–1015.

Dulay, M. F., & Busch, R. M. (2012). Prediction of neuropsychological outcome after resection of temporal and extratemporal seizure foci. *Neurosurgical Focus, 32,* E4.

Finn, S. E., & Kamphuis, J. H. (2006). Therapeutic assessment with the MMPI-2. In J. N. Butcher (Ed.), *A practitioner's guide*. Washington, DC: APA Books.

Foran, A., Bowden, S., Bardenhagen, F., Cook, M., & Meade, C. (2013). Specificity of psychopathology in temporal lobe epilepsy. *Epilepsy & Behavior, 27,* 193–199.

Gargaro, A. C., Sakamoto, A. C., Bianchin, M. M., Geraldi, C. d. V., Scorsi-Rosset, S., Coimbra, É. R., Velasco, T. R. (2013). Atypical neuropsychological profiles and cognitive outcome in mesial temporal lobe epilepsy. *Epilepsy & Behavior, 27,* 461–469.

Hinton-Bayre, A. D. (2010). Deriving reliable change statistics from test-retest normative data: Comparison of models and mathematical expressions. *Archives of Clinical Neuropsychology, 25,* 244–256.

Hocking, J., Thomas, H. J., Dzafic, I., Williams, R. J., Reutens, D. C., & Spooner, D. M. (2013). Disentangling the cognitive components supporting Austin Maze performance in left versus right temporal lobe epilepsy. *Epilepsy & Behavior, 29,* 485–491.

Ives-Deliperi, V. L., & Butler, J. T. (2012). Naming outcomes of anterior temporal lobectomy in epilepsy patients: A systematic review of the literature. *Epilepsy & Behavior, 24,* 194–198.

Jewsbury, P. A., Bowden, S. C., & Strauss, M. E. (2015). Confirmatory factor analysis of executive function models: A Cattell-Horn-Carroll based reanalysis. *Submitted for publication.*

Kanner, A. M. (2008). Can fMRI replace the Wada test in predicting postsurgical deterioration of verbal memory? *Nature Clinical Practice Neurology, 4,* 364–365.

Kaufman, A. S. (2013). Intelligent testing with Wechsler's fourth editions: Perspectives on the Weiss et al. studies and the eight commentaries. *Journal of Psychoeducational Assessment, 31,* 224–234.

Kaufman, A. S., & Lichtenberger, E. O. (1999). *Essentials of WAIS-III assessment.* Hoboken: Wiley.

Kaufman, A. S., & Lichtenberger, E. O. (2005). *Assessing adolescent and adult intelligence.* Hoboken: Wiley.

Larrabee, G. J. (2000). Association between IQ and neuropsychological test performance: Commentary on Tremont, Hoffman, Scott, and Adams (1998). *The Clinical Neuropsychologist, 14,* 139–145.

Lee, G. P. (2010). *Neuropsychology of epilepsy and epilepsy surgery.* New York: Oxford University Press.

Lichtenberger, E. O., & Kaufman, A. S. (2012). *Essentials of WAIS-IV assessment.* Hoboken: Wiley.

Loughman, A., Bowden, S., & D'Souza, W. (2014). Cognitive functioning in idiopathic generalised epilepsies: A systematic review and meta-analysis. *Neuroscience & Biobehavioral Reviews, 43,* 20–34.

McGrew, K. S. (2009). CHC theory and the human cognitive abilities project: Standing on the shoulders of the giants of psychometric intelligence research. *Intelligence, 37,* 1–10.

Nunnally, J. C., & Bernstein, I. (1994). *Psychometric theory.* New York: McGraw-Hill.

Rausch, R., & Babb, T. L. (1993). Hippocampal neuron loss and memory scores before and after temporal lobe surgery for epilepsy. *Archives of Neurology, 50,* 812–817.

Reilly, R. E., Bowden, S. C., Bardenhagen, F. J., & Cook, M. J. (2006). Equality of the psychological model underlying depressive symptoms in patients with temporal lobe epilepsy versus heterogeneous neurological disorders. *Journal of Clinical and Experimental Neuropsychology, 28,* 1257–1271.

Sawrie, S. M., Chelune, G. J., Naugle, R. I., & Lüders, H. O. (1996). Empirical methods for assessing meaningful neuropsychological change following epilepsy surgery. *Journal of the International Neuropsychological Society, 2,* 556–564.

Saykin, A. J., Gur, R. C., Sussman, N. M., O'Connor, M. J., & Gur, R. E. (1989). Memory deficits before and after temporal lobectomy: effect of laterality and age of onset. *Brain and Cognition, 9,* 191–200.

Seidenberg, M., Hermann, B., Wyler, A. R., Davies, K., Dohan, F. C., Jr., & Leveroni, C. (1998). Neuropsychological outcome following anterior temporal lobectomy in patients with and without the syndrome of mesial temporal lobe epilepsy. *Neuropsychology, 12,* 303.

Sellbom, M., Ben-Porath, Y., McNulty, J. L., Arbisi, P. A., & Graham, J. R. (2006) Elevation differences between MMPI-2 clinical and restructured clinical (RC) scales: Frequency, origins, and interpretative implications. *Assessment, 13*, 430–441.

Sherman, E., Wiebe, S., Fay-McClymont, T. B., Tellez-Zenteno, J., Metcalfe, A., Hernandez-Ronquillo, L., Jetté, N. (2011). Neuropsychological outcomes after epilepsy surgery: Systematic review and pooled estimates. *Epilepsia, 52*, 857–869.

Spielberger, C. D. (1989). *State-Trait Anxiety Inventory: A comprehensive bibliography* (2nd ed.). Palo Alto: Consulting Psychologists Press.

Spreen, O., & Strauss, E. (1998). *A compendium of neuropsychological tests: Administration, norms, and commentary* (2nd ed.). New York: Oxford University Press.

Tombaugh, T. N., Kozak, J., & Rees, L. (1999). Normative data stratified by age and education for two measures of verbal fluency: FAS and animal naming. *Archives of Clinical Neuropsychology, 14*, 167–177.

Tulsky, D., Zhu, J., & Ledbetter, M. (1997). *WAIS-III/WMS-III technical manual*. San Antonio: Psychological Corporation.

Wechsler, D. (1997a). *WAIS-III/WMS-III administration and scoring manual: WAIS-III and WMS-III scoring assistant supplement*. San Antonio: The Psychological Corporation.

Wechsler, D. (1997b). *WMS-III administration and scoring manual*. San Antonio: The Psychological Corporation.

Wechsler, D. (2008). *Wechsler adult intelligence scale–Fourth edition (WAIS–IV)*. San Antonio: NCS Pearson.

Wiebe, S., Blume, W. T., Girvin, J. P., & Eliasziw, M. (2001). A randomized, controlled trial of surgery for temporal-lobe epilepsy. *New England Journal of Medicine, 345*, 311–318.

Chapter 6
Neuropsychological Assessment of Medico-Legal Capacity in the New Zealand Context

Kay L. Cunningham

Legal and Clinical Principles

In New Zealand, The Protection of Personal and Property Rights Act 1988 (PPPR Act) operates alongside the Mental Health Compulsory Assessment and Treatment Act 1992. While there may be some legal differences in legal capacity determination in other countries, fundamental principles are likely to be similar or same, and in particular the process of clinical evaluation will hold the same challenges regardless of country.

Legal capacity (also referred to as competence) refers to characteristics the person possesses either relative to a particular decision or in regards to all decision-making situations, that is, capacity can be described as on a continuum from full capacity to full incapacity. Clinicians can only provide opinion on capacity, whereas the Courts provide a legal judgement and determination of the need for a designated substitute decision-maker. Personal Orders relate to the specific area/s in which the Courts have deemed a different decision-maker to the individual is required for up to a period of 3 years, after which reapplication to Court is required. Personal orders may be in the form of a Welfare Guardianship or Property Management. In the instance of partial capacity related to Welfare Guardianship, the individual retains limited decision-making ability and ideally has input from trusted others within a supported decision-making process (Church and Watts 2007). Partial capacity may be dependent on the individual in question being willing to accept supported decision-making through others.

There is a considerable difference in the clinical depth to which capacity assessments are undertaken, with this ranging from simplistic (whereby only a very basic cognitive screen is used during a short doctor's visit) to a more in-depth assessment utilizing multiple sources of information. When cognitive impairment is severely profound, then simple methods may well be sufficient. However, given the impact

K. L. Cunningham (✉)
PO Box 15280, Miramar, Wellington 6243, New Zealand
e-mail: kay.cunningham@xtra.co.nz

J. A. B. Macniven (ed.), *Neuropsychological Formulation*,
DOI 10.1007/978-3-319-18338-1_6

to the individual of loss of rights, employing a neuropsychological formulation approach is recommended in situations where capacity may not be as obviously determined. Providing clear justification for opinion for capacity or incapacity is also important regardless of the extent of testing employed.

Guiding principles behind relevant legislations (New Zealand Protection of Personal and Property Rights Act 1988 (PPPR Act); Mental Capacity Act, England and Wales, 2005) indicate that:

1. There is an assumption of capacity unless proved otherwise.
2. It is necessary to enable and support the person to develop or exercise capacity wherever and whenever possible.
3. A person is not to be treated as unable to make a decision because decisions may be unwise, but must be due to actual incapacity, that is, the risk of harm to the individual or to others outweighs the benefits of preserved autonomy.
4. Any decisions on behalf of the individual must be in their best interests and must be the least restrictive of the person's rights and freedom of action.

The primary determinants for assessment of mental capacity are defined as having the:

1. Ability to understand relevant information, and including the ability to retain information relevant to the decision.
2. Ability to appreciate the consequences of a decision.
3. Ability to act voluntarily and autonomously (i.e., to freely make a decision without undue influence).
4. Ability to communicate decisions.

Capacity can be fluctuating in nature or at different levels of ability at different points of time (either improving or declining). Even a person with a significant and global cognitive impairment may still have the capacity to make simple decisions. Clinical capacity is usually limited to a particular decision, so that persons who have temporary incapacity are not deemed incapable beyond the period of their incapacity. However, when a condition exists that is either permanent and stable or deteriorating (such as dementia), then lack of capacity may be deemed to go beyond specific decisions. It is generally accepted that the person being assessed has a disability that can potentially result in poor decision-making, as a necessary "threshold requirement" (Australian Psychological Society Submission (2010)).

Relevant Issues in Clinical Evaluation of Capacity

Studies such as by Sullivan (2004) provide some understanding on the strengths and difficulties inherent in general evaluation of mental capacity. Sullivan notes that there is a lack of consistency in assessment between professionals. Historically, medical staff have conducted capacity assessments using very brief status examinations which are not universally considered to be adequate for opinions on capacity. When a more multidisciplinary approach has been applied, opinion has often been based on subjective appraisal and very limited objective measures, potentially leading to an underestimation of the extent of incapacity. There are also significant differences between clinical versus legal interpretations of capacity, with the former not being a unitary concept in contrast to the latter requiring a more black and white definition. Difficulties become most apparent when cases reflect borderline impaired incapacity as opposed to more obvious incapacity. Even when objective tests are employed within assessments, they may not necessarily cover the range and type of abilities crucial to capacity determination. Additional complexity arises when people make decisions that are generally considered as unwise and perhaps unsafe. The assessment will need to determine whether these decisions are based on cognitive lack of understanding of the (long-term) consequences or simply individual choice that may be unwise.

There is a dearth of specific capacity measures available. Of those that are available, they are most commonly relevant to aging and/or dementia patients, thus they often have less applicability for other patient groups. Moye et al. (2006) state that clinical judgement is still the "gold standard" for capacity determination. However, as there is no clear consensus on what constitutes capacity assessment then variability between raters within and between specialities can often occur, and clinical judgement can, therefore, be particularly flawed. As noted by Mullaly et al. (2007) there is a relative lack of training for many (neuro)psychologists in this area. This can result in both a stressful and difficult process even for clinicians considered to have some of the most in-depth knowledge in this area (Sullivan 2004).

Nevertheless, the determination of loss of mental capacity is in some situations complex and in these instances neuropsychological assessment can provide additional information to assist the court and others in these matters. Neuropsychologists can provide an in-depth assessment that involves clinical judgement based on information from a range of sources combined with tests that evaluate relevant cognitive processes. Ecological validity of neuropsychological tests in predicting decisional ability has been questioned by some (e.g., Moberg and Kniele 2006), and certainly in isolation this is a valid concern. As noted by Crowe (2005), impairment is what can be measured by testing whereas disability is the actual handicap that impairment causes in the real world. It would seem, therefore, that a formulation which clearly integrates objective testing with multiple information sources and clinical judgement becomes particularly crucial in the determination of capacity versus incapacity.

Capacity to self-manage finances is an area that has been largely neglected in rehabilitation research (Hoskins and Crowe 2005). One available study is by Hoskins et al. (2005). They found that prediction of specific money management behaviors (i.e., problematic impulsive spending and paying bills/rent late) was more reliable using specific neuropsychological measures than attempting a prediction of overall money management.

Decision-making around consent to sexual acts is another area which requires a careful and in-depth clinical approach. Individuals with intellectual/cognitive disability have the same rights as others to have sexual intimacy within their relationships. It is, however, also imperative that potential harm and exploitation are minimized, and the reader is referred to studies such as by Brown and Turk (1992),

Niederbuhl and Morris (1993), Morris et al. (1993), Murphy (2003), McCarthy (2003), Murphy and O'Callaghan (2004), Eastgate (2005), Benedet and Grant (2007) to provide relevant consideration of sexual consent and capacity to consent.

Assessment Considerations

While not without potential problems it is possible to undertake neuropsychological assessments that provide systematic and evidence-based evaluation. Based on the "best practice" models suggested in various research and reviews of capacity assessment (e.g., Moberg and Kniele 2006; Herbert 2013), the following approach was employed for the three case studies described.

1. Consideration of both legal and clinical standards based on guiding principles and determinants of capacity and incapacity.
2. Consideration of whether the evaluation and conclusions reached are in respect to a specific decision or is appropriate to all major decisions.
3. Identification and implementation of any adaptations and environmental supports to ensure a valid assessment (e.g., communication aids, ethical considerations including informed assent/consent).
4. Detailed interview of the individual (if possible on more than one occasion) and collateral information from reliable informants.
5. Functional assessment through both observations of behavior and other measures to provide ecologically valid representations of the individual's capacity.
6. Neuropsychological and psychological assessment using appropriate methods of evaluation.
7. Interpretation and formulation of results and functional relationship based on both an understanding of the person's condition, relevancy of particular skills in decision-making (including qualitative information), and consideration of the dynamic relationship between cognitive strengths and weaknesses.
8. Within the psychological assessment, gaining knowledge of the individual's values and preferences are important as part of the capacity assessment, for example, if incapacity is determined then the individual's preference for who may be a named guardian or where they may wish to live.

Additionally, it is important to take into account relevant cultural, religious and personal, and social factors which may affect the interpretation of behavior and responses in regards to capacity.

Case 1: Susan—A Person Presenting with a Congenital Intellectual Disability

Susan was referred for assessment to determine her capacity to understand the nature and foresee the consequences of decisions relating to her personal care and welfare as well as self-management in relation to property. Susan was a 35-year-old woman with Down syndrome. She had a benign heart murmur identified in infancy, but had maintained reasonably good health throughout her life. She could not speak until between the ages 4–5 years (other than occasional words such as "no"), but was reported by her parents as being able to understand a reasonable amount of language, despite expressive language limitation. She gained functional language skills over time and was able to hold a simple conversation effectively.However with information and instructions that went beyond a singular amount, she did require repetition and simplification. She adapted well to school where she was in special needs classes with some mainstreaming. Due to learning difficulties she did not gain any formal academic qualifications and left school at the age of 21. She developed friendships with others with disabilities and had a loving and supportive family. Through the support of family and relevant agencies, independent living skills were taught and reinforced with Susan able to manage some basic routine tasks which had become very well learnt.

Ethical Issues—The Question of Consent

There is a fundamental presumption that a person has capacity until proven otherwise, therefore consequent consideration needs to be given to the question of obtaining informed assent/consent in persons undergoing capacity assessment. Assent/consent, where possible, is needed before proceeding with any assessment or intervention that can affect a person's well-being. When incapacity is suspected prior to an assessment, then measures must be taken to engage persons who are known to have the person's best interests at heart (e.g., family members) and are trusted to the person. If they are not available, then a designated support or advocate would need to be advised of the purpose of the assessment. Susan's parents, her primary supports, were informed and gave assent for the assessment to proceed. Susan also gave her assent to completing the tasks.[1] Her father was present during the first session. After the initial clinical interview Susan and her father indicated that they were comfortable with (and preferred) the testing being undertaken without her father present, with this reflecting her desire to be as independent as possible.

The purpose of the assessment needs to be explained to the person at a level they can understand and then repeated at each meeting. In Susan's case, some initial time was spent developing a working relationship with her as well as allowing opportunity to gain familiarity with Susan's expressive and receptive language skills. Language was simplified to an expected level of ability. Susan was able to say back in her own words what she understood as to why the assessment/interview was occurring, as well as her understanding of the limits to confidentiality. Further clarification was provided as required, and her father also provided additional explanation to Susan, based on his knowledge of her level of understanding. She was

[1] Assent refers to a willingness to participate, whereas consent refers to permission. While these are mostly synonymous, where there is potential for an individual not to have capacity to understand in a fully informed manner, then only assent rather than consent can be assumed. Others may therefore provide assent on the individual's behalf in situations whereby incapacity may be an issue.

specifically informed of how information would be used, who was likely to have access to it, and what the information might be used for—for example, for the Judge making a decision about whether she was able to make all decisions/choices about what she could do for herself, or whether she may need someone else to make, or help her make, important decisions for her.

The conversation was then led into different matters, with this serving as a brief interference process. Susan was then asked what she recalled of the prior discussion around assessment process. This approach ensured her response was not automatically copying what had been said to her.

Specific comprehension of certain keywords used (e.g., "decision") were checked out by asking her if she knew what was meant by the word "decision." She was then asked to say in her own words and/or in a sentence of her choice so that it was clear she understood both the meaning and the context. She was asked how she felt about doing the assessment (e.g., did she feel worried, scared, upset, ok, happy, etc.) and also that was it okay for her to talk about her feelings and concerns. It was stressed that neither the assessor nor others would be upset or angry with her if she did not want to talk and answer the questions—it was her choice and there was no pressure to make her do so. Because there is a likelihood that information discussed in one conversation may not be remembered at a later time, or may become distorted through poor memory encoding/retrieval, the process was repeated as necessary. Her father was able to clarify that he felt Susan had a basic and appropriate level of understanding about the purpose and process of assessment.

Adaptive Living Skills Ratings

An adaptive rating scale was used to measure daily functioning skills with the Adaptive Behaviour Assessment System-Second Edition (ABAS-II; Harrison Oakland 2003) being the scale available at that time. Susan's father and her support worker each filled in the ABAS-II with strong consistency between the two raters. Susan had some areas of relative skill, however, the General Adaptive Composite (GAC) scale, scores for both raters indicated that Susan's overall abilities for adaptive living were within the borderline functioning range. On the Conceptual Composite scale, the two raters' scores placed her within the borderline functioning range for receptive and expressive language, reading and writing, money concepts, and self-direction. On the Practical Composite scale, Susan's overall score for both raters placed her within the extremely low range of abilities compared to age peers, for skills relating to basic maintenance activities of daily living (e.g., eating, mobility, self-cares, dressing), instrumental activities of daily living (e.g., meal preparation, housekeeping, transportation, taking medications, money management, telephone use) together with occupation skills and maintenance of safe environments. On the Social Composite scale, the raters' scores placed her within the borderline functioning range of abilities compared to age peers, for skills required for interpersonal relationships, responsibility, self-esteem, gullibility/naiveté, following rules, obeying laws, and avoiding victimization. Individual analysis of specific skill sets indicated communication and social skills were relative strengths (borderline functioning to average range) with health and safety, self-care, self-direction, and functional academics the lowest ratings (extremely low range). Relevant information from the occupational therapist involved with Susan was consistent with raters' impressions of Susan's functional abilities.

Presentation and Behaviors During Interviewing and Testing

Susan presented as a casually dressed and tidily groomed woman. There were no signs of personal neglect. She had a very pleasant, polite, and cooperative manner. She showed basic but appropriate social etiquette, with appropriate eye contact and length of gaze. She showed a sense of humor and a keenness to please. Susan's speech was generally intelligible, but at times it was necessary to ask her to repeat a word or phrase, when pronunciation was not clear. When asked to repeat, she did so willingly and would repeat a word or phrase until it could be understood. When speaking to Susan, it was necessary to use simple words and phrases, presented in a slightly slowed pace. If she could not understand or was unsure she would spontaneously say "I don't understand," thus allowing the assessor to rephrase the question. Questions or verbal information given to Susan had to be at a concrete level, that is, at a literal level whereby vocabulary was simplistic and she was not required to make inferences. During the testing phase (occurring over two sessions), Susan attempted the tasks well and did not require prompting to stay on task. She persisted with tasks even when they were difficult and to the point where she clearly could not do the item. There was no overt anxiety; rather she showed a strong desire and eagerness to do her best. She was well within the acceptable threshold on the Test of Memory Malingering (TOMM; Tombaugh 1997) that evaluates for an appropriate level of effort (Simon 2007). A psychological screen was completed based on clinical interview (questions and observations) and information from others who saw her on a daily basis. Susan has no history with mental health services and there were no concerns in regards to her mental wellness at the time of the assessment.

Tests Administered and Assessment Results

Wechsler Adult Intelligence Scale-Fourth Edition (WAIS-IV; core subtests) Australian/NZ adaptation (Wechsler 2008)

Wechsler Memory Scale-Fourth Edition (WMS-IV: Logical Stories) (Wechsler 2009)

Delis–Kaplan Executive Function System (D-KEFS: Sorting and Proverbs) (Delis et al. 2001)

The following provides the test results combined with relevant research to aid in formulation.

Table 6.1 Wechsler Adult Intelligence Scale (Fourth edition) composite scores

WAIS-IV	Composite score		Percentile rank	95 % confidence interval	Qualitative description
Verbal comprehension	VCI	61	<1	57–68	Extremely low
Perceptual reasoning	PRI	60	<1	56–68	Extremely low
Working memory	WMI	60	<1	56–69	Extremely low
Processing speed	PSI	56	<1	52–69	Extremely low
Full scale	FSIQ	53	<1	50–58	Extremely low

General Intellectual Functioning and Adaptive Living Skills

Global deficits in intelligence are a key feature of Down syndrome. Impairments are present in expressive communication and explicit memory, and cognitive functions most affected are subserved by structures that mature relatively late in development, such as the prefrontal cortex (executive function (EF) skills), hippocampus (memory), and cerebellum (which contributes to coordination and accurate timing in movement).

Based on the WAIS-IV, Susan's general intellectual abilities were within the extremely low range. Full Scale IQ was 53 which met the criteria for moderate to mild intellectual disability (Table 6.1). The ABAS-II rating results were consistent with mild intellectual disability.

Specific Test Analysis

(i) Attention and Speed of Information Processing

The speed with which information can be mentally processed is typically slower in Down syndrome, particularly when information is in the auditory/verbal mode. Studies have shown significant time delay in sensory information arriving to cortical areas which suggests abnormal subcortical processing (Maraj et al. 2002).

Susan's ability on tasks that measure attention and the speed with which she could process information was within the extremely low range. She had a limited capacity to process information even when it is in simple form, and a very limited capacity to hold and manipulate information (i.e., in working memory; Table 6.2).

(ii) Memory and Learning

Based on research findings, there is clear evidence that Down syndrome is associated with particularly poor verbal short-term memory performance and a deficit in verbal short-term memory, with likely negative effects on aspects of language acquisition, particularly vocabulary development. Individuals with Down syndrome also show impaired explicit long-term memory for verbal information, and may also have particular problems in explicit long-term memory for visual-object as-

Table 6.2 WAIS-IV Working Memory and Processing Speed subtest scores

WAIS-IV subtests	SS and percentile	Range	Descriptions
Digit span total	SS: 1, < 1st percentile	Extremely low	
Digit span forwards	SS: 2,< 1st percentile	Extremely low	Susan had a limited capacity to process and rote recall sets of simple verbal information (digit span of 4)
Digit span backwards Digit span sequences	SS: 2, < 1st percentile SS: 2, < 1st percentile	Extremely low Extremely low	She also had a limited capacity to hold and mentally reorder sets of simple verbal information (digit span of 3)
WAIS-IV Arithmetic	SS: 4, 2nd percentile	Extremely low	When required to complete verbally presented arithmetic items, Susan was able to complete only very basic numerical problems involving simply counting or subtracting items from a pictorial presentation of simple familiar objects
WAIS-IV Coding	SS: 3, 1st percentile	Extremely low	Susan was able to visually scan, find, and accurately copy simple symbols, indicating she had basic visual discrimination skills. However, the number of reproductions she could produce in the set time indicated a slow ability to process information
WAIS-IV Symbol search	SS: 1, < 1st percentile	Extremely low	Susan was able to visually scan and match simple symbols, indicating she had basic visual discrimination skills. However, the number she could produce in the set time frame again indicated a slow ability to process information

sociations (Jarrold et al. 2009), particularly as information goes beyond very simple units of information.

Susan had significant difficulties with processing and retaining verbal information for immediate recall even when it was presented in a well-associated and contextual form (i.e., narrative, as occurs in conversation). When each story was read to her, not only was she unable to recall more than a few details but also what she did recall was incorrect. Her responses showed that when she was mentally overwhelmed by information she was unable to recall the main "gist" (as she could not

Table 6.3 Wechsler Memory Scale (Fourth Edition)

WMS-IV logical stories	SS and percentile	Range	Qualitative
Immediate recall	SS: 1, < 1st percentile	Extremely low	Only two accurate details were recalled from each story, and these were provided in a sentence by Susan. Her recall showed she had confused the context of the information, resulting in her being unable to comprehend and encode the main "gist" of the story
Delayed	SS: 1, < 1st percentile	Extremely low	After a 30-min delay, the two accurate details she previously managed to recall were lost. Instead she recalled details which showed confusion between the first and second story (interference effect)
Recognition	< 2nd percentile	Extremely low	When provided with prompts in the form of "yes/no" questions for each story, Susan still had a very poor performance, indicating difficulties were with her ability to encode the information effectively during the initial learning process

effectively process and integrate what she had heard). Information became confused on recall with little association with what had been presented (i.e., distortion was evident) (Table 6.3).

(iii) Language Expressive and receptive language difficulties are part of the cognitive pattern for Down syndrome. People with Down syndrome are less able to understand grammatically difficult sentences—a limitation that may reflect, in part, a general difficulty with precisely remembering sequences of spoken words (Marcell et al. 1990).

Susan had only a basic understanding and comprehension of language, and frequently required instructions and words to be repeated so she could work out what was required of her (Table 6.4). This need for repetition was not only due to limited attention skills (capacity and speed of processing ability) but also due to limitations in her depth of understanding of what words meant. Her very limited ability to think abstractly meant that she was not able to independently make inferences to work out what a phrase, term, or instruction may have meant (i.e., she had only a very concrete/literal perspective). Her expressive language was unsophisticated in terms of content and this was consistent with her reasoning abilities. While she had a basic knowledge and use of grammar, her verbal expression was interspersed with some grammatical errors.

Table 6.4 WAIS-IV Verbal Comprehension subtests

WAIS-IV subtests	SS and percentile	Range	Qualitative
Vocabulary	SS: 4, 2nd percentile	Extremely low	Susan was able to recognize and describe words when they were at a basic level, but was unable to do so when vocabulary became less concrete and more abstract (for example, she could not describe words such as curious or assemble)
Information	SS: 3, 1st percentile	Extremely low	Susan had a very limited knowledge of general factual knowledge (e.g., related to history, geography, and other subjects typically learnt during schooling)

Speech production was affected by speech motor difficulties (a typical Down syndrome characteristic). This resulted at times in the need for others to ask her to repeat and further clarify what she was trying to say. Susan had some reading and writing skills, but at a very basic (primary school) level. Written expression was consistent with oral expressive skills (i.e., unsophisticated with basic phraseology and some grammatical errors). Spelling errors were also evident and indicative of limited literacy skills.

(iv) Visuo-Spatial-Constructional Studies of visuospatial cognition in individuals with Down syndrome have suggested that visual memory, visual-motor integration, and visual imitation seem to be areas of relative strength within visuospatial processing, whereas spatial memory and visuoconstructive abilities seem to be areas of relative weakness (Fidler 2005).

Susan showed a relative strength for simple processing of visuospatial information on one task, but could not work out how to integrate information beyond this simplistic level (Table 6.5).

Table 6.5 WAIS-IV Perceptual Reasoning tasks

WAIS-IV subtests	SS and percentile	Range	Qualitative
Block design	SS: 4, 2nd percentile	Extremely low	Susan had a limited (basic) ability to mentally then manually work out how parts of a design could be integrated to create a complete matching "whole"
Visual puzzles	SS: 5, 5th percentile	Borderline impaired	On a multiple-choice task that required her to have the ability to mentally integrate several parts to make a complete whole, she again had a limited ability. She could complete items that were simple, but was unable to complete any as complexity increased

(v) Executive Functioning EF is the term for a range of skills which develop over childhood through brain maturation in cerebral-neural networks and particularly within frontal-subcortical circuitry. In normal development, full maturation typically occurs around the age of 25 years (Brocki and Bohlin 2004). EF refers to a range of complex skills (Willner et al. 2010a; Bailey et al. 2011). These include the capacity to:

- Reason abstractly, make decisions by analysing information in situations, and consider or foresee wider consequences/repercussions.
- Undertake mental operations through sufficient working memory functioning.
- Effectively engage in goal setting, prioritising of tasks, managing time, and structuring steps to achieve the goal or the decision.
- Problem solving through creatively generating ideas and alternative perspectives.
- Regulate emotions and behaviors.
- Have flexibility in thought and behavior when needed in response to changing needs or situations.
- Learn from situations and errors with effective application of this learning into similar or new situations.

Research suggests that when there is an intellectual disability, EF skills may develop to a lower mental age than other intellectual skills. This is possibly because the maturation of EF skills occurs later than other areas of cognition, and brain maturation in intellectual disability does not go beyond a certain maturational level (Rowe et al. 2006). One of the aspects of limited EF in intellectual disability is impairment in the person's ability to "weigh up" information—and this deficit in reasoning becomes increasingly apparent when there is a need to integrate information from two or more sources.

Susan showed very limited EF ability. She was able to solve the problem and reason at a very basic level (i.e., when solutions were provided and/or obvious). However, she lacked the ability to reason beyond this level, and had a rigid and limited level of cognitive flexibility (Table 6.6).

Formulation

Determining Susan's capacity has been based on her ability to:

a. Understand relevant information, and including the ability to retain information relevant to the decision,
b. Appreciate the consequences of a decision,
c. Act voluntarily and autonomously (able to freely make a decision without undue influence),
d. Communicate decisions.

Table 6.6 WAIS-IV and DKEFS subtests

Subtest	SS and percentile	Range	Qualitative
WAIS-IV Similarities	SS: 3, 1st percentile	Extremely low	This task required Susan to work out how two verbal concepts were related to each other (verbal reasoning). She was only able to complete some initial items, whereby the concepts were very basic and required minimal inferential skills
WAIS-IV Matrix reasoning	SS: 1, < 1st percentile	Extremely low	On a multiple-choice nonverbal reasoning task involving visual pattern matching and analogy problems (without time limits) Susan was only able to accurately reason when very simplistic items were involved. As greater complexity in deductive reasoning was required, she was unable to produce an accurate response (and was unaware her responses were errors)
WAIS-IV Comprehension	SS: 3, 1st percentile	Extremely low	On a task that assesses theoretical comprehension of social situations and evaluates for some aspects of social judgement, Susan had a very limited ability. She was only able to answer some very basic questions, but had no capacity to extrapolate a response on questions that she did not have immediate knowledge and familiarity with (i.e., she was unable to undertake an abstract reasoning process)
DKEFS Sorting free sort condition Sort recognition	SS: 2, < 1st percentile SS: 1, < 1st percentile	Extremely low Extremely low	Susan was unable to identify more than one correct sort for each condition showing very limited flexibility in thinking beyond a very basic level. Sorting the groups for her, thereby reducing the need for her to find the various groups, did not improve her score
DKEFS: Proverbs	SS: 1, < 1st percentile	Extremely low	When required to work out the underlying meaning from proverbs, Susan was unable to correctly work out any of the items (0 score, < 1st percentile, extremely low range), indicating a very literal interpretation. Providing multiple-choice options did not improve Susan's score (also < 1st percentile)

The following outline is in consideration of each of these functions. The process of determining these has been based on the neuropsychological assessment (quantitative and qualitative), semi-structured interviewing of Susan, observations, and information gathered from persons in her life who knew her well. Within clinical interviewing, language was simplified to minimize communication difficulties and vignettes used as a means to provide evaluation of Susan's likely responses in "real life" type situations. A range of social factors were also evaluated in regards to Susan's likely suggestibility, deference/acquiescence, and social skills/assertiveness/communications skills.

(a) Understanding Relevant Information, and Including the Ability to Retain Information Relevant to the Decision and (b) Appreciate the Consequences of a Decision

As stated by Bonardi (2009), in order to "think carefully" about choices, relevant information needs to be made available, and people need to be able to use the information. As outlined in the Submission to the Productivity Commission (2010), it may require additional time from others to carefully communicate information (i.e., on more than one occasion). The assisted person is then able to make a decision. Supported decision-making has been established as the most appropriate way to empower an individual with intellectual disability (or cognitive impairment) in their decision-making processes. This potentially can be provided by family, friends, or any trusted others who become part of the conversation with providers and others when decisions are made. Decision-making processes involve a number of cognitive skills, and in particular EF and memory skills, which include:

- The capacity to process and attend to available information, often in multiple form, and to integrate it together to give it meaning and structure (i.e., attention span and working memory ability).
- Flexibility in thinking in order to generate and consider options from various perspectives, as well as being able to change thinking when new or conflicting information becomes available.
- Cognitive estimation—ability to use information to make reasonable judgements or deductions about the world (to go beyond the literal, to make inferences about what cannot be seen).
- Goal-directed behavior—being able to (a) keep a goal in mind, (b) figure out which sequence of actions, and which strategy, best suits the approach to decision-making and, (c) initiate the action required.
- The ability to identify and prioritize what is most important with an appreciation of the "big picture" (going beyond the immediate, to consideration of future needs and consequences).
- Memory skills—being able to hold in mind all the relevant factors, how they interplay together, and recall them accurately, and as necessary, in a logical form.
- Reasoning ability, which involves a process of inductive and deductive reasoning in order to reach a conclusion, and the capacity to evaluate the decision made (i.e., inductive reasoning is the process of making simple observations of a certain kind and applying these observations through generalization to a different problem to make a decision).
- The ability to understand and "resist" emotional factors that may affect a process of logical deduction.

As decision-making increases in complexity, so do the cognitive requirements to engage effectively in this processing. The ability to appreciate consequences of a decision requires the same skills involved in the initial decision-making process itself. Susan had significant limitations in all the necessary cognitive areas outlined above in respect to making decisions, apart from those that involve very concrete/simplistic level skill. Assessment findings showed that without appropriate support, she was vulnerable to:

- Being unable to process all relevant factors, to identify relevance of information, and to consider all aspects in an integrated fashion.
- Being readily confused or unable to understand information beyond a very simplistic/literal level, and therefore was unable to "make sense" of it in a way that could effectively inform decision-making.
- Being unable to make effective associations and inferences, or to generate appropriate options/alternatives.
- Impairment in her ability to effectively encode, retain, and recall information in an accurate form.

(c) Act Voluntarily and Autonomously (Able to Freely Make a Decision Without Undue Influence)

Undue influence can be present in various forms. In reference to testamentary capacity, Quinn et al. 2010 state that virtually any act of persuasion that overcomes the free will and judgement of another may amount to undue influence. This differs from duress whereby there is an intentional use or threat of force to coerce another. For undue influence to be established, it needs to be demonstrated that the individual had some form of condition (mental, physical, psychological) which showed there was susceptibility. Additionally there needed to be an opportunity for undue influence to occur, for example, through a confidential relationship.

Undue influence can also take the form of controlling weaker persons' environments and social interactions by imposing isolation, insulating them from outside supervision and advisors, poisoning their relationships with others by "bad mouthing" them, and invoking fear of others. An outline of the elements of undue influence (i.e., types of victim and influencers' characteristics, actions, or tactics, and unethical transactions) is provided by Quinn et al. (2010a).

(i) Susan's Characteristics That Contribute to Vulnerability from Undue Influence Susan's personality trait was to please others and acquiesce in the face of pressure and/or conflict (perceived or actual). She became distressed and would quickly "give in" if she felt others were getting angry at her. She was highly suggestible. For example, in a situation in which she was given only minimal or distorted information and the intention of the person interacting with her was dubious, she would believe what she was told without the capability to consider questioning it.

(ii) Influencers' Characteristics, Sources of Power, and Opportunities Susan had been in a situation whereby a male acquaintance had been showing a sexual interest in her. This had resulted in her parents feeling very concerned because of Susan's naivety and vulnerability to being exploited. For a period of time the person attempted to socially isolate Susan by telling her that others were saying bad things about her. This caused Susan to become upset, confused, and initially to reject others, such as her support carers and parents, thus leaving her very vulnerable to the emotional and sexual manipulation of this dubious individual.

(iii) Actions or Tactics, Including Emotional, Psychological, and Legal Manipulation Social isolation and disconnection from primary personal and agency supports is a powerful method of psychological manipulation. In Susan's case her naivety and lack of understanding of relationships meant her desire for friendship was taken advantage of, with a sexual relationship occurring without her recognising the implications of this.

(iv) Unfair, Improper, "Unnatural" or Unethical Transactions, or Outcomes The outcome was that Susan was constantly under stress, and she developed significant trust issues with the previously most significant relationships in her life. Her limited judgement and decision-making, combined with her vulnerability to undue influence, led to deterioration in her personal care and health. Her capacity to understand and protect herself from sexual exploitation was impaired, resulting in her being at risk of exposure to sexually transmitted diseases and emotional distress. A complaint was made to police by Susan's parents with the man in question given a warning that charges could be brought in regards to sexual exploitation. This resulted in him no longer having contact. Susan underwent psychological counselling support and this assisted her to deal with the emotional impact around the relationship as well as her reconnecting effectively with her primary supports.

(d) Communicate Decisions

The ability to communicate decisions is determined by the capacity to conceptualize decisions, and the rationale within them. Communication is not necessarily dependent on having strong expressive language skills, as even persons with significant expressive language difficulties (e.g., after stroke) can communicate decisions when provided with the appropriate technological aids and when they have supports that assist rather than control or influence what they are trying to convey.

Susan's ability to conceptualize and communicate decisions was significantly impaired. Her responses were very simplistic and indicative of what she liked/wanted, rather than reflective of her communicating a decision based on a rationale that involved a "weighing up" of information. Therefore, while she could verbally express a very simple choice she did not have the ability to form and thus communicate decisions at a level of adequate knowledge and understanding.

Acceptance of Supported Decision-Making

Part of competency is to have the insight and recognition that limitations are present and to utilize appropriate supports to aid in maintaining independence. Susan had some acceptance of supported decision-making, however, this was variable with her rejecting this when required based on how she was feeling and whether there was undue influence from others. Consequently, Susan did not have insight at a level that would ensure she relied, or could utilize the support from those with her best interests at heart when she was at her most vulnerable.

Assessment of Capacity to Manage Own Property and Finances

A second part of the assessment was to assess Susan's capacity to manage her own affairs in relation to her finances and property. In the study by Suto (2005a) the author noted that there has been a growing recognition of the importance of enabling people with intellectual disabilities to be more directly involved in managing their own financial affairs. However, to date little is known about this aspect of their decision-making. In a second study Suto (2005b) further proposed a model of three factors which affect financial decision-making abilities. The model contends that:

1. Intellectual ability contributes to the acquisition of basic financial understanding.
2. There exists a direct and potentially reciprocal relationship between basic financial understanding and decision-making opportunities in everyday life.
3. There exists a direct and potentially reciprocal relationship between such decision-making opportunities and financial decision-making abilities.

As outlined in the article by Bailey et al. (2010) decision-making is only possible if the decision-maker has the mental ability to engage in reasoning and manipulate information rationally, in order to weigh the pros and cons of alternative outcomes. They describe how weighing up two items is very simple when expressed in the same dimensions (such as the choice between paying £10 or £100 for the identical outcome. The task becomes more problematic when there are more sources of information expressed in different dimensions. Willner et al. (2010) proposed that individuals with intellectual disability typically base decisions on a single item of information, and while such decisions may appear rational they may often be irrational because of a lack of weighing up evidence.

To assess Susan's financial decision-making abilities, several approaches were used. First, formal testing of arithmetic skills (i.e., understanding and application of numerical operations) was assessed on the WAIS-IV Arithmetic subtest. Susan's overall score was in the extremely low range. She had a very limited understanding of even basic numerical operations, that is, she was only able to complete items involving some simple addition and subtraction equations whereby she could visually see simple pictorial representations (e.g., objects). However, she was not able do any numerical operations when entirely dependent on working memory capacity. This would affect her ability to undertake calculations and understand the complexities of money management. Second, Susan was asked about her understanding of what income she regularly received, where it came from, and where money was spent or was needed to be spent on necessary utilities etc. Susan was quite confused by some of this, and when she gave figures of outgoings versus incoming finances these were incompatible. She was unable to understand, correct, or rationalize the anomalies involved. Third, she was given vignette examples (based on the principles outlined in the study by Willner et al. 2010). Susan clearly had difficulties with estimation of the value to objects/services when they went beyond familiar items (and involved larger amounts of money). She was not able to rationalize how to "split" up money to afford things in the future. She lacked ability to hold and manipulate concepts and information necessary for financial decision-making, and to retain this in memory to utilize or recall later. She was also very vulnerable to being taken advantage of for the reasons already outlined.

Conclusions

(a) Clinically Defined Capacity to Make Informed Decisions
Retaining rights should not mean that either people themselves or the community will be at a greater risk (Submission to the Productivity Commission 2010). For Susan to be without the oversight and intervention where necessary by trusted others meant that her welfare was at significant risk. Taking all the factors into consideration and based on the criteria of legal definitions of incapacity the assessment determined that from a clinical perspective Susan wholly lacked capacity in regards to making decisions in managing her own welfare. She did not have the capacity to accept and engage effectively in supported decision-making processes, therefore, substitute decision-making was more appropriate. It was, however, important that she was engaged in understanding why and what decisions were being made for her, and the reasons for this at a level she was most likely to comprehend. Ascertaining her wants and desires was also of relevance so that these could also be taken into account where possible.

(b) Clinically Defined Capacity to Manage Own Property and Finances
Based on poor numeracy and memory skills, impairment in understanding financial concepts, inability to weigh up information and consider consequences, and probable vulnerability to undue influence, it was concluded that Susan wholly lacked the capacity to manage her own affairs in relation to property and finances.

Case 2: Stephen—The Effects of Traumatic Brain Injury on Capacity

Challenges exist in determining capacity in cases whereby cognitive skills presents as largely intact on formal testing, but behavior observed and reported by others are at odds with seemingly adequate cognition. The importance of evaluation beyond clinical setting presentations are particularly emphasized when capacity is to be determined. In this following case, the discrepancy between formal testing results and other sources of information are discussed.

Background Information

Stephen was a 50-year-old man who suffered a traumatic brain injury at age 25 years as the result of a fall from a horse which was galloping at speed. Glasgow Coma Scale was 3/15 at the accident scene. He remained in a coma for several weeks and in post-traumatic amnesia for further 3 weeks. CT imaging identified diffuse cerebral injury with cerebral oedema and contusions to bilateral temporal and frontal regions. He developed seizures 15 years after the accident and continued on anti-convulsant medication for management of the post-traumatic epilepsy. He subsequently only had very occasional seizures (tonic-clonic) when he omitted to take his medication.

Relevant background history included Stephen completing 3 years of secondary schooling and passing exams relevant to that level. Work history was primarily in office and sales positions. Stephen had started consuming alcohol at about the age of 16, and from this time he had been a relatively heavy drinker for some years, whereby two nights each week he would drink up to a bottle of wine in one sitting. There was no reported history of drink-driving convictions or alcoholic blackouts and he denied any history of substance abuse. Stephen said he had not consumed any alcohol since the accident. His wife, Sandra, subsequently confirmed the accuracy of Stephen's statements.

Presentation

Stephen presented as a casually dressed man with no signs of personal neglect, apart from missing some of his front teeth from previous poor oral hygiene. There was some dysarthria (speech production difficulties) making speech initially hard to understand. With increasing familiarity it became possible to understand him with minimal need for repetition. He had some gait unsteadiness due to left-sided weakness, but was able to walk unaided.

Stephen was friendly and pleasant in his manner, and showed a sense of humour during lighter moments in the assessment. At the beginning of the session he seemed perplexed about needing to have an assessment, but he did not show any overt signs of reluctance to engage in testing. With his wife present the purpose and limits of confidentiality were explained to him, using the process described for Case 1. During both sessions seen he showed the ability to maintain social etiquette, at least within this assessment context. He responded to all questions, although, at times his first reaction was that he did not know the answer or could not say how he felt. With some gentle encouragement he was at times able to expand on an answer but at other times could not, instead repeating his initial response. He reported at the end of the session that he had enjoyed the testing and felt he had done well.

Self-Description of Difficulties

During interviewing Stephen was able to acknowledge (albeit at quite a superficial level) that he had problems with remembering things, had effortful speech, and had remaining weakness on his left side. Stephen completed the Behavior Rating Inventory of Executive Functioning-Adult Version (BRIEF-A; Roth et al. 2005) self-report scale, with items read out to him. The BRIEF-A identifies behaviors related to EF and includes assessment of insight. The same scale was completed by his wife, Sandra, for the purposes of providing an informant perspective.

On the self-report scale, several of the individual BRIEF-A scales were elevated, suggesting that Stephen was able to self-identify some areas of difficulty with EF. In particular he rated problems with modulating emotions, monitoring his own social behavior, initiating problem solving or activity, sustaining working memory, and planning and organizing problem-solving approaches. He did not describe having problems with his ability to inhibit impulsive responses, adjust to changes in routine or task demands, attend to task-oriented output, and organize environment and materials. However, while Stephen's responses suggested reasonable insight getting his responses required some prompting for completion of the rating scale. Additionally, based on the reporting of his wife and also his support worker, this apparent theoretical insight did not translate into him appreciating when difficulties actually arose in daily life, or in him having the ability to respond to them in any effective form.

Informant Information

Sandra's ratings of Stephen on the BRIEF-A Informant measure indicated several of the individual scales were elevated. Concerns were noted by Sandra with Stephen's ability to inhibit impulsive responses, to monitor his own social behavior, to sustain working memory, and to sustain concentration. His ability to adjust to changes in routine or task demands, modulate emotions, initiate problem solving or activity, plan and organize problem-solving approaches, and organize environment and materials were not described by Sandra as being problematic.

When comparing Stephen and Sandra's ratings, the primary differences were Sandra rating Stephen as having problems with impulse regulation and being able to attend (maintain concentration), whereas Stephen rated these as within normal limits. Stephen rated himself as having problems with being able to organize a problem-solving approach, whereas Sandra rated him as not having a problem in this area.

Table 6.7 WAIS-IV composite measures

WAIS-IV	Composite score		Percentile rank	95% confidence interval	Qualitative description
Verbal comprehension	VCI	83	13	78–89	Low average
Perceptual reasoning	PRI	82	12	77–89	Low average
Working memory	WMI	100	50	93–107	Average
Processing speed	PSI	62	1	57–74	Extremely low
Full scale	FSIQ	78	7	74–83	Borderline impaired (however significant variation between composite scores)

In separate interviewing both Sandra and Stephen's support worker described Stephen as being very preservative in his thinking and actions, with him frequently becoming fixated on a particular topic. He had poor safety awareness resulting in him being unable to be left alone. He typically would forget what he had been told and often confused information he was given. In one-to-one situations he could be, generally, socially appropriate, but difficulties in this area become evident when he was in social groups with him becoming easily agitated and unaware of how his comments and behaviors could offend others.

Tests Administered and Assessment Results

Wechsler Adult Intelligence Scale, Fourth Edition (WAIS-IV; core subtests)— Australian/New Zealand adaptation (Wechsler 2008).
Wechsler Memory Scale-Fourth Edition (WMS-IV: Logical Stories) (Wechsler 2009)
California Verbal Learning Test-Second Edition (CVLT-II) (Delis et al. 2002)
Rey Complex Figure Test (RCFT: Meyers & Meyers 1995)
Delis–Kaplan Executive Function System (D-KEFS: Trails, Colour-Word Interference, Word Fluency, Sorting, 20 Questions) (Delis et al. 2001)
Behavioural Assessment of Dysexecutive Syndrome (BADS: Zoo map test) (Wilson et al. 1996)
Wechsler Test of Adult Reading (WTAR) (The Psychological Corporation 2001)
Neuropsychological Assessment Battery (NAB: Language module) (Stern and White 2003)
Test of Memory Malingering (TOMM) (Tombaugh 1997)

WAIS-IV composite scores showed significant variance (Table 6.7). On the full range of tests administered, Stephen achieved individual scores largely within the low average to average range indicating abilities within the expected (premorbid) range, based on his scores on tasks of well-established knowledge. Specifically, these were on simple span of attention and working memory tasks (WAIS-IV Digit Span and Arithmetic tasks), word knowledge (WAIS-IV Vocabulary), visuoconstructional abilities (WAIS-IV Block Design), some speed of information tasks

(DKEFS Trails), on a response inhibition task (DKEFS Colour Word Interference), verbal fluency and naming retrieval (DKEFS Word Fluency and Colour Word), and some aspects of reasoning, problem solving, and planning ability (DKEFS 20 Questions and Sorting; BADS Zoo map test).

Scores reflecting impaired performance (i.e., two standard deviations below premorbid estimate) were on two visual attention tasks that required perceptual matching of items combined with speed of response (WAIS-IV Coding and Symbol Search), poor organizational approach to the copying of the complex design (RCFT) with subsequent poor recall, and on a verbal reasoning task (WAIS-IV Similarities). On two verbal memory tasks (WMS-IV Logical Stories and CVLT-II) difficulties were evident in both the amount and accuracy of information retrieved. A high number of repetition errors were present during the free recall of the word list (CVLT-II), suggesting that he was having difficulty in keeping mental track of what he had already said.

The NAB Language Module was used to assess aspects of receptive and expressive language including the ability to complete simple bill payment tasks. On tasks of verbal, reading, and written communication abilities, the overall performance was within the low average range with subtests ranging from borderline impaired to average. He had low average range scores for tasks involving speech and with comprehension of more complex questions or instructions. On a task requiring him to follow instructions and make sense of how to complete a bill payment task, the score was within the extremely low range. The approach for assessing capacity to manage personal property and finances in Case 1 was applied to Stephen. He was unable to understand the complexities of money management with similar difficulties identified.

Formulation and Conclusions

In Stephen's case, while there were areas of low score the presence of relative strengths suggested Stephen had areas of functioning that might have allowed him to have the capacity to make informed decisions. Formal testing did indicate poor organizational skills and limited memory abilities with vulnerability for inaccurate recall. Assessment also highlighted impairments that would indicate difficulties with money management. On their own these test results could not be considered sufficient for determining clinical incapacity in relation to welfare guardianship. However, on further examination of his adaptive living functioning, his difficulties became more apparent. While his responses on the BRIEF-A rating scale suggested he had insight, in reality Stephen had minimal insight whereby he could not fully appreciate his difficulties, nor how his behavior affected others and consequently he was unable to change or self-regulate behavior when necessary. The rating scale items became a structured form of prompting whereby Stephen tended toward a "yes" bias, rather than him truly showing awareness of deficit. Normal range scores on two specific tests suggested there were no issues in regards to valid performance (TOMM and CVLT-II Forced Choice).

Cases such as Stephen's emphasize that formal cognitive testing is only one part of assessing the effects of injury. Stephen had a primarily behavioral variant of dysexecutive syndrome. While for some individuals EF problems are notably evident, in test performance for others such as Stephen the primary difficulties become most apparent in daily life. He could manage within structured environments where he was guided, prompted, or had learnt basic routines and expectations. However, if supports that oversaw his care were removed then Stephen would not have had the capacity to cope independently. He was reliant upon others, such as his wife, to make important decisions as Stephen was not able to consider all aspects to a situation and weigh up that information in an effective way. This was confirmed through reporting from two separate informants observing Stephen in two different environments. Fortunately, there were no issues of undue influences with Stephen having appropriate care from those providing support.

In conclusion, based on the principles of formulation for assessment of capacity, Stephen was not able to understand all relevant information, or to retain information relevant to decisions. He was also not able to appreciate the consequences of a decision, nor did he have effective insight into the limitations he had. Stephen was at significant risk of self-neglect and potential harm without the direct oversight and decision-making capacity being undertaken by others. It was, therefore, concluded that he wholly lacked the capacity for self-determination in regards to his own welfare and property management. The length of time since the injury was 25 years and the information obtained from multiple sources indicated a consistent and permanent state.

Case 3: Emily—Childhood Meningitis Causing Intellectual Impairment

Emily contracted meningitis at the age of 5 years with subsequent learning difficulties throughout her schooling years, resulting in her requiring additional learning support. She also had physical limitations whereby she had impaired gait and at times needed to use a wheelchair. As an adult she had attended life skills courses for individuals with intellectual disability. She had lived with her parents prior to moving to a supported living community at the age of 32. There was no history of any mental health issues. Apart from the meningitis she had maintained good health. Emily described having a very supportive family and she maintained regular contact with them.

Presentation

Emily was supported by her sister within the assessment process and this including during informing of the purpose of the assessment, with assent given by both. Emily was very well groomed and clearly took pride in her personal appearance.

She readily engaged into the assessment process, with her spontaneously offering information and asking questions when she was unsure. During interviewing, her expressive language was without impediment and she was able to articulate her thoughts and feelings clearly with no verbosity or tangentially evident. She was reciprocal in conversation, with appropriate social etiquette, including eye contact.

Psychological screening did not identify any her issues and this was consistent with information obtained from her care supports and sister.

Within testing Emily engaged fully and applied herself well. There were no signs of perseveration, distractibility, or impulsivity. Concentration was maintained well over 2 h of interviewing and testing, with two short breaks in between. She took a careful and considered approach to tasks, persisting even when faced with difficulty. She showed effective self-monitoring skills during task execution whereby she noticed errors when they occurred and either self-corrected, or attempted to self-correct errors made. She showed a good awareness of her limitations and rather than showing frustration or anxiety she kept herself calm and tried as best she could. She achieved normal range scores on two specific performance effort tests.

Adaptive Living Skills Ratings

At the time of the assessment Emily lived in a small flat within the assisted community and was able to complete household tasks, including cooking of simple meals, without the need for prompting or assistance. She managed her own finances with the support and input of her sister. Adaptive living skills ratings (ABAS-II) by two raters (her sister and her support worker where Emily lived) identified a number of relative strengths (borderline functioning to low average range) in the areas of communication, community use, social, and self-direction. Ratings for functional academics, home living, self care, health and safety, and leisure were within the extremely low range. Information obtained from informants provided context to the functional limitations, whereby Emily required support but showed an awareness of and willingness to follow instructions. She was cautious and, therefore, preferred to wait or check with others she trusted before engaging in a task. She did not always know how to initiate an activity, hence low scores in some areas, but with support could manage reasonably effective.

Table 6.8 WAIS-IV Composite scores

WAIS-IV	Composite score		Percentile rank	95 % confidence interval	Qualitative description
Verbal comprehension	VCI	72	3	67–79	Borderline impaired
Perceptual reasoning	PRI	69	2	64–77	Extremely low
Working memory	WMI	69	2	64–78	Extremely low
Processing speed	PSI	62	1	57–74	Extremely low
Full scale	FSIQ	63	1	60–68	Extremely low

Tests Administered and Assessment Results

Wechsler Adult Intelligence Scale-Fourth Edition (WAIS-IV; core subtests) Australian/NZ adaptation) (Wechsler 2008)
Wechsler Memory Scale-Fourth Edition (WMS-IV: Logical Stories) (Wechsler 2009)
Delis-Kaplan Executive Function System (D-KEFS: Sorting and 20 Questions) (Delis et al. 2001)
Test of Memory Malingering (TOMM) (Tombaugh 1997)

On WMS-IV composite measures ranged from extremely low to borderline with FSIO indicating mild intellectual disability (Table 6.8). Immediate and delayed recall of the WMS-IV logical stories was within the low average and borderline impaired ranges, respectively. A qualitative analysis showed Emily was able to recall the main plot of the story, in simple form, with no distortion. On the recognition format she had an average range score, indicating with simple cueing her retrieval of information was enhanced. Her scores on the DKEFS Sorting task was within the borderline impaired range for the free sorting condition, but with an average range score achieved for the second condition in which the information was structured for her. She achieved a borderline impaired range score on the DKEFS 20 Questions task, indicating some basic skills in logical reasoning involving hypothesis testing and deduction, as well as keeping mental track of responses already given.

Summary of Formulation and Conclusions

In Emily's case her WAIS-IV scores suggested she might have intellectual limitations to an extent that capacity would be an issue. However, Emily's ability to recognize her own limitations, to have self-regulatory capacity, and to be willing to take on board support and guidance indicates she had partial capacity. Her cognitive limitations meant she did require a supported decision-making process, but provided this was available she had the capacity to make appropriate decision in regards to her own welfare. Her acknowledgement and acceptance of this need for support was also evident for property and financial management, consequently she was able to give consent for support in this area also. Based on the primary determinants for assessment of mental capacity, and provided she had access to an appropriate supported decision-making process, Emily is able to retain most of her independence in decision-making. While there was some susceptibility to being taken advantage of and therefore undue influence, Emily confided in her primary supports and sought advice in new situations and when meeting new people, therefore, modifying this risk.

Final Comments

Comparison of these three case studies shows that impairment in cognitive functioning does not automatically indicate incapacity. Equally, test performance which produces age-expected range scores does not necessarily mean the individual has capacity to self-manage personal finances or to be able to make informed decisions in regards to welfare. Capacity is dependent upon adequate functioning in particular aspects of cognition, self-regulation, and insight which may show up within neuropsychological testing, but cannot be reliably determined by testing alone.

Neuropsychological assessment which involves multiple sources of information and includes both quantitative and qualitative measures, is able to consider the range of multifactorial factors and influences underlying capacity. This is regardless of whether the individual in question is affected by a developmental or an acquired brain related condition. Assessment is based on how best to identify relevant strengths and weakness appropriate to each case, rather than there being a set test battery in a "one size fits all" approach. An in-depth neuropsychological formulation as outlined ensures that the individual's unique cognitive, psychological, and (where relevant) personality trait profile is evaluated in the context of personal vulnerabilities and strengths along with the integrity of their social supports. Integrating clinical considerations with legal requirements, therefore, becomes a more robust process based on responding specifically and effectively to the cognitive abilities underlying capacity functioning.

References

Australian Psychological Society Ltd. (2010). Submission to the Victorian Law Reform Commission's Guardianship and Administration Act Review.

Bailey, R., Willner, P., & Dymond, S. (2010). Evaluation of the ability of people with intellectual disabilities to 'weigh up' information in two tests of financial reasoning. *Journal of Intellectual Disability Research, 54*(4), 380–391.

Bailey, R., Willner, P., & Dymond, S. (2011). A visual aid to decision-making for people with intellectual disabilities. *Research in Developmental Disabilities, 32*, 37–46.

Benedet, J., & Grant, I. (2007). Hearing the sexual assault complaints of women with mental disabilities: Consent, capacity and mistaken belief. *McGill Law Journal, 52*, 243–289.

Bonardi, A (2009). *The balance between choice and control: Risk management in new zealand intellectual disability services*. Wellington: Fulbright NZ.

Brocki, K. C., & Bohlin, G. (2004). Executive functions in children aged 6 to 13: A dimensional and developmental study. *Developmental Neuropsychology, 26*(2), 571–593.

Brown, H., & Turk, V. (1992). Defining sexual abuse as it affects adults with learning disabilities. *Mental Handicap, 20*(2), 44–55.

Church, M., & Watts, S. (2007). Assessment of mental capacity: A flow chart guide. *The Psychiatrist, 31*, 304–307.

Crowe, S. (2005). *The parallel universe: Does neuropsychological assessment tell us anything about the real world?* Australian Psychological Society. Inpsych, June 2005.

Delis, D. C., Kaplan, E., & Kramer, J. H. (2001). Delis-Kaplin executive function system (D-KEFS). The Psychological Corporation: San Antonio, TX.
Delis, D. C., Kramer, J. H., Kaplan, E., & Ober, B. A. (2002). *California verbal learning test—2nd Edition (CVLT-II)*. San Antonio: Psychological Corporation
Eastgate, G. (2005). Sex, consent and intellectual disability. *Australian Family Physician, 34*(3), 163–6.
Fidler, D. J. (2005). The emerging Down syndrome behavioural phenontype in early childhood. *Infants & Young Children, 18*(2), 86–103.
Harrison, P., & Oakland, T. (2003). Adaptive behaviour assessment system- Second edition (ABAS II). Minneapolis: Pearson Assessment.
Herbert, C. (2013). Mental capacity. In L. H. Goldstein & J. E. McNeil (Eds.), *Clinical Neuropsychology: A practical guide to assessment and management for clinicians* (pp. 445–462). United Kingdom: Wiley.
Hoskins, K., & Crowe, M. (2005). Money management after acquired brain dysfunction: The validity of neuropsychological assessment. *Rehabilitation Psychology, 50*(4), 355–365.
Hoskin, K. M., Jackson, M., & Crowe, S. F. (2005). Money management after brain injury: The validity of neuropsychological assessment. *Rehabilitation Psychology, 50*(4), 355–365.
Jarrold, C., Nadel, L., & Vicari, S. (2009). Memory and neuropsychology in Down syndrome. *Down Syndrome Research and Practice, 12*(3), 68–73.
Lotan, G., & Ells, C. (2010). Adults with intellectual and developmental disabilities and participation in decision making: Ethical considerations for professional-client practice. *Intellectual and Developmental Disabilities, 48*(2), 112–125.
Maraj, B. K. V., Robertson, S. D., Welsh, T. N., Weeks, D. J., Chua, R., Heath, M., Roy, E. A., Simon, D. A., Weinberg, H., & Elliot, D. (2002). Verbal-motor behaviour in persons with Down syndrome. In M. Cuskell, A. Jobling, & S. Buckley (Eds.), *Down syndrome across the lifespan*. United Kingdom: Whurr Publishing.
Marcell, M. M., Coren, P. S., & Sewell, D. H. (1990). *Language comprehension in Down syndrome and other trainable mentally handicapped individuals*. Paper presented at the Biennial Conference on Human Development (11th, Richmond, VA, March 29–31, 1990).
McCarthy, M. (2003). Drawing a line between consented and abusive sexual experiences: The complexities for women with learning difficulties. *The Journal of Adult Protection, 5*(3), 34–40.
Meyers, J. E., & Meyers, K. R. (1995). *Rey complex figure and recognition trial: Professional manual*. Odessa: Psychological Assessment Resources.
Moberg, P. J., & Kniele, K. (2006). Evaluation of competency: Ethical considerations for neuropsychologists. *Applied Neuropsychology, 13*(2), 101–114.
Morris, C. D., Niederbuhl, M. M., & Maher, J. M. (1993). Determining the capability of individuals with mental retardation to give informed consent. *American Journal in Mental Retardation, 98*(2), 263–272.
Moye, J., Gurrera, R. J., Karel, M. J., Edelstein, B., O'Connell, C. (2006). Empirical advances in the assessment of the capacity to consent to medical treatment: Clinical implications and research needs. *Clinical Psychological Review, 26*(8), 1054–1077.
Mullaly, E., Kinsella, G., Berberovic, N., Cohen, Y., Dedda, K., Froud, B., Leach, K., & Neath, J. (2007). Assessment of decision-making capacity: Exploration of common practices among neuropsychologists. *Australian Psychologist, 42*(3), 178–186.
Murphy, G. H. (2003). Capacity to consent to sexual relationships in adults with learning disabilities. *Journal of Family Planning and Reproductive Health Care, 29*(3), 148–149.
Murphy, G., & O'Callaghan, A. C. (2004). Capacity of adults with intellectual disabilities to consent to sexual relationships. *Psychological Medicine, 34*, 1347–1357.
Niederbuhl, J. M., & Morris, C. D. (1993). Sexual knowledge and the capability of persons with dual diagnosis to consent to sexual contact. *Sexuality and Disability, 11*(4), 295–307.
Quinn, M. J., Goldman, E. G., Nerenberg, L., & Piazza, D. (2010a). *Undue influence: Definitions and applications*. Final Report to the Borchard Foundation on Law and Aging. California Administrative Office of the Courts.

Quinn, M. J., Goldman, E., Nerenberg, L., & Piazza, D. (2010b). *A project supported by the Borchard Foundation Centre on Law and Aging: Final report*. California Administrative Office of the Courts.

Roth, R. M., Isquith, P. K., & Giola, G. A. (2005). *Behavior rating inventory of executive functioning-adult version (BRIEF-A)*. Lutz: Psychological Assessment Resources.

Rowe, J., Lavender, A., & Turk, V. (2006). Cognitive executive function in Down syndrome. *British Journal of Clinical Psychology, 45*(Part 1), 5–17.

Simon, M. J. (2007). Performance of mentally retarded forensic patients on the test of memory malingering. *Journal of Clinical Psychology, 63*(4), 339–344.

Stern, R. A., & White, T. (2003). *Neuropsychological assessment battery: Language module (NAB-L)*. Lutz: Psychological Assessment Inc.

Sullivan, K. (2004). Neuropsychological assessment of mental capacity. *Neuropsychology Review, 13(*3), 131–142

Submission to the productivity commission. 2010. Inquiry into disability care and support office of the public advocate south Australia, August.

Suto, W., Clare, I. C. H., Holland, A. J., & Watson, P. C. (2005a). Capacity to make financial decisions among people with mild intellectual disabilities. *Journal of Intellectual Disability Research, 49*(3), 199–209.

Suto, W. M. I., Clare, I., Holland, A., & Watson, P. C. (2005b). The relationships among three factors affecting the financial decision-making abilities of adults with mild intellectual disabilities. *Journal of Intellectual Disability Research, 49*(3), 210–217.

The Psychological Corporation. (2001). *Wechsler test of adult reading (WTAR)*. San Antonia: Harcourt Assessment.

Tombaugh, T. N. (1997). *The test of memory malingering (TOMM)*. New York: Multi-Health Systems, Inc.

Wechsler, D. (2008). *Wechsler adult intelligence scale-Fourth edition. (WAIS IV: Australian/New Zealand adaptation)*. San Antonio: Pearson Assessment.

Wechsler, D. (2009). *Wechsler memory scale—fourth edition (WMS IV)*. San Antonio: The Psychological Corporation.

Willner, P., Bailey, R., Parry, R., & Dymond, S. (2010a). Evaluation of executive functioning in people with intellectual disabilities. *Journal of Intellectual Disability Research, 54*(4), 366–379.

Willner, P., Bailey, R., Dymond, S., & Parry, R. (2010b). Coins and costs: A simple and rapid assessment of basic financial knowledge. *Journal of Applied Research in Intellectual Disabilities, 24*, 285

Willner, P., Bailey, R., Parry, R., & Dymond, S. (2010c). Evaluation of the ability of people with intellectual disabilities to 'weigh up' information in two tests of financial reasoning. *Journal of Intellectual Disability Research, 54*(4), 380–391.

Wilson, B. A, Alderman, N., Burgess, P. W., Emslie, H. C., & Evans, J. J. (1996). *The behavioural assessment of the dysexecutive syndrome*. Flempton: Thames Valley Test Company.

Chapter 7
Neuropsychological Assessment of an American Indian with a Ruptured Right Carotid Aneurysm and Associated Subarachnoid Hemorrhage

Vicky T. Lomay and George P. Prigatano

Introduction

Clinical neuropsychological assessment is a process by which several sources of information regarding a patient have to be reviewed and integrated in order to adequately describe disturbances in brain–behavior relationships and the implications of those findings for patient care. The process by which clinicians formulate their neuropsychological understanding of a patient can be a complicated one.

While age and educational experiences clearly influence performance on neuropsychological tests (Heaton et al. 2009), the patient's cultural background, present language skills, and occupational history may also influence test performance (see Lezak et al. 2004). Furthermore, the questions asked in the clinical interview help clarify or confuse the patient's symptom picture. Finally, the clinical training and experiences of the examiner greatly influence clinical formulations and decision-making.

In this chapter, we attempt to describe the various steps involved in performing a clinical neuropsychological examination of a 62-year-old American Indian male with 9 years of formal education, who suffered a subarachnoid hemorrhage (SAH) and later clipping of a right carotid bifurcation aneurysm. The patient was followed up for a 2-year period with repeat examinations. We describe his initial presentation (as documented in the medical records) and his subsequent neuropsychological performance. We summarize the interview process with this patient and his family

The author would like to thank Mary Henry and Anthony Tran for their help in preparing this manuscript. Funding to George P. Prigatano obtained from the Newsome Chair allowed time to prepare portions of this manuscript.

V. T. Lomay (✉)
Tsinajini Psychology Services, 1146 N. Mesa Drive, Suite 102-251, Mesa, AZ 85201, USA
e-mail: vlomay@tsinajinipsych.com

G. P. Prigatano
Barrow Neurological Institute, 222 W Thomas Rd, Suite 315, Phoenix, AZ 85013, USA
e-mail: george.prigatano@dignityhealth.org

J. A. B. Macniven (ed.), *Neuropsychological Formulation,*
DOI 10.1007/978-3-319-18338-1_7

and how the information obtained from neuropsychological testing was used to clarify for the patient and family our understanding of his neuropsychological difficulties and the implications for him in his everyday life. We will also attempt to make explicit our view of how various factors influenced our clinical understanding of this patient.

Before proceeding, however, we will review demographic information concerning American Indians and Alaska Natives relevant for neuropsychologists. We will also review a sparse literature pertinent to the neuropsychological examination of this group of individuals.

A Brief Review of Demographics

According to the 2010 US Census, 1.7% (5.2 million) of the US population were identified as American Indian/Alaska Native (AI/AN) alone or in combination with another race (U.S. Census Bureau 2012). Nearly half of the population reported multiple races, in combination with AI/AN. The largest proportion of AI/AN lived in the Western USA, followed by the South, the Midwest, and the Northeast, respectively. The largest reported populations of AI/AN were in California (14%), followed by Oklahoma, Arizona, Texas, and New York (U.S. Census Bureau 2012). Between 2000 and 2010, the AI/AN alone or in-combination population grew in nearly every state. Cities with the largest AI/AN populations were New York, NY, followed by Los Angeles, CA; Phoenix, AZ; Anchorage, AK; and Albuquerque, NM. The majority of the AI/AN population was reported living outside their respective reservations or AI/AN areas. The largest tribal groupings included Cherokee, Navajo, and Choctaw. The AI/AN population has grown in the past decade and they reside in every state and region of the USA. The likelihood of encountering a person of American Indian and/or Alaska Native heritage should be expected, especially in the West.

Neuropsychological Test Findings with AI/AN and Navajos

Review of the literature reveals a paucity of studies regarding the neuropsychological examination of American Indians and Alaska Natives (King and Fletcher-Janzen 2000; Vanderpool and Catano 2008). The majority of published studies on neuropsychological measures/diagnostic issues with the American Indian groups focus on children (Common and Frost 1988; Diessner and Walker 1986; McLellan and Nellis 2003; McShane and Plas 1984; McShane and Berry 1988; Plank 2001; Ross 1982; Tsethlikai 2011; Vocate 1984), adolescents (Sidles et al. 1987; Wright et al. 1996; Wiseley 2001), or older adults (Griffin-Pierce et al. 2008; Jervis et al. 2007; Jervis et al. 2010; Spencer and Cruz 1989; Whyte et al. 2005; Verney et al. 2008). A common recommendation was that further research is needed.

Studies with adults often focus on specific diagnostic questions and do not address broad conceptualization/examination issues. For example, Halpern et al. (2005) studied the neuropsychological effects of peyote, which is used in specific American Indian ceremonies. They found no significant neuropsychological impairments in those who used peyote in a religious context, whereas a former alcoholic comparison group showed deficits on visuospatial memory and learning.

Jervis et al. (2010) examined predictors of performance, the Mini-Mental Status Exam (MMSE) and Mattis Dementia Rating Scale (2nd Edition) (DRS-2), with elders from an American Indian tribe in the Plains area. She and her colleagues found, in general, education and indicators of economic need predicted higher scores. Having more formal education and qualifying for assistance such as food stamps or utilizing Social Security or Supplemental Security Income were related to better performance on both measures. An explanation of these findings remained unclear.

Indigenous populations of the South and Central America share many similarities to US tribal groups with respect to culture, education levels, and difference in acculturation to outside/mainstream cultures. Ostrosky-Solis et al. (2004) examined the influence of culture and education on neuropsychological tests with a group of Mexican Mayan and Pame Indians. They found that level of education significantly correlated with higher verbal and working memory test scores. In addition, the illiterate group of participants was found to have better performance on visuoperceptual and constructive tasks. In a study of neuropsychological assessment of Aruaco Indians of Colombia, Ardila and Moreno (2001) also found significant correlation between test performance and years of school. Exposure to formal education usually leads to acquisition of expected skill levels in reading and writing, as well as learning contextual skills emphasized in standardized neuropsychological testing (i.e., speed, attention, and following directions).

While current research of neuropsychological assessment with AI/AN is limited (see Lomay and Hinkebein 2006), there is a broad cross-cultural literature relevant to this discussion (Ardila 1995, 2005; Puente and Ardila 2000; Rosselli and Ardila 2003). Teng and Manly (2005), for example, highlighted the usefulness of a neuropsychological evaluation for differential diagnosis, detecting changes over time and consultations relevant to patient care. They emphasize the importance of considering the patient's education level, reading skill level, their typical approach to test-taking, as well as the ecological validity and appropriateness of neuropsychological test items. The need for normative data for different cultural groups is further emphasized. Wong et al. (2000) have offered practical suggestions when conducting a neuropsychological examination, which are relevant when evaluating American Indians.

1. Recognize, understand, and, if necessary, train for cross-cultural diversity and sensitivity.
2. Be aware of cultural nuances, consider sociocultural influences on the patient's behavior, and try to offer a culturally sensitive environment.

3. Utilize a thorough clinical interview to help in identifying and understanding cultural nuances and differences.
4. If the primary language of the patient is unfamiliar to the neuropsychologist, they should make an earnest effort to refer to a neuropsychologist competent in evaluating that language.
5. A referral should be considered if, even when language is not an issue, other cultural issues may be a hindrance to a competent evaluation.
6. If at all possible, the use of translators or interpreters should be avoided.
7. Avoid the use of translated text or instruments unless test score interpretations have been validated in the translated form.
8. A set of tests chosen judiciously with cross-cultural considerations in mind should be used.
9. Cross-cultural issues should be elucidated clearly in the evaluation report.

Neuropsychological Consequences of SAH Secondary to a Ruptured Aneurysms

Cognitive morbidity after SAH associated with ruptured cerebral aneurysms is common. Prigatano and Henderson (1997) noted that the deficits tend to cluster around eight factors (depending on the location and severity of the hemorrhage). They are increased mental fatigue, impaired memory, reduced problem-solving skills, language dysfunction, visual-spatial disturbances, and reduced speed and efficiency of information processing. In addition, disturbances in personality which are difficult to define can occur, which influence personal and social judgment. Emotional liability and irritability are often commonly observed, especially in the acute and subacute phases following an SAH. More recent reviews describe similar findings but utilize the term "executive dysfunction" when describing disturbances in problem-solving, personal and social judgment, and associated changes in personality (see Lezak et al. 2004; Towgood et al. 2004; Sheldon et al. 2013).

Psychometric studies often emphasize cognitive deficits, particularly memory and working memory disturbances (Hillis et al. 2000; Preiss et al. 2011; Sheldon et al. 2012; Sheldon et al. 2013; Vieira et al. 2011). Clinical interviews of patients, however, often reveal a complex interaction of cognitive, personality, and physical difficulties. Mental fatigue and "confusion" are often described by the patient. In addition, family members may be unclear as to how a person has changed and what to do to help them.

Culture and Language Considerations

While neuropsychologists initially looked for "biological markers of intelligence" (Halstead 1976), it became quite obvious that the higher integrative brain functions do not develop independently of the person's educational and cultural environment.

Luria (1966) emphasized this point in his writings and made a cogent argument for the central role of speech and language in the development of cognitive functioning (also see Scott et al. 1979). Since that time, many authors have emphasized, and provided data, supporting these observations. For example, educational level/experiences clearly influence neuropsychological test findings (e.g., Ardila 1995, 2005; Heaton et al. 2009).

These findings, and many others, lead to the common practice of developing normative databases that take into consideration the person's cultural and educational background. This type of information helps determine if the level of performance on specific tests is within or outside the average range for different subgroups of individuals. Unfortunately, there is no adequate normative database for American Indians who are raised within their particular cultural background (King and Fletcher-Janzen 2000). Thus the examining clinical neuropsychologist must often interpret the neuropsychological test findings cautiously, looking for patterns of findings that would be compatible with the known medical/neurological findings. The neuropsychologist should also be familiar with how to ask certain questions when interviewing a person different from their own cultural background. This can be a challenging task as several authors have pointed out (e.g., King and Fletcher-Janzen 2000; Prigatano and Leathern 1993; Wong et al. 2000).

In the case example provided below, one of the examiners was an American Indian woman from a Southwest tribe undergoing training in clinical neuropsychology. She helped guide the interview process and assisted in test administration and interpretation. She also helped provide feedback to the patient's family in a manner that facilitated their understanding of the patient's clinical condition.

Case Presentation and Formulation

Medical History and Findings At age 61, a right-handed American Indian male with 9 years of formal education was hospitalized after a 5-day history of severe headaches. He was originally cared for in a regional Indian Health Center in New Mexico. He subsequently was transferred to Phoenix, AZ. Radiology studies revealed an SAH in the basal cisterns and sylvian fissure, particularly on the right side of the brain. This bleed was thought to be related to a ruptured right carotid bifurcation aneurysm (for a review of the anatomy of such aneurysms and associated SAH, see Bederson 1997). In addition, it was noted that he had severe ventriculomegaly and a focal high-density lesion in the right basal ganglia.

When evaluated in an inpatient neurorehabilitation center approximately 1 month after the onset of his SAH, he was described as easily fatigued and demonstrated bilateral motor weakness and blurred vision. He was tangential in his free speech, preservative, and noted to quickly forget new information. He voiced several times that he was "sick of the hospital" and wanted to go home.

Demographic Considerations Including Occupational and Educational Considerations The patient had lived his life on his tribe's reservation and worked as a diesel mechanic for many years. He was right-handed. He had a history of poor academic achievements, particularly in math and history. He had, however, no history of special education. He was bilingual in English and his native language, but spoke native language in his home. He was working up until the time he became ill. He was married to his wife for over 40 years. His wife was of the same tribal heritage as he and she also mainly spoke their native language.

Cultural Considerations for This Patient This gentleman identified himself by his tribal affiliation, which has a large population in the USA. The reservation from which he originates, spans across a large area in the Southwestern USA. Its remoteness contributes to several key cultural issues that need to be considered in his evaluation. The first issue is his language of preference. Even today, many older generation members of his tribe continue to communicate in their native language. English was often learned as a second language. Many elders were monolingual native speakers until they were introduced to the school system. Their English fluency can range from excellent to functional, depending on their life, work, and educational experiences.

For this gentleman, it seems he understood both his native language and English well, but preferred his native language with other speakers. His opportunity to use or learn an extensive English vocabulary was probably limited. The majority of his family and community spoke their native language. Thus it would have been ideal to examine him in his native language. It should be expected that he would have a limited English vocabulary and limited English verbal reasoning skills prior to his SAH.

The second issue to consider is the level of his formal education. Learning a second language coupled with trying to complete a standard education in English was most likely difficult for this man. Thus, his reading level prior to his SAH was most likely functional and fluent enough to accomplish general activities, such as reading the paper, doing his banking, and filling out applications. It would be expected that his formal English reading skills would be no higher than the typical 8th grade level prior to his SAH.

The third issue is closely tied to the first two. Given the remoteness of his reservation, the access to many services including adequate healthcare was most likely limited. Grocery stores and clinics are often spread far apart, usually resulting in 1–3-h drives. In addition, the land is often rural, with a heavy emphasis on a ranching, off-the-grid lifestyle. Independence and self-reliance are key characteristics to living in this kind of area and are key aspects to this man's sense of self-worth and purpose in life. If his family has livestock, it would be important for him to contribute to the care of the animals as well as general upkeep of the ranch or home. Riding horses would be an essential skill to contribute to a ranch. On horseback, a rider can get to places a vehicle cannot. In addition, he may have learned to ride at an early age; in some areas this was the only mode of transportation. Understanding these cultural influences is important to the examination and interview with this gentleman. They also have to be considered when giving him feedback regarding his neuropsychological functioning and the implications for his returning back to his old lifestyle.

Clinical Presentations at Different Time Periods Following the SAH This patient was examined, from a neuropsychological perspective, on five different occasions over a 2-year period of time. The first examination was relatively brief, given the acuteness of his clinical condition. That examination occurred approximately 1 month after his SAH and surgical repair of his aneurysm. While cooperative, he was easily confused and demonstrated severe memory impairments. He was also easily fatigued and in a hypo-aroused state.

When examined 5 months later, on an outpatient basis, he was frail and weak. He continued to be cooperative, but often spoke in a very quiet voice. It appeared, at times, he did not fully understand some of the questions asked of him. His verbal responses were often difficult to understand. Family members, who were seen when he was interviewed, provided much of the information concerning his present and past functioning.

During this time, the patient was asked to make ratings about his self-perceived level of functioning in a number of cognitive and affective domains. This was challenging for him to do. Both he and his family rated his cognitive functioning as being mildly impaired. In retrospect, these questions perhaps should have not been asked at this point, since this type of self-rating and family rating would be somewhat unusual, given their cultural background.

The patient was re-examined 6 months later, which was approximately 1 year post the onset of his ruptured aneurysm and SAH. At that time he had gained back some lost weight and appeared to have more energy. He continued, however, to be thin. He had a better, but not yet completely accurate understanding of the questions asked in the clinical interview. For the first time he appeared mildly disinhibited. He acknowledged memory difficulties, but felt his memory had improved. His wife reported he was still forgetful, as reflected in his inability to correctly identify the day of the week. She noted that his energy level had improved, but was still a problem.

The patient was again asked to rate his level of difficulties in a number of cognitive and affective domains. It should be emphasized at this point, however, that a therapeutic alliance had been established with both the patient and family. At this time, the patient's self-ratings indicated that he believed he was mildly to moderately impaired in a number of areas. His wife's ratings were similar, despite his obvious severe impairments (to the examiner). We did not ask him to rate levels of anxiety and depression (which is a common practice when assessing American individuals with a Western European culture). We thought this would be inappropriate, given his cultural background. The patient and his wife, however, spontaneously noted that he was more irritable (a common and perhaps non-direct effect of brain injury).

The patient was then re-examined 6 months later. He, his wife, and his daughter were again conjointly interviewed. Physically, the patient looked stronger and continued to gain weight. He was now eager to return to riding a horse and driving a car. He was frustrated over the limitations that had been imposed on him. He also wanted to return to work. The family wanted to have him consider retirement. He was less interested in doing so.

A very good rapport had been established with the patient and his family by the time of this examination. Thus he was asked to make self-ratings about perceived areas of difficulty in multiple domains. He and his family now reported moderate difficulties with fatigue and memory difficulties. Both the patient and his family now reported elevated anxiety, but neither knew how to rate (or answer) questions about depression (which would be difficult to do in his culture). The patient and his wife, however, both agreed that irritability was high and attributed this to his inactivity and restricted lifestyle.

The patient was seen for his fourth and final neuropsychological examination 6 months later, which was approximately 2 years post the onset of his neurological condition. Again he was interviewed in the presence of his wife and daughter. On this examination, the patient appeared more somber. At this time, he had not been cleared to return to riding a horse due to safety reasons. This was very difficult for this man, given the cultural and practical importance of this activity and his previous lifestyle. Horseback riding provided both an exciting recreational experience and a sense of personal competency. Also the patient was not able to return to work, which he obsessed about according to his family members.

The patient's perception was that his memory was continuing to improve, but this was not the perception of his wife or daughter. Due to insurance reasons, they could not obtain outpatient rehabilitation services to help teach him memory compensations by an experienced occupational therapist who was in private practice.

By this time, notable neuropsychological recovery had taken place (see psychometric test findings listed below) but severe impairments in cognitive functioning compatible with his known medical condition continued to be observed. The postdoctoral fellow who was involved in his repeated examinations was an American Indian from the Southwestern USA, and helped refer the patient for appropriate psychological services at a native health clinic in New Mexico where he resided. From a neuropsychological perspective, no further assessments were needed, but long-term help in adjusting to his disabilities was now considered necessary.

Repeated and Changing Neuropsychological Test Findings Table 7.1 summarizes selected neuropsychological test findings over the five examinations. During the first four examinations, he was administered the Barrow Neurological Institute (BNI) screen for higher cerebral functions (Prigatano et al. 1995). His overall level of performance was in the severe range during the first year following his SAH. By 18 months post SAH, his performance on this screening test was within the lower range of normal, compared to non-American Indian males of similar age (i.e., *T*-score of 41).

Even though this gentleman was an accomplished diesel mechanic, on the Wechsler Scale of Intelligence, his Block Design age-adjusted scaled score remained severely impaired up until 18 months post SAH.

Perhaps one of the most important observations was that rote verbal learning appeared to improve by 6 months post SAH, while visuospatial rote learning remained impaired for 1 year post onset. This is clearly compatible with his known neurological history. By 18 months post onset, visual learning and memory appeared

Table 7.1 Summarized neuropsychological test findings obtained over time from a 62-year-old Navajo male with a history of SAH secondary to a rupture aneurysm. See text for details

	Inpatient	Exam #1 (5 months)	Exam #2 (11 months)	Exam #3 (18 months)	Exam #4 (23 months)
BNI screen	21/50 T>1	29/50 T=4	31/50 T=15	38/50 T=35	–
WAIS-III					
Information	–	–	–	–	SS=5
Coding	–	SS=5	SS=6	SS=5	SS=6
Vocabulary	–	SS=4	SS=4	SS=4	SS=5
Picture completion	–	SS=4	SS=5	SS=6	SS=6
Digit span	–	SS=3	SS=5	SS=4	SS=5
Arithmetic	–	–	–	–	SS=4
Block design	–	SS=3	SS=4	SS=8	SS=8
Similarities	–	–	–	–	SS=5
Picture arrange	–	–	–	–	SS=6
Symbol search	–	------	–	–	SS=3
Trails A	–	T=23	T=24	T=41	T=25
Trails B	–	D/C	D/C	D/C	D/C
RAVLT					
Trials 1–5 (RS)	–	3, 8, 8, 11, 11	6, 10, 8, 8, 9	5, 10, 12, 9, 12	5, 8, 9, 11,14
Total	–	T=53	T=53	T=61	T=60
SD	–	T=47	T=50	T=60	T=67
LD	–	T=53	T=59	T=56	T=64
BVMT-R					
Trial 1	–	T=24	T=34	T=38	T=29
Trial 2	–	T<20	T=22	T=41	T=27
Trial 3	–	T=40	T<20	T=45	T<20
Delay	–	T=34	T=20	T=43	T=25
WMS-R					
LMI	–	–	–	44th percentile	–
LMII	–	–	–	48th percentile	–
VRI	–	–	–	48th percentile	–
VRII	–	–	–	20th percentile	–
ROCF					
Copy	–	–	–	–	>16th percentile
Delay	–	–	–	–	12th percentile
Finger tapping					
DOM (R)	T=15	T=25	T=44	T=45	T=45
NONDOM (L)	T=11	T=26	T=44	T=44	T=44

to approach the lower range of average performance. However, using an alternative form of the test at 2 years post onset, the reality of ongoing severe visuospatial learning and memory was clearly in evidence.

Speed of finger tapping was bilaterally slow during the first 6 months after his SAH. At this time, he was confused in his thinking and had a generalized reduction in overall cognitive functioning, with perhaps limited self-awareness of his cognitive limitations. Bilaterally slow speed of finger movement has been observed in patients with severe traumatic brain injury who are severely cognitively impaired at 1 year post injuries (Dikmen et al. 1995). Thus, this finding is also compatible with his known neurological condition.

Interpretation of Those Findings During the serial neuropsychological assessments of this gentleman, his age, educational level, occupational history, cultural background, and known neurological conditions were kept in mind when interpreting his responses during clinical interviews and his performance on various neuropsychological tests that were not normed on a Southwest American Indian population. His clinical presentation of severe mental confusion and fatigue were thought to be caused by his acute SAH that influenced brain functions, particularly those mediated primarily from the right cerebral hemisphere.

His performance on memory tests and speed of finger tapping was thought to primarily reflect his neuropsychological status and not be greatly influenced by his native culture or educational and occupational history. His occupational history, however, influenced our view of his performance on the Block Design subtest. Being a mechanic, we assumed that his visuospatial skills would be at least average (a scaled score of 10) before the onset of his SAH. His very low scores during the second and third examinations were interpreted as reflecting severe visuospatial problem-solving disturbance. While his scaled score reached 8 by 1 year post onset, it appeared to us to still not return to premorbid estimates. This conclusion (i.e., formulation) was based not only on his occupational history, but his continued poor visuospatial memory performance.

Another important observation was his slow speed of new learning reflected by very low Digit Symbol or Coding scores. Slow performance on these tests has repeatedly been related to overall severity of cognitive dysfunction and unlikely successful return to gainful employment, at least for the Caucasian population (see Prigatano et. al. 1986). It is not known, however, how his American Indian cultural background may influence this particular measure.

While other neuropsychological tests were administered and were included in our diagnostic formulations, the findings presented greatly influenced our understanding of this man's neuropsychological status over time. The findings suggested improvement of neurocognitive function with time, but severe residual impairments most compatible with right hemisphere dysfunction.

Another important point is that his vocabulary level remained considerably below average over every examination period in which it was sampled. We interpreted this finding as reflecting pre-injury level of below average knowledge of the meaning of English words used in present day American society, and not reflecting the knowledge of words used within the tribal cultural setting in which he was raised and worked. At no time did his family report any aphasic disturbance, but he did present early with "confused speech."

Given our analyses of these findings, we felt this person was not in a position to return to gainful employment. We also did not feel he was safe to ride a horse during the various occasions we examined him. We felt he was clearly in need of psychological help in dealing with his normal depression over his clinical condition and its implications for the rest of his life.

Feedback Given to Patient and Family at Different Time Periods The process of giving feedback to the patient and family regarding the patient's neuropsychological status was clearly a delicate one. We attempted to assess the patient's ability to understand what was being said and to choose language that was respectful of this person's age and cultural values and beliefs. The feedback was concise but also attempted to provide direction as to the next steps of his care (see Prigatano and Gray 2011 for an elaboration of these points).

During the first examination, which occurred within a month of his SAH, limited verbal feedback was given to the patient because of his confused clinical state. The family was informed that he showed many of the cognitive difficulties expected after an SAH. His confused thought process and speech was described as a common sequela of this condition and they should improve with time and therapies. In fact they did. This helped build a therapeutic relationship with family members who were understandably cautious when accepting the help of individuals outside of their cultural world.

During the second examination, which was about 5–6 months post onset, the patient showed significant cognitive impairments, but the patient's wife did not report her husband having significant cognitive impairments. This had to be handled cautiously. It was stated (given culturally appropriate methods of respectfully communicating) that patients with her husband's condition may have cognitive impairments that the patient may not perceive and the family members may not recognize. It was suggested that helping patients who have a similar medical history not return to normal activities too soon would be eventually helpful to them. It was also stated that individuals with such a history could benefit from further therapies. Presented in this manner, the patient and his wife experienced a helpful consultation and returned for repeated evaluations.

On the remaining examinations, findings were reviewed and areas of improvement were first described. Areas of continued difficulty were then mentioned. On each occasion, it was emphasized that it would take time to determine what the ultimate level of recovery would be and the implications for work and riding a horse (both of which were very important to the patient). Effort was taken to make sure that the findings were presented in a concise manner and the family asked if they noticed the same type of strengths and limitations in everyday life. It was emphasized that the test findings were limited, but provided one source of information that would help us be objective about the patient's recovery patterns.

This manner of interaction proved very helpful, as in part witnessed by the family and patient never missing an appointment and being eager to learn what each neuropsychological examination finding revealed.

Having the patient's daughter present for many of the examinations was also helpful for two reasons. She spoke more fluent English than her mother and felt she could interpret to both parents the findings in a manner they could better understand. Second, when speaking to her and her mother privately (while the patient was being tested), she spoke a little more directly regarding her father's cognitive difficulties, without being disrespectful of him. This gave the patient's wife an opportunity to also express herself with less caution.

While the patient seemed to have diminished self-awareness of his cognitive limitations, both the daughter and mother were reasonably aware, but often reported fewer difficulties in the clinical interview when the patient was present. Here, cultural influences seem to greatly influence how relatives described the patient and this greatly influences our understanding of the patient and his cultural background. We did not see the family "denying" his limitations, but being cautious and respectful in what they reported about.

Concluding Comments

The neuropsychological examination and interpretation (i.e., formulation) of test findings is a complicated process that requires the examining clinical neuropsychologist to be sensitive to how many variables may influence test performance. In this chapter, we have tried to make explicit how we went about this process when examining a 62-year-old American Indian man who suffered an SAH following a ruptured right carotid aneurysm.

We have tried to emphasize what factors seem to influence the level of test performance observed in several domains observed over time. We have attempted to highlight how we conducted our interview of the patient and family to obtain useful information, but doing so in a manner respectful of the person's age, educational level, occupational background, primary language, and, most importantly, culturally based and valued skills and attitudes.

Having one examiner of American Indian heritage and similar background was clearly very helpful in knowing how to speak with the patient and his family in a manner that made them comfortable and fostered a good working relationship. This, of course, was crucial for obtaining useful clinical information regarding the patient's neuropsychological status and conveying that information that appeared helpful to the patient and his family.

References

Ardila, A. (1995). Directions of research in cross-cultural neuropsychology. *Journal of Clinical and Experimental Neuropsychology, 17*(1), 143–150.

Ardila, A. (2005). Cultural values underlying psychometric cognitive testing. *Neuropsychology Review, 15*(4), 185–195.

Ardila, A., & Moreno, S. (2001). Neuropsychological test performance in Aruaco Indians: An exploratory study. *Journal of the International Neuropsychological Society, 7*(4), 510–515.

Bederson, J. B. (Ed.) (1997). Subarachnoid hemorrhage: Pathophysiology and management. *The American Association of Neurological Surgeons*. Park Ridge: Thieme.

Common, R. W., & Frost, L. G. (1988). The implications of the mismeasurement of Native students' intelligence through the use of standardized intelligence tests. *Canadian Journal of Native Education, 15*(1), 18–30.

Diessner, R., & Walker, J. L. (1986). A cognitive pattern of the Yakima Indian students. *Journal of American Indian Education, 25*(2), 39–41.

Dikmen, S. S., Machamer, J. E., Winn, H. R., & Temkin, N. R. (1995). Neuropsychological outcome at 1-year post head injury. *Neuropsychology, 9*(1), 80–90.

Griffin-Pierce, T., Silverberg, N., Connor, D., Jim, M., Peters, J., Kaszniak, A., & Sabbagh, M. N. (2008). Challenges to the recognition and assessment of Alzheimer's disease in American Indians of the southwestern United States. *Alzheimer's & Dementia, 4*(4), 291–299.

Halpern, J. H., Sherwood, A. R., Hudson, J. I., Yurgelun-Todd, D., & Pope, H. G., Jr., (2005). Psychological and cognitive effects of long-term peyote use among native Americans. *Biological Psychiatry, 58*(8), 624–631.

Halstead, W. C. (1976). *Brain and intelligence.* Chicago: The University of Chicago Press. (Original work published 1947).

Heaton, R. K., Ryan, L., & Grant, I. (2009). Demographic influences and the use of demographically corrected norms in neuropsychological assessment. In I. Grant & K. M. Adams (Eds.), *Neurological assessment of neuropsychiatric and neuromedical disorders* (pp. 127–155). New York: Oxford University Press.

Hillis, A. E., Anderson, N., Sampath, P., & Rigamonti, D. (2000). Cognitive impairments after surgical repair of ruptured and unruptured aneurysms. *Journal of Neurology, Neurosurgery, and Psychiatry, 69,* 608–615.

Jervis, L., Beals, J., Fickenscher, A., & Arciniegas, D. (2007). Performance on the Mini-Mental State Examination and Mattis Dementia Rating Scale among older American Indians. *The Journal of Neuropsychiatry and Clinical Neurosciences, 19*(2), 173–178.

Jervis, L., Fickenscher, A., Beals, J., Cullum, C., Novins, D., Manson, S., & Arciniegas, D. (2010). Predictors of performance on the MMSE and the DRS-2 among American Indian elders. *The Journal of Neuropsychiatry and Clinical Neurosciences, 22*(4), 417–425.

King, J., & Fletcher-Janzen, E. (2000). Neuropsychological assessment and intervention with Native Americans. In E. Fletcher-Janzen, T. L. Strickland, & C. Reynolds (Eds.), *Handbook of cross-cultural neuropsychology* (pp. 105–122). New York: Kluwer Academic.

Lezak, M. D., Howieson, D. B., & Loring, D. W. (2004). *Neuropsychological assessment* (4th en.) New York: Oxford University Press.

Lomay, V. T., & Hinkebein, J. H. (2006). Cultural considerations when providing rehabilitation services to American Indians. *Rehabilitation Psychology, 51*(1), 36.

Luria, A. R. (1966). *Higher cortical functions in man.* New York: Basic Books.

McLellan, M. J., & Nellis, L. (2003). Using the WISC-III with Navajo children: A need for local norms. *Journal of American Indian Education, 42*(2), 50–60.

McShane, D., & Berry, J. W. (1988). 15 Native North Americans: Indian and Inuit abilities. In S. H. Irvine & J. W. Berry (Eds.), *Human abilities in cultural context* (pp. 384–426). Cambridge: Cambridge University Press.

McShane, D. A., & Plas, J. M. (1984). The cognitive functioning of American Indian children: Moving from the WISC to the WISC-R. *School Psychology Review, 13*(1), 61–73.

Ostrosky-Solis, F., Ramirez, M., & Ardila, A. (2004). Effects of culture and education on neuropsychological testing: A preliminary study with indigenous and nonindigenous population. *Applied Neuropsychology, 11*(4), 186–193.

Plank, G. A. (2001). Application of the cross battery approach in the assessment of American Indian children: A viable alternative. *American Indian and Alaska Native Mental Health Research, 10*(1), 21–33.

Preiss, M., Koblihová, J., Netuka, D., Bernardová, L., Charvát, F., & Beneš, V. (2011). Verbal memory capacity after treatment for ruptured intracranial aneurysm—the outcomes of three psychological tests: Within a month, 1 year after and 5–7 years after treatment. *Acta Neurochirugica, 154,* 417–422.

Prigatano, G. P. (1986). *Neuropsychological rehabilitation after brain injury*. Baltimore: Johns Hopkins University Press.

Prigatano, G. P., & Gray, J. A. (2011). Conducting feedback for pediatric neuropsychological assessments. In A. S. Davis (Ed.), *Handbook of pediatric neuropsychology* (pp. 495–499). New York: Springer.

Prigatano, G. P., & Henderson, S. (1997). *Cognitive outcome after subarachnoid hemorrhage. Subarachnoid hemorrhage: Pathophysiology and Management* (pp. 27–40). Park Ridge: Thieme.

Prigatano, G. P., & Leathern, J. M. (1993). Awareness of behavioral limitations after traumatic brain injury: A cross-cultural study of New Zealand Maoris and non-Maoris. *The Clinical Neuropsychologist*, 7(2), 123–135.

Prigatano, G. P., Amin, K., & Rosenstein, L. D. (1995). *BNI screen for higher cerebral functions*. Phoenix: Barrow Neurological Institute.

Puente, A. E., & Ardila, A. (2000). Neuropsychological assessment of Hispanics. In E. Fletcher-Janzen, T. L. Strickland, & C. Reynolds (Eds.), *Handbook of cross-cultural neuropsychology* (pp. 87–104). New York: Kluwer Academic.

Ross, A. C. (1982). Brain hemispheric functions and the Native American. *Journal of American Indian Education, 21*(3), 2–5.

Rosselli, M., & Ardila, A. (2003). The impact of culture and education on non-verbal neuropsychological measurements: A critical review. *Brain and Cognition, 52*(3), 326–333.

Scott, S., Hynd, G. W., Hunt, L., & Weed, W. (1979). Cerebral speech lateralization in the native American Navajo. *Neuropsychologia, 17*(1), 89–92.

Sheldon, S., Macdonald, R. L., & Schweizer, T. A. (2012). Free recall memory performance after aneurysmal subarachnoid hemorrhage. *Journal of the International Neuropsychological Society, 18,* 334–342.

Sheldon, S., Macdonald, R. L., Cusimano, M., Spears, J., & Schweizer, T. A. (2013). Long-term consequences of subarachnoid hemorrhage: Examining working memory. *Journal of the Neurological Sciences, 332,* 145–147.

Sidles, C., MacAvoy, J., Bernston, C., & Kuhn, A. (1987). Analysis of Navajo adolescents' performance on the Raven Progressive Matrices. *Journal of American Indian Education, 27*(1), 1–8.

Spencer, J., & Cruz, M. (1989). Neuropsychological performance changes in a bilingual patient following an infarct at the left thalamic level. *Archives of Clinical Neuropsychology, 4*(2), 138–139.

Teng, E. L., & Manly, J. J. (2005). Neuropsychological testing: Helpful or harmful? *Alzheimer Disease & Associated Disorders, 19*(4), 267–271.

Towgood, K., Ogden, J. A., & Mee, E. (2004). Neurological, neuropsychological, and psychosocial outcome following treatment of unruptured intracranial aneurysms: A review and commentary. *Journal of the International Neuropsychological Society, 10,* 114–134.

Tsethlikai, M. (2011). An exploratory analysis of American Indian children's cultural engagement, fluid cognitive skills, and standardized verbal IQ scores. *Developmental Psychology, 47*(1), 192.

U.S. Census Bureau. (2012). The American Indian and Alaska native population: 2010. http://www.census.gov/prod/cen2010/briefs/c2010br-10.pdf. Accessed 11 Nov 2013.

Vanderpool, M., & Catano, V. M. (2008). Comparing the performance of Native North Americans and predominantly White military recruits on verbal and nonverbal measures of cognitive ability. *International Journal of Selection and Assessment, 16*(3), 239–248.

Vieira, A. C., Azevedo-Filho, H. R., Quinino, S., Souza, M. L., Camara, D. J., Leitao, L., et al. (2011). Language, memory, and verbal fluency changes in patients with aneurysmal subarachnoid hemorrhage: Results of a preoperative investigation. *World Neurosurgery, 75*(5), 653–659.

Verney, S. P., Jervis, L. L., Fickenscher, A., Roubideaux, Y., Bogart, A., & Goldberg, J. (2008). Symptoms of depression and cognitive functioning in older American Indians. *Aging and Mental Health, 12*(1), 108–115.

Vocate, D. R. (1984). Differential cerebral speech lateralization in Crow Indian and Anglo children. *Neuropsychologia, 22*(4), 487–494.

Whyte, S. R., Cullum, C. M., Hynan, L. S., Lacritz, L. H., Rosenberg, R. N., & Weiner, M. F. (2005). Performance of elderly Native Americans and Caucasians on the CERAD neuropsychological battery. *Alzheimer Disease & Associated Disorders, 19*(2), 74–78.

Wiseley, M. C. (2001). Non-verbal intelligence and Native-American Navajo children: A comparison between the CTONI and the WISC-III (unpublished doctoral dissertation). The University of Arizona, Tucson, AZ.

Wong, T. M., Strickland, T. L., Fletcher-Janzen, E., Ardila, A., & Reynolds, C. R. (2000). Theoretical and practical issues in the neuropsychological assessment and treatment of culturally dissimilar patients. In E. Fletcher-Janzen, T. L. Strickland, & C. Reynolds (Eds.), *Handbook of cross-cultural neuropsychology* (pp. 3–18). New York: Kluwer Academic/Plenum.

Wright, S. C., Taylor, D. M., & Ruggiero, K. M. (1996). Examining the potential for academic achievement among Inuit children: Comparisons on the raven coloured progressive matrices. *Journal of Cross-Cultural Psychology, 27*(6), 733–753.

Chapter 8
Paediatric Neuropsychological Formulation of a Traumatic Brain Injury with Special Reference to Culture

Cathy Grant and Arleta Starza-Smith

Introduction

There is a sizable literature on the neuropsychological effects of traumatic brain injury (TBI) in children (see Yeates 2010 for a review). In brief, TBI, especially when severe, is associated with widespread deficits in intellectual function, language, visuospatial skills, motor skills, attention, memory and executive skills (Catroppa et al. 2011; Donders 1993; Yeates et al. 2005). Behavioural difficulties are common after TBI and impact upon family function (Anderson et al. 2005). Social function, adaptive function and academic attainments are often compromised (Ewing-Cobbs et al. 2004; Yeates et al. 2004). In young children, who have few established skills, the impact of TBI may prevent skill acquisition or may seriously alter the developmental course (Anderson et al. 2011). Moreover, the full effects of TBI are not seen until the brain has fully matured, so some difficulties may emerge and become apparent only later in development (Muscara et al. 2008).

This case study illustrates the importance of cultural considerations in relation to neuropsychological assessment, formulation and rehabilitation. In the UK, there is an increasing and evolving cultural and linguistic diversity that has considerable

The authors would like to acknowledge Dr. Daniel Smith, Lincoln College Oxford, for his invaluable assistance in the proofreading of this chapter.

C. Grant (✉) · A. Starza-Smith
Department of Clinical Psychology and Neuropsychology, Nottingham University Hospitals NHS Trust, QMC Campus, Derby Road, Nottingham, Nottingham NG7 2UH, UK
e-mail: cathy.grant@uhl-tr.nhs.uk

A. Starza-Smith
e-mail: Arleta.starza-smith@nuh.nhs.uk

J. A. B. Macniven (ed.), *Neuropsychological Formulation*,
DOI 10.1007/978-3-319-18338-1_8

implications for specialist paediatric neuropsychology services. The 2011 census reported that 7.7% of the population did not have English (or Welsh in Wales) as a first language. Polish, Punjabi, Urdu, Bengali (including Sylheti and Chatgaya) and Gujarati were the most common 'other' languages spoken, and accounted for almost 1 million of the 63.2 million people estimated to live in the UK (Office for National Statistics 2011). Furthermore, there are differences in the geographical distribution of cultures and language use across the UK. For instance, there is a clustering of some cultures. In specific areas, the population of that culture may be relatively large whilst being practically nonexistent in other parts of the UK. The issues relating to the complexity of providing culturally appropriate neuropsychology services are similar worldwide, although the origins and cultures of the minority populations who need to be considered vary. The rate of change in cultural and linguistic diversity may also vary by country. The UK has experienced rapid changes in cultural and linguistic diversity in recent years. As a profession that is relatively small in number, often it is not possible to find a paediatric neuropsychologist who is able to conduct an assessment in a child's first language.

The difficulties of working with a child and their family where English is not their first language is clearly a significant factor for assessment and rehabilitation. However, cultural issues go beyond the language barrier to include the belief systems and cultural practices of a given community. Determination of which belief systems are most powerful in a family is often not straightforward. There may be intergenerational issues where the child's identity may be very much 'British', but the family identity remains rooted elsewhere. In some cases, the family may prefer input from within their own community. Conversely, even if the child was born in the UK, their identity may be 'country of roots'. Cultural issues have a powerful influence on how the child and their family respond to stress, illness or injury that impact approaches and response to assessment, rehabilitation and outcome. Often within the wider culture, specific societies or subcultures exist, and it is essential for the clinician to consider how the beliefs of the family may influence rehabilitation. Some children and families are refugees who may have complex and traumatic experiences from both their country of origin and the asylum-seeking processes in the UK.

Approach to Assessment

The purpose of neuropsychological assessment is to understand brain–behaviour relationships and how these relate to a child's cognitive strengths and weaknesses, emotional regulation and behaviour, and to use this understanding to inform medical management and/or rehabilitation (Baron 2010). Assessment is guided by what is known about the individual child with respect to their developmental level at the time of injury, current developmental level, injuries sustained and theory regarding TBI, including anatomy most vulnerable to injury and the neuropsychological and developmental effects of injury. The child's environment, including support available to the family, socioeconomic status (SES) and culture, has a powerful influence upon typical development and is likely to exert an effect upon the long-term outcome in children with brain injury (Breslau 1990; Taylor and Schatschneider 1992). Furthermore, specific genetic conditions, birth history or early developmental factors related to malnutrition, trauma or access to learning and education may need to be taken into account when considering differential diagnosis.

The interpretation of psychometric assessments used with a child from a minority population requires careful consideration as the normative sample may not have included people from minority backgrounds or may have included only a small sample. For instance, the Wechsler Intelligence Scale for Children-Fourth Edition (WISC-IV) UK standardisation sample included 4.2% Asian children (children from India, Pakistan and Bangladesh as well as other Asian countries) which was representative of the UK population. However, this equates to only 33 children in a sample of 780 (Wechsler 2004). The literature addressing the impact of culture and ethnicity on test performance in children is sparse and does not exist for many standardised tests (Byrd et al. 2008). One of the most researched tests is the US WISC-IV standardisation sample, where typically developing children from some minority backgrounds have been reported to perform below nonminority children. For instance, Prifitera et al. (2005) reported that within the US WISC-IV standardisation sample, not only did children from minority ethnic backgrounds perform below nonminority children but there was also variation between the minority ethnic groups, with the African-American children showing a greater discrepancy (almost 12 points) than the Hispanic children (10 points). They also reported that the effect was not uniform across indexes, with the Working Memory Index and Processing Speed Index showing less difference between groups. Moreover, differences between groups were reduced (to 5–9 points) if SES was taken into account (Prifitera et al. 2005). Differences between groups became more pronounced with age, with younger children showing the smallest difference. The authors interpreted this finding as reflecting the impact that social, economic and educational opportunities have upon intellectual development. Similar studies do not exist on the WISC-IV UK standardisation sample.

Garrett and Kelly (2007) have examined the impact of bilingualism on performance on the NEPSY, a developmental neuropsychological assessment battery for children. In a sample of typically developing children aged 6–7 years who lived in the UK, they found few differences among groups on the domains of attention/executive functioning, sensorimotor, visuospatial and memory. It was only on the language domain (i.e. testing knowledge of the native language of the country in which the test was being administered/the English language) that the bilingual children performed lower than the monolingual comparison group.

Separating out the effects of brain injury from the effects of SES, bilingualism and minority background is complex but important for predicting long-term prognosis. Whilst early studies suggested that bilingualism hindered language development (e.g. Barke and Williams 1938), more recent research suggests that bilingual children produce their first words at about the same time as monolingual children (e.g. Patterson and Pearson 2004). Although vocabulary acquisition may initially be below age expectations in each language spoken (Oller et al. 2007), total vocabulary across languages combined is age appropriate in bilingual children (e.g. Marchman et al. 2009; Poulin-Dubois et al. 2012).

Neuropsychological assessment and formulation in children is usually serial rather than based on a one-off assessment, as the child is in the process of development, and neuropsychological strengths and weaknesses emerge across development. In young children, it is not easy to separate out the various neuropsychological functions of memory, language, attention and executive function in the way that is possible with older children and adults. Neuropsychological abilities are heavily interdependent early in development, and many tests remain largely experimental (see special issue on preschool assessment edited by Anderson and Baron (2012)).

Case Background/Referral Details

Hassan sustained a moderate to severe brain injury as the result of a fall of approximately 15 ft from an overhanging grassy ledge onto flat rock below, when he was aged 3 years. He was on a day trip to a local country park with his aunt and uncle when the accident happened. When the ambulance arrived, his Glasgow Coma Scale was 15, but this decreased to 7 in the ambulance and was recorded as 3 on arrival at hospital. He was found to have jaw clenching and tonic-clonic jerking of his legs and arms. A computerised tomography (CT) scan showed a subdural haemorrhage in the right frontal and parietal areas, right hemisphere contusions and a wide fracture of the right frontal and parietal bone with some extension to the left parietal bone and associated intraventricular haemorrhage. Hassan was admitted to the Paediatric Intensive Care Unit (PICU) where he remained for 11 days. He experienced seizures whilst in PICU. He was treated for raised intracranial pressure with external ventricular drain, sedation, cooling and intubation. Hassan was transferred onto the specialist Paediatric Neurosciences Ward where he remained for 6 weeks. He had a left-sided weakness in his arms and legs which responded well to physiotherapy, but he had a residual mild left-sided hemiplegia and some difficulties with balance. Hassan returned to wearing nappies for a year post-injury and had to relearn how to speak.

Hassan was first seen by neuropsychology at 6 months post discharge from in-patient care. A neuropsychological evaluation was requested by the medical team to document the extent and nature of any difficulties resulting from the brain injury and the likely prognosis. His parents were seen at this appointment along with an interpreter as the referral letter noted that Hassan's mother did not speak English. At that time, his parents did not want to pursue an assessment as they thought things were getting 'back to normal'.

Hassan was re-referred at 5 years of age, after a diagnosis of epilepsy had been made and parents were concerned that Hassan was experiencing behavioural difficulties. Hassan was also seen for reassessment at transition to junior school and again 3 years later to prepare for transition to secondary school. Hassan and his family were seen within a regional neurosciences service.

At the time of the re-referral for neuropsychological assessment, Hassan lived with his mother and father, siblings (a brother who was 6 years older than Hassan and a sister who was 10 years older than Hassan) and paternal grandparents. Hassan's father was born in Pakistan but he had lived in the UK since he was a young child. He spoke English and Urdu fluently. Hassan's mother had grown up in Pakistan and had lived in the UK after she married. She spoke Urdu fluently and was learning to speak English. Hassan's grandparents spoke Urdu only. His father worked in a garment factory and his mother was a housewife. Prior to the accident, Hassan had been typically developing. He walked by the age of 12 months. He had a good understanding of language but did not say his first word until 24 months of age. By 30 months he was reported to be using two-word phrases both in English and Urdu.

Medical records indicated that Hassan had been assessed by a physiotherapist, occupational therapist and speech and language therapist in preparation for entry into nursery school. The physiotherapist reported that he was unsteady on his feet and was neglecting to use his left arm. Hassan improved after strategies were put in place. He subsequently attended nursery with no additional support. At age 5 years, Hassan developed tonic-clonic seizures, which he experienced almost weekly. Hassan's seizures typically lasted for 5 min, but he had one prolonged seizure of 30 min. His seizures became well controlled on carbamazepine.

At the time of re-referral, the history was taken with an interpreter present to support Hassan's mother. Hassan's parents reported concerns about his ability to concentrate and noted that even when watching his favourite TV programmes, he was constantly 'on the go' and unable to sit down. He had difficulties with pronunciation of words in both English and Urdu. He also had difficulties with writing. Parents felt that Hassan was able to express his needs but he experienced regular temper tantrums 2–3 times per week. He had little understanding of risk and would climb on furniture, putting himself in danger. Hassan was reported to have difficulties with everyday skills such as getting himself dressed. He struggled with buttons, toileting and brushing his teeth.

Hassan had transferred from nursery to mainstream school with no additional needs identified. In the school setting, Hassan was reported by his teachers to be very bubbly, talkative and 'full of beans'. He was academically behind and was noted to have speech difficulties, whereby he would have difficulties with certain sounds, for example 'T' would be replaced with 'G'. He had an intensive reading programme, but he seemed to have difficulties retaining information. For example, teachers noted that one day he was able to write his name, but the next day he would miss out letters and write some letters upside down. They noted that letters would be confused and gave the example that 'f' would be mistaken for 't' and 'v' would be mistaken for 'n'. Hassan was receiving some help with speech through a speech group run by speech and language therapy, but the school had few details from this service as to how best to support Hassan. Parents said that he was often very tired at the end of the school day and regularly fell asleep on the journey home from school.

Serial Assessment

Hassan was assessed on three different occasions at age 5, 7 and 10 years.

Age 5 Years
Hassan was right-handed. English was judged by parents to be Hassan's first language. Hassan was noted to have difficulties with pronouncing words and he said 'dod' for 'dog' and 'tar' for 'car'. He also had difficulties understanding instructions, even if these were brief and there was the opportunity for repetition. The use of interpreters in psychometric testing is fraught with difficulty and potentially undermines the validity of the evaluation (Harris and Llorente 2005). The interpreter was used on one occasion to explore if Hassan was more able to understand instructions in Urdu, which was not the case, so the assessment was undertaken in English. He showed good effort throughout the neuropsychological assessment, although he required short assessment sessions of a maximum of 1 hour, with breaks, as he became fidgety.

Tests Administered
Wechsler Preschool and Primary Scale of Intelligence-Third UK Edition (WPPSI-III^{UK})
A Developmental Neuropsychological Assessment (NEPSY)
Children's Memory Scale (CMS)
Wechsler Non-Verbal Scale of Ability (WNS)
Wechsler Objective Reading Dimensions (WORD)

Intellectual Function
Hassan's intellectual function, as measured by the WPPSI-III^{UK}, is summarised in Table 8.1. Hassan was able to understand test instructions on the majority of WPPSI-III^{UK} subtests but only after some repetition of information. Hassan's verbal and performance skills were evenly developed and both fell within the Borderline range of ability. On the Verbal Index, Hassan's performance was similar across subtests. On the Performance Index, Hassan performed better on picture concepts than other subtests, which is a reported strength in children with acquired brain injury (Donders et al. 2013).

Processing Speed
Slowed processing speed is a common consequence of paediatric TBI. Hassan's Processing Speed Index as measured by the WPPSI-III^{UK} fell within the Lower Extreme.

Attention
Observations of Hassan throughout the assessment suggested significant attention difficulties. Attention was measured using the Attention Index on the CMS. Hassan obtained an index score that fell within the Low Average range. The tests that contribute towards this are Digit Span (forwards and backwards) and Sequences. Hassan's longest digits forward span was four and he was unable to complete any digits backwards, even after explanation and practice. On Sequences, he was able

Table 8.1 Neuropsychological test scores at age 5 years (Index scores italicised)

	Test result	Percentile	Qualitative descriptor
General intellectual abilities			
WPPSI-III verbal	*74*	*4th*	*Borderline*
WPPSI-III performance	*75*	*5th*	*Borderline*
WPPSI-III processing speed	*60*	*0.4th*	*Lower Extreme*
WPPSI-III subtest information	4	2nd	Lower Extreme
WPPSI-III subtest vocabulary	6	9th	Low Average
WPPSI-III subtest word reasoning	5	5th	Borderline
WPPSI-III subtest block design	5	5th	Borderline
WPPSI-III subtest picture concepts	8	25th	Average
WPPSI-III subtest matrix reasoning	5	5th	Borderline
WPPSI-III subtest picture completion	4	2nd	Lower Extreme
WPPSI-III subtest coding	2	<1st	Lower Extreme
WPPSI-III subtest symbol search	4	2nd	Lower Extreme
Language			
WPPSI-III general language	*72*	*3rd*	*Borderline*
WPPSI-III subtest receptive vocab	5	5th	Borderline
WPPSI-III subtest picture naming	5	5th	Borderline
Memory			
CMS subtest stories immediate	5	5th	Borderline
WNS subtest recognition memory	5	5th	Borderline
Attention			
CMS attention/concentration index	*82*	*12th*	*Low Average*
Visuospatial skills			
NEPSY subtest design copying	6	9th	Low average
NEPSY subtest visuomotor precision	4	2nd	Lower Extreme
Sensorimotor skills			
NEPSY subtest imitating hand positions	4	2nd	Lower Extreme

to count from 1 to 10 forwards and backwards, but was unable to complete any of the other items.

Language

The General Language Index from the WPPSI-III^{UK} measures receptive (pointing to correct picture) and expressive (picture naming) language. Hassan performed similarly on both expressive and receptive measures, both falling within the Borderline range.

Visual Motor Integration and Visuoperceptual Skills

The NEPSY Design Copying assesses visual motor integration, where the child copies two-dimensional geometric figures on paper. Hassan's performance fell within the Low Average range.

The NEPSY Block Construction assesses the ability to reproduce, from models and from pictures, block constructions in three dimensions. Hassan's performance fell within the Borderline range.

Sensorimotor Functions

The NEPSY Imitating Hand Positions assesses the ability to imitate a hand position from a model. The examiner models a hand position, and the child attempts to reproduce it. Hassan obtained a score that fell within the Lower Extreme.

The NEPSY Visuomotor Precision assesses fine motor skills and hand/eye coordination. The child draws a line inside a track as quickly as possible. Hassan's performance fell within the Lower Extreme.

Memory

On the CMS, it was unclear if Hassan had understood the instructions on Dot Locations and Faces, so these subtests were discontinued. Some subtests were not completed as the assessment was too difficult for him. On Stories, Hassan was only able to recall two pieces of information from the first story and nothing from the second story. For this reason, delayed recall was not attempted. On Word Pairs, Hassan was unable to recall the sample items despite repetition and multiple attempts. He was only able to recall the first letter of a word, for instance, 'd' for down and 'f' for farm and this subtest was discontinued. Hassan was able to complete the subtests that contribute to the Attention Index and he scored within the Average range on these items.

Recognition Memory from the WNS was used to further assess memory whilst reducing the language demands of the task. Hassan's performance fell within the Borderline range.

Reading and Spelling

The Wechsler Objective Reading Dimensions (WORD) was attempted. Hassan was unable to complete even the initial items on the WORD which addresses the understanding of phonemes. Although Hassan was able to understand the concepts of the beginning and end of a word, he was unable to detect the sounds and the assessment was discontinued.

Age 7 Years and Age 10 Years

Similar tests were used at age 7 and 10 years. These assessments have been collapsed so that progress across assessments can be considered.

Hassan was reassessed at age 7 when he transferred into primary school. Hassan attended this assessment accompanied by his mother and an interpreter to support communication with his mother. At the time of the assessment, he was receiving small group teaching and one-to-one support but this was done without a Statement of Special Educational Needs in place. His teachers said that Hassan found it difficult to pay attention, although he was very motivated and keen to learn. He tended to fiddle with materials and was distracted by his surroundings.

Hassan's mother reported that he was very active at home and he found it difficult to sit still. This was evident in the clinic when he was left to his own devices, but he responded well to direction and was able to stay seated and calm when occupied. Hassan had a busy life, combining a full day at school with 1.5 hours each evening at mosque school. Hassan's seizures had been fairly well controlled, but he had experienced two seizures whilst he was alone in his bedroom. This had raised his mother's anxiety to the point where she did not want to leave the house during the day in case she missed a call from the school informing her that Hassan had experienced a seizure (although this had never happened). She was reluctant to leave him to sleep alone at night and would usually sleep in the room with him.

Hassan was reassessed in preparation for his transition to secondary school at age 10 years. Hassan attended these sessions with his mother without the aid of an interpreter as she was now able to communicate in English and had indicated that she did not want an interpreter to be present. Hassan's mother reported that he continued to be hyperactive at home and he regularly experienced tantrums when he could not get his own way. Hassan remained busy, attending school full time and mosque school for 2 hours per night on weekdays. Hassan said that he liked to play on his Xbox and he was worried about being behind at school. He found both school and mosque school challenging. It was difficult for him to express how he felt emotionally, but he was able to describe difficulties coping with the brightness and noise at school and mosque school.

Family life was also busy and challenging at times. Hassan's grandparents had developed significant health issues. Their role within the family had altered from a supportive role to one where they required care. Hassan's mother continued to find it difficult to allow him to sleep alone for fear of seizures. At the assessment when Hassan was aged 10, she shared that she was experiencing nightmares and intrusive thoughts relating to the time of the accident and Hassan's hospitalisation.

The school staff were concerned that Hassan was not making the gains he had previously been making. He required one-to-one support to help him focus on tasks. He showed variability in performance across days, seeming brighter on some days and 'not with it' on others. He sometimes fell asleep at school. He had started to have seizures that seemed to occur only at school. Investigations by neurology diagnosed these to be non-epileptic attacks.

Tests Administered

Wechsler Intelligence Scale for Children-Fourth UK Edition (WISC-IV^{UK})
Children's Memory Scale (CMS)
Wechsler Individual Achievement Test-Second UK Edition (WISC-IV^{UK})
Test of Everyday Attention for Children (TEA-Ch)

Intellectual Function

At age 7, Hassan was outside of the age range for reassessment using the WPPSI-III^{UK}. Consequently, intellectual function was assessed using the WISC-IV^{UK} short index form (Crawford et al. 2009). Hassan was able to comprehend instructions more easily than on the previous assessment, although he did still require some repetition. He was noted to have difficulties retaining instructions and found it difficult to work on tasks even just for a couple of minutes without support. Hassan was reassessed on the WISC-IV^{UK} at age 10.

Verbal and nonverbal abilities were evenly developed at both 7 and 10 years, which was consistent with Hassan's profile at 5 years (see Fig. 8.1). Hassan's abilities were at the Borderline/Lower Extreme at age 7, but at age 10 his verbal and nonverbal abilities fell firmly within the Lower Extreme. Hassan's lower index scores reflected that he was making a small amount of progress, but at a much slower pace than his peer group.

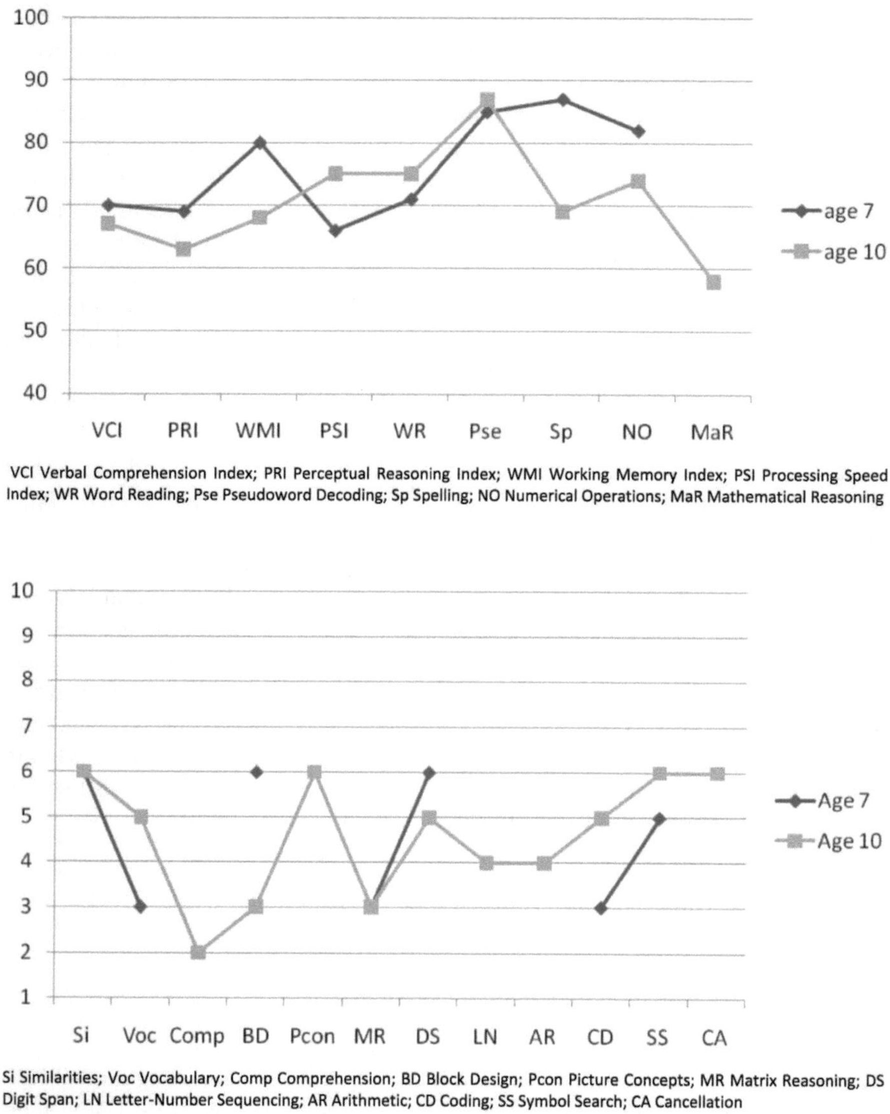

Fig. 8.1 WISC-IV^{UK} Index *(upper)*, subtest scaled scores *(lower)* and WIAT-II standard scores *(upper)* at age 7 and 10 years

Processing Speed

At age 7, Hassan's processing speed fell within the Lower Extreme (Processing Speed Index 66, <0.1 percentile), although this score resulted from nonstandardised administration of subtests, as Hassan found it difficult to work unaided. On Coding, he needed help and reminders of where to start on the task, even though he had just been told moments before. He also needed reminders to carry on once he got to the end of the line repeatedly throughout the task, even though the instruction had only been given relatively recently. On Symbol Search, he needed help with turning the page and remembering what he was supposed to do. On one occasion he turned the page so that it was upside down and he seemed unaware that the page was the wrong way round.

At age 10, and in contrast to other index scores falling back relative to peers, Hassan made some improvements in his ability to process information. The standardised administration could be followed on this occasion and Hassan had developed a verbal technique to keep himself on task. For instance on Coding, he would say under his breath '1 is … 3 is …' and then use his finger to locate the required symbol. His performance at age 10 fell within the Borderline range, whereas on previous assessments, it had been within the Lower Extreme.

Working Memory

At age 7, Hassan's auditory working memory, as measured Digit Span on the WISC–IV^{UK}, fell within the Low Average range. At age 10, Hassan was able to complete Letter Number sequencing in addition to Digit Span. These assessments, along with Hassan's performances on arithmetic, suggested that his working memory remained largely unchanged across assessments. Hassan's longest digits forwards span was four items on both assessments and his longest digits backwards was two items on both assessments. It is notable that Hassan's longest digits forwards span was four when he was assessed at 5 years, meaning that his span had not altered across 5 years of development.

Attention

Attention was formally assessed at 7 years only. Selective visual focused attention as measured by Sky Search on the TEA-Ch identified that Hassan had difficulty identifying targets, was slow to identify targets and that difficulties remained even when motor slowness was accounted for, with all of his performances falling within the Lower Extreme. On the SCORE subtest, which measures sustained attention, Hassan required several practice trials before he understood the requirements of the task, but his performance fell into the Low Average range. Creature Counting was abandoned as, although on the practice trial with support he could do the task, when unsupported he was unable to hold the task requirements in mind. On dual attention, as measured by Sky Search DT, Hassan's performance was Borderline.

Visual Motor Integration and Visuoperceptual Skills

This was informally assessed at age 10 years. Hassan was asked to draw a clock, a bicycle and a house which are shown in Fig. 8.2. Hassan's drawings were immature and lacking in detail.

Memory

When assessed at age 7, Hassan's memory, as measured by the CMS, fell within the Lower Extreme, and his abilities across verbal and visual memory were similar (see Table 8.2). On subtests where multiple learning trials were presented, his learning curve remained flat and he was only able to retain one or two pieces of information on any one trial. On recall after a delay, he was able to recall the same one or two pieces of information that he had encoded across trials. On Stories, in which mate-

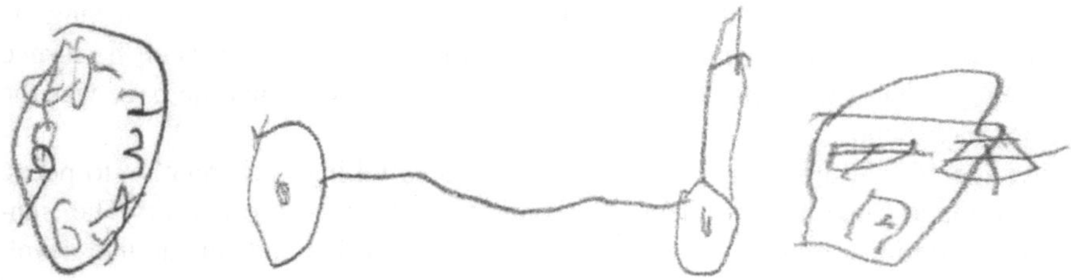

Fig. 8.2 Drawings of a clock, a bicycle and a house

Table 8.2 Performance on Children's Memory Scale at age 7 and 10 years

	Age 7	Age 10
General Memory Index	*< 50, < 0.1st percentile*	–
Verbal Immediate Memory Index	*60, 0.4th percentile*	–
Stories immediate	5	3
Word pairs	2	1
Verbal Delayed Memory Index	*66, 1st percentile*	–
Stories delayed	5	–
Word pairs delayed	4	–
Delayed Recognition Index	*60, 0.4th percentile*	–
Stories delayed recognition	2	–
Word pairs delayed recognition	5	–
Visual Immediate Memory Index	*60, 0.4th percentile*	–
Faces immediate	4	–
Dot locations	3	6
Visual Delayed Memory Index	*57, 0.2nd percentile*	–
Faces delayed	1	–
Dot locations delayed	5	–
Learning Index Score	*54, 0.1st percentile*	–
Dot locations learning score	3	6
Word pairs learning score	2	3

rial was only presented once, Hassan found it difficult to encode the information, although what he did encode was retained for later recall. In the immediate recall condition of Stories, he recalled the animal in the story as being a cow rather than a cat and could only recall a small amount from the beginning and end of both stories. On Story Recognition, he became easily confused about which details were parts of the story and which details were not and he performed no better than chance. His recognition of materials that he had learnt across multiple trials was better and he recognised correctly 25 out of 30 word pairs, which is a performance that is better than chance.

When Hassan was reassessed at age 10, the CMS was discontinued as it was evident that he continued to have severe difficulties with encoding information. Hassan was aware of his difficulties at this stage and completing the assessment was distressing for him. Similar to the assessment at age 7, Hassan was able to recall only one or two items of verbal information but it was notable that competing information had large interference effects. For visual materials, he was able to encode only two to three items at a time. The test was discontinued and delayed recall was not administered as Hassan became upset.

Memory was further assessed at age 10. Hassan completed the Rey-Osterrieth Complex Figure Test (Meyers and Meyers 1996) in a separate session which he engaged with well and completed without becoming distressed. Hassan's copy trial, along with immediate and delayed recall trials, is shown in Fig. 8.3. Hassan's performance fell at or below the 1st percentile on copy and below the 1st percentile on immediate and delayed recall.

Reading, Spelling and Numeracy

At age 7, Hassan's literacy and numeracy skills fell within the Low Average range (see Fig. 8.1) and his performance was consistent with what would be predicted from his overall levels of intellectual function. At age 10, well-established skills such as phonetic decoding remained within the Average range. Word Reading and

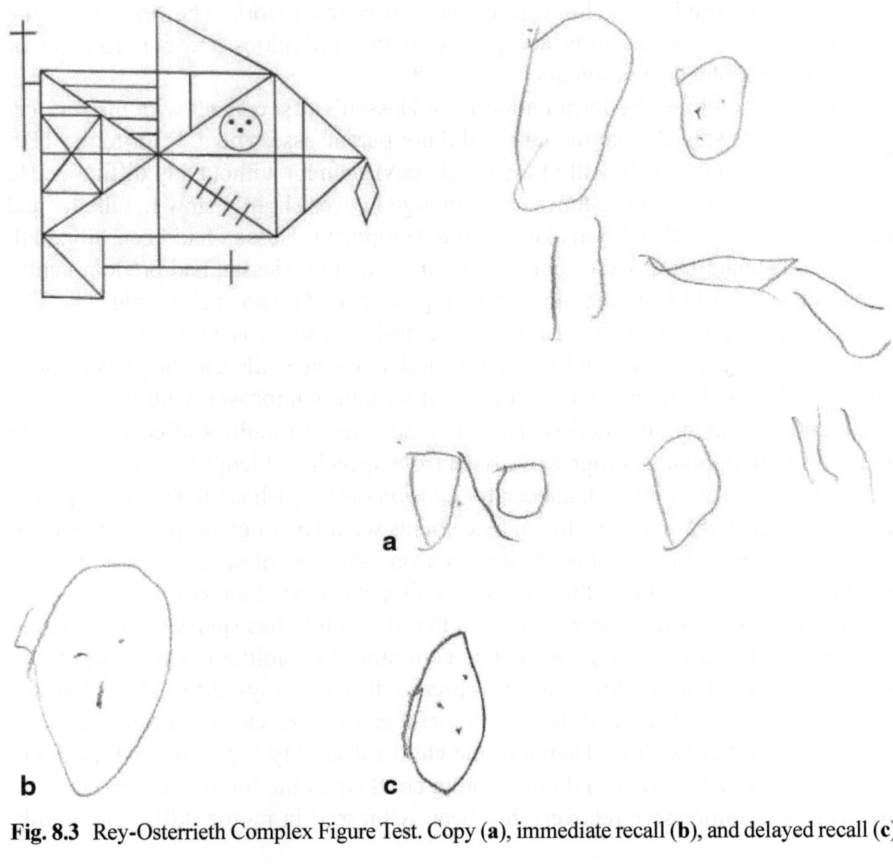

Fig. 8.3 Rey-Osterrieth Complex Figure Test. Copy (**a**), immediate recall (**b**), and delayed recall (**c**)

Spelling, on which continued success requires building up sight vocabulary to manage irregular words, were areas in which Hassan began to fall behind. Hassan's Word Reading, which fell in the Borderline range, was commensurate with his level of intellectual function. In contrast, Spelling, which fell into the Lower Extreme, was significantly below what would be predicted. Hassan's performance on Numerical Operations, which fell into the Borderline range, was also commensurate with intellectual function. However, his ability to apply this knowledge (mathematical reasoning), such as understanding time, money, calendars, graphs etc., was significantly below what would be predicted from his intellectual function.

Formulations

Anderson et al. (2001a) presented a stage model of issues that children and families face following TBI. In the acute stage, issues revolve around survival, with families experiencing fear, guilt and helplessness. In the subacute stage, families try to balance the needs of the injured child with the needs of the rest of the family, adjust to changes in the child, and manage rehabilitation and other practical issues such as time for required extra childcare or time away from work. The final stage, the chronic stage, is about family acceptance of the difficulties and management of behaviour and physical problems.

Figure 8.4 outlines the formulation from Hassan's first contact with the service, in the subacute stage, when the family did not pursue assessment. Prior to the TBI, his development unfolded within the family environment without any difficulty. He achieved all his motor milestones and although he was slightly slow to talk, he had been progressing well with his language development. Hassan had been bilingual. Both English and Urdu were spoken at home, although Hassan had predominantly been in the care of his mother and paternal grandparents who spoke Urdu. The TBI necessitated the input of the health service and education. Hassan's parents were initially alarmed at the loss of his toileting and language skills and the physical left-sided weakness. Toileting and the left-sided weakness improved with professional input and the parents normalised Hassan's language difficulties after he began to make a small amount of progress. Advice from speech and language therapy in the post-acute stage after injury had been to focus on his English language development as Hassan's nursery and educational placements would be English speaking. Hassan was considered as being at high risk of neuropsychological sequelae as a result of the TBI and it was predicted that this would disrupt his development. This phase can be difficult for families who are relieved that their child has survived and is home from hospital, but are trying to balance community rehabilitation with the desire to get back to a 'normal' life. Families react in different ways at this stage depending upon their own coping styles and sometimes families cannot accept that there will be residual difficulties. Denial of the child's disability is part of an adjustment process and may be easier to do in a young child when the focus is on maximising recovery and impressive recovery has been witnessed in motor skills. The family

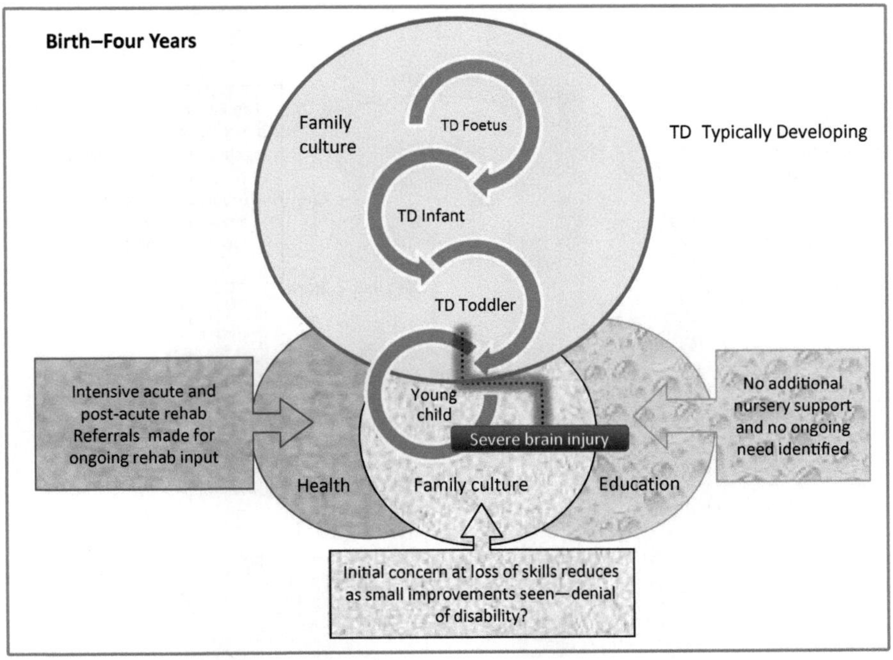

Fig. 8.4 Formulation in the post-acute stage

largely disengaged from health services as they believed that things were getting back to normal and that Hassan would recover without any ongoing difficulties.

Figure 8.5 outlines the formulation at age 5, when Hassan was re-referred. Using Anderson et al.'s (2001) model, the family had moved towards the chronic stage where they were adjusting expectations to some degree, but they had not fully moved from denial of disability. However, the family lacked an understanding of the nature of the difficulties and how to manage these as health services had not succeeded in having the ongoing communication and liaison that is usually required to ensure that the child's deficits are fully understood. The family re-engaged with health services when Hassan developed seizures. His parents were concerned about Hassan's behaviour at this time but they were not necessarily relating this to his brain injury and had a narrative that he was a wilful child who, as the youngest child, may have been spoilt. English was Hassan's reported first language and he had little understanding of Urdu. Although his parents recognised that Hassan had some language problems, they had no suspicion that he had learning difficulties and they did not fully understand the nature, causes and treatment of his epilepsy. A complicating factor was that an interpreter was used in these early assessments. It is not clear whether the family may have been minimising issues through concern that the difficulties would be shared with their community by the interpreter. Parents sought out traditional treatments and took Hassan to Pakistan for help with his seizures and restlessness. This resulted in him missing 3 months of school. Teachers were aware that Hassan had difficulties and

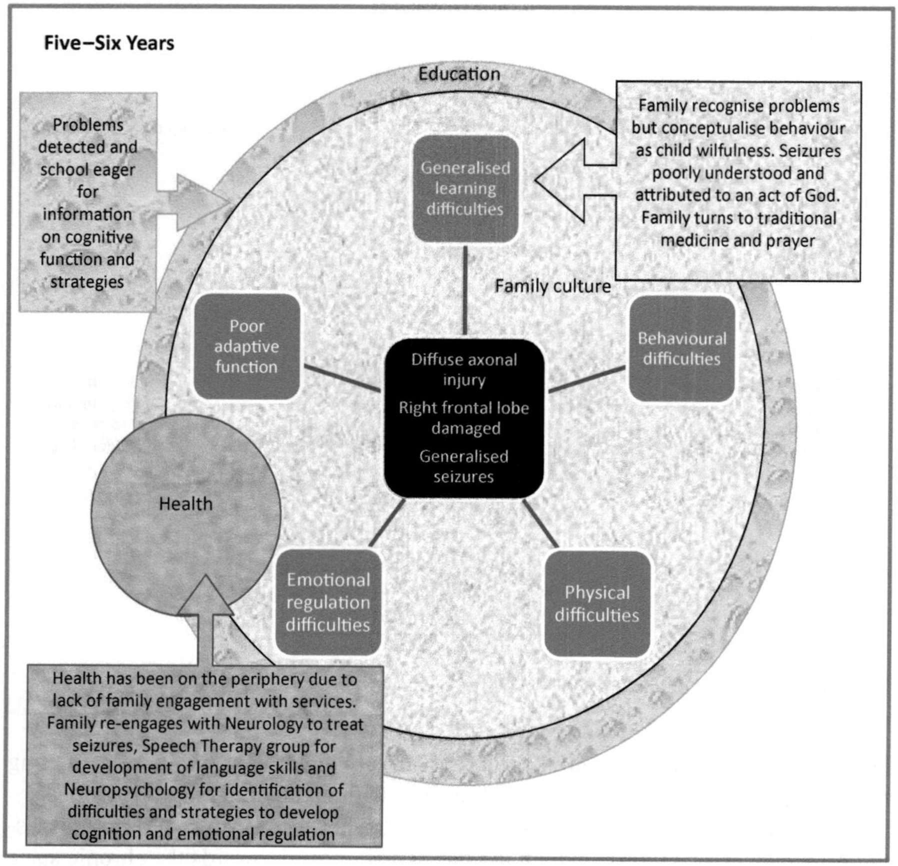

Fig. 8.5 Formulation at age 5–6 years

suspected that he had a learning difficulty. However, they were unclear how many of the difficulties may have related to his language problems or even to missed school.

Hassan's performance on the standardised assessments suggested significant neuropsychological sequelae. His presentation was generally consistent with the commonly reported effects of TBI in a young child, such as generalised learning difficulties, memory impairment, attention and executive functioning difficulties. Under some circumstances, the young brain shows impressive recovery of function after brain injury. For example, language skills can show significant recovery in focal injury in young children (see Anderson et al. 2011 for a discussion). This 'plasticity' or the ability of the brain to recover may result from the child's brain being less functionally committed than the adult brain and therefore having more capacity to transfer functions to undamaged areas (Kolb and Gibb 2011). However, when injury is more diffuse and widespread, plasticity may be reduced as there is less undamaged tissue to take over function and the white matter tracts connecting different regions of the brain are also disrupted. The widespread effect of the TBI on Hassan's brain is therefore likely to have resulted in limited plasticity.

Vulnerability models, which stress the detrimental impact of brain injury at a young age when there are few established skills, may be more informative when considering Hassan's prognosis. Vulnerability models postulate that skills undergoing rapid development at the time of insult may be particularly prone to disruption and derailment of further development (Dennis 1989). Many of Hassan's skills were undergoing rapid development at the time of his injury. In particular, he was slow to talk, having just started the period of rapid vocabulary acquisition in both Urdu and English. Consequently, language skills may have been particularly vulnerable. This may account for why his language skills were so severely affected in the acute and post-acute stages. There is a strong body of evidence which suggests that a younger age at the time of the TBI is associated with poorer recovery of cognitive function back to pre-morbid levels and slower developmental progress post-injury (Anderson et al. 2000; Ewing-Cobbs et al. 1997). A longitudinal study by Jaffe et al. (1995) suggested that children have a relatively short period of recovery from brain injury compared to adults (12 months compared with 2 years for adults), which means that Hassan was likely to have recovered to the full extent possible from his brain injury at the time of his assessment at age 5 years.

The school and family were provided with information about Hassan's cognitive level and strategies to support him. The service was able to prepare handouts and leaflets for the family in Urdu. Recommendations were made that school should seek the advice of educational psychology and speech and language therapy. It was crucial to engage the rehabilitative health services that the family had disengaged from to ensure that Hassan's development was maximised. Although Hassan was receiving some support for his language difficulties through a group, one-to-one sessions were recommended due to the severity of his difficulties and the importance of school being provided with strategies to help support Hassan in developing his skills. Referral to occupational therapy was also recommended to help with developing Hassan's daily living skills such as dressing and toileting.

Hassan's parents were unable to accept that he had learning difficulties and expected that he would improve once his language improved. They were in agreement with a referral to speech and language therapy but were reluctant to have occupational therapy involvement as they thought that he did not need this support. Parents recognised that Hassan was experiencing significant reading delay and welcomed the targeted intervention to help him work on letter sounds and phonological awareness that school had put into place, but they were viewing these problems as relating solely to Hassan's language difficulties. The news that Hassan was already falling behind his peers in his cognitive development and academic attainments was not taken on board and the recommendation that Hassan was assessed for a Statement of Special Educational Needs to ensure that appropriate provision was in place to support him at school was not welcomed. The school had already put into place a small amount of extra classroom support, which was accepted by parents, so teachers decided against starting the process for a Statement of Special Educational Needs in accordance with parents' wishes. Regular breaks were introduced at school to manage fatigue, but Hassan was still tired and fell asleep at school. Hassan's parents were reluctant to have part-time attendance at school as they did not believe that

Hassan needed it. They were given ongoing support on managing behaviour and advised that Hassan would need to be supervised as he was at risk of injury due to his impulsiveness and lack of understanding of risk. Hassan had little appreciation of his difficulties at this stage and was generally happy at school.

Figure 8.6 outlines the formulation at age 7. Hassan's developmental experiences were still primarily rooted within his family, although there were other systems around Hassan that helped to manage his difficulties. Hassan had difficulties falling asleep, which may have resulted from his brain injury, his environment or an interaction of these factors. Brain injury is commonly associated with sleep initiation difficulties (Beebe et al. 2007). Hassan's mother usually stayed with him as he fell asleep, which may also have impacted upon him becoming independent with sleep. Hassan's mother worried that he may have a seizure and she would usually sleep in his room throughout the night. Worry around Hassan having seizures also meant that his mother continued to stay home when Hassan was at school in case he needed her. The impact of the brain injury upon the emotional wellbeing of Hassan's mother had the potential to negatively affect Hassan's development. Hassan's

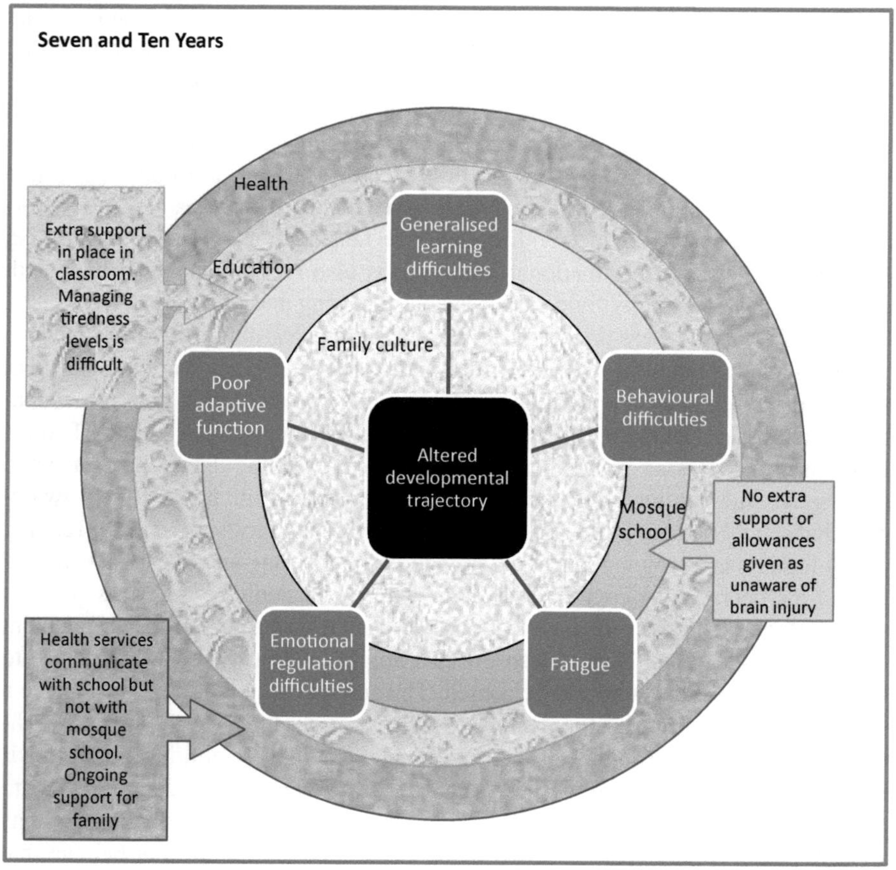

Fig. 8.6 Formulation at age 7 and 10 years

father worked long hours and his mother was the main carer, along with support from paternal grandparents. As grandparents spoke only in Urdu, bilingual communication would have been expected from Hassan.

At age 7, school was also exerting a powerful influence upon Hassan's development. The experience of participating in focused activities was improving his ability to sit and engage in work for a longer duration. In addition, the extra support that school had given Hassan, with basic strategies for improving attention and listening skills, was also likely to have helped. In a quiet setting with one-to-one support, Hassan could attend much better than he could previously; although clearly it is not possible to separate out the effects of maturation from the effects of intervention. On tests of attention and in unstructured settings, a significant weakness in attention was still evident. With intensive support, Hassan had made good progress with literacy and numeracy. His progress was better than may have been expected given his learning difficulties.

Hassan was still tired at the end of a school day. There was now the additional expectation that he attended mosque school for 1.5 hours each evening to study Islam and the Koran. Hassan sometimes fell asleep at mosque school, which embarrassed his parents. Hassan's parents had not disclosed to the community that he had experienced a brain injury. It was important to the family that Hassan attended mosque school not only for his own development but also to avoid stigma within the community. His parents were beginning to appreciate that Hassan had some difficulties with learning and that these were not temporary or confined to language difficulties. Hassan liked to attend mosque school as he wanted to engage in similar activities to his older brother. He found the teachings difficult to understand. However, he took pride in beginning to read the Koran in Arabic script. Hassan strongly identified with his brother and father and he wanted to be included in traditional male activities.

Recommendations were made for improving sleep and the family was given advice about local community services that could help them implement a behavioural sleep programme. This was not accessed as Hassan's mother did not necessarily want to leave Hassan to sleep alone. The family and school were given information about brain injury, fatigue and its management. It was highlighted that full-time school and mosque school would be too much for Hassan to cope with and that activities needed to be reduced to allow more time for rest. The school introduced breaks for Hassan but his attendance at mosque school remained unchanged. It was recommended that the school continued to support Hassan with one-to-one and small group teaching, and it was highlighted that this was going to be required throughout his academic career. It was again suggested that a Statement of Special Educational Needs would be required to support him appropriately, but this was not initiated, in accordance with parents' wishes. Hassan's severely impaired encoding and learning was highlighted and the family and school were advised that he could process only small amounts of information at any one time. The school was advised that Hassan would need information to be overlearnt through regular review and revision and that he would be unable to learn at a similar pace to his peer group. Ultimately Hassan was going to struggle to retain information and therefore the demands upon learning needed to be reduced, targeted and simplified. The families were given suggestions for visual supports to help Hassan become more independent in his activities of daily living.

Although the family did not always implement the advice given by health services, they did remain engaged. The school was also engaged with health services and sought advice on an ad hoc basis and through annual reviews. Ultimately, it had been difficult to reach a balance between the parents' understandable wish for normality for their child and the need for life to change due to Hassan's severe cognitive difficulties. Hassan's parents were planning ahead to his adolescence and adult years. In traditional Pakistani families, marriage and family are of paramount importance and males are viewed as the providers for the family. Hassan's parents believed that he would be able to marry and have a life as an independent adult. They imagined that they could arrange a marriage for him, and that his life as an adult would be normal.

When Hassan was 10 years old, his mother's English was good enough that she requested sessions without an interpreter. She disclosed that she was experiencing flashbacks and nightmares relating to the time of his accident and she understood these as being God's way of punishing her for not taking better care of Hassan. She had been experiencing these symptoms since Hassan's accident but had not disclosed this information earlier as interpreters were used and she feared that her difficulties would get back to the community. She would not discuss these experiences with her family and consequently they were unaware of these symptoms. A session was undertaken to educate her about anxiety and post-traumatic stress but onward referral for help was refused.

The neuropsychological assessment at age 10 indicated that Hassan continued to make slow progress but his teachers were reporting that his progress had stalled. Fatigue management at school had fallen off somewhat and Hassan was experiencing significant variability in his performance across days that was the likely result of fatigue. The demands of mosque school had gone up to 2 hours a day during the week and Hassan had been busy learning to read the Koran in Arabic. Parents reported he was able to read the words of the Koran, although he could not understand what he read. Hassan had developed more awareness of his difficulties and he worried that he was behind at school. His peer group was more mature in the games they wanted to play and Hassan was now socially isolated. He no longer enjoyed school and found it overwhelming. Fatigue and Hassan's emotions were likely to be contributing to the lack of progress reported at school.

In addition to Hassan developing greater awareness of his difficulties, he had also developed some simple compensatory strategies to help him manage his poor attention which he was able to use spontaneously. In view of Hassan's flat learning curve, school was supporting Hassan with his learning through simplifying information and reducing the amount of information to be remembered. Given the range of cognitive difficulties he had, it was judged unlikely that Hassan would benefit from the introduction of more complex compensatory memory strategies. A referral to occupational therapy was recommended to work on helping Hassan become more independent in his activities of daily living.

Plans were being made for Hassan's transition to secondary school and he wanted to go to the same mainstream school as his brother. This was also his parents' preference. The school had discussed with his parents the issue of whether Hassan may be better supported in a specialist placement. The neuropsychologist had also expressed doubts about whether Hassan would cope with a mainstream school. The family thought that mainstream school was the best option for Hassan and that his older brother would be able to help him at break times, if necessary.

Shortly after the assessment was completed, Hassan developed non-epileptic seizures, which seemed to be the turning point in his management and a major shift occurred in the family's acknowledgement and acceptance of his difficulties. It was challenging initially for the family and school to understand the concept of non-epileptic seizures but once they did, both systems realised that the demands on Hassan were too great. Within a few weeks, the family disclosed Hassan's difficulties to the community. They ceased sending him to mosque school, instead arranged for an elder to come to their home to complete prayers with him. The school implemented regular scheduled breaks throughout the day and reduced his school hours (Hassan missed registration). The family discussed seriously whether Hassan would cope in a mainstream school and visited several specialist provision schools to consider what may be the best placement for him. The family agreed to school applying for a Statement of Special Educational Needs. The school and family took on board that Hassan needed to build in fun and sociable activities into his schedule, and that the development of satisfying peer relationships had to be given as much importance as academic and religious activities. The family seemed to have moved into the acceptance stage of Anderson et al.'s (2001) model which allowed for more open and realistic goals and supports to be put in place.

Conclusion

Neuropsychological impairment is common in children who have experienced a moderate to severe TBI. The associated widespread damage to the brain has the potential to alter the developmental course of the child and it can permanently alter how the family functions.

Serial assessment of neuropsychological function is required in children who have sustained a TBI. If an injury was sustained in early childhood, this may mean that the child is assessed on four or five different occasions across their childhood and adolescence. Formulation is a working hypothesis that is revised with each new assessment. Assessments of neuropsychological function are used as a component part of formulation and reformulation along with other information surrounding how the child is managing within the school and home environment. Family function is an important factor to consider in the prognosis of a child after TBI. Families who understand their child's needs can advocate for their child and are in a stronger position to optimise their child's environment than families who are unable to appreciate the difficulties that their child is experiencing and how to negotiate services. It is important for neuropsychologists to appreciate the underlying beliefs and cultural factors that may play a role in whether families engage with services and the type of support that will be acceptable to them.

Continual support and intervention was likely to be ongoing for Hassan throughout his adolescence. Some families and schools are able to utilise the neuropsychological formulation to provide an optimal learning environment for the child and may only require support at times of transition. In contrast, other families require support that is continuous, especially when the child has more severe cognitive or behavioural difficulties, which was the case for Hassan.

References

Anderson, J. P., & Baron, I. S. (Eds.). (2012). Special section: Neuropsychological assessment of preschoolers. *Neuropsychology Review, 22*(4), 311–312.

Anderson, V., Catroppa, C., Morse, S., Haritou, F., & Rosenfeld, J. (2000). Recovery of intellectual ability following TBI in childhood: Impact of injury severity and age at injury. *Pediatric Neurosurgery, 32,* 282–290.

Anderson, V., Anderson, P., Northam, E., Jacobs, R., & Catroppa C. (2001a). Development of executive functions through late childhood and adolescence in an Australian sample. *Developmental Neuropsychology, 20,* 385–406.

Anderson, V., Northam, E., Hendy, J., & Wrennall, J. (2001b). *Developmental neuropsychology: A clinical approach.* New York: Psychology Press.

Anderson, V., Catroppa, C., Haritou, F., Morse, S., & Rosenfeld, J. (2005). Identifying factors contributing to child and family outcome 30 months after traumatic brain injury in children. *Journal of Neurology, Neurosurgery and Psychiatry, 76,* 401–408.

Anderson, V., Spencer-Smith, M., & Wood, A. (2011). Do children really recover better? Neurobehavioural plasticity after early brain insult. *Brain, 134,* 2197–2221.

Barke, E. M., & Williams, D. E. P. (1938). A further study of the comparative intelligence of children in certain bilingual and monoglot schools in South Wales. *British Journal of Educational Psychology, 8,* 63–77.

Baron, I. S. (2010). Maxims and a model for the practice of pediatric neuropsychology. In K. O. Yeates, M. D. Ris, H. G. Taylor, & B. F. Pennington (Eds.), *Pediatric neuropsychology*. London: Guilford.

Beebe, D. W., Krivitizky, L., Wells, C. T., Wade, S. L., Taylor, G. H., & Yeates, K. O. (2007). Brief report: Parental report of sleep behaviors following moderate or severe paediatric traumatic brain injury. *Journal of Pediatric Psychology, 32,* 845–850.

Breslau, N. (1990). Does brain dysfunction increase children's vulnerability to environmental stress? *Archives of General Psychiatry, 47,* 15–20.

Byrd, D., Arentoft, A., Schneiner, D., Westerveld, M., & Baron, I. S. (2008). State of multicultural neuropsychological assessment in children: Current research issues. *Neuropsychology Review, 18,* 214–222.

Catroppa, C., Anderson, V., Godfrey, C., & Rosenfeld, J. V. (2011). Attentional skills 10 years post-paediatric traumatic brain injury (TBI). *Brain Injury, 25,* 858–869.

Crawford, J. R., Anderson, V., Rankin, P. M., & MacDonald, J. (2009). An Index-based short-form of the WISC-IV with accompanying analysis of the reliability and abnormality of differences. *British Journal of Clinical Psychology, 49,* 235–258.

Dennis, M. (1989). Language and the young damaged brain. In T. Boll & B. K. Bryant (Eds.), *Clinical neuropsychology and brain function: Research, measurement and practice*. Washington: American Psychological Association.

Donders, J. (1993). Memory functions after traumatic brain injury in children. *Brain Injury, 7,* 421–437.

Donders, J., Elzinga, B., Kulpers, D., Helder, E., & Crawford, J. R. (2013). Development of an eight-subtest short form of the WISC-IV and evaluation of its clinical utility in children with traumatic brain injury. *Child Neuropsychology, 19,* 662–670.

Ewing-Cobbs, L., Fletcher, J. M., Levin, H. S., Francis, D. J., Davidson, K., & Miner, M. E. (1997). Longitudinal neuropsychological outcome in infants and preschoolers with traumatic brain injury. *Journal of the International Neuropsychological Society, 3,* 581–591.

Ewing-Cobbs, L., Barnes, M., Fletcher, J. M., Levin, H. S., Swank, P. R., & Song, J. (2004). Modeling of longitudinal academic achievement scores after pediatric traumatic brain injury. *Developmental Neuropsychology, 25,* 107–133.

Garrett, L. C., & Kelly, T. P. (2007). To what extent does bilingualism affect children's performance on the NEPSY? *Child Neuropsychology, 14,* 71–81.

Harris, J. G., & Llorente, A. M. (2005). Cultural considerations in the use of the wechsler intelligence scale for children-fourth edition (WISC–IV). In A. Prifitera, D. H. Saklofske, & L. G. Weiss (Eds.), *WISC-IV clinical use and interpretation.* London: Elsevier.

Jaffe, K. M., Polissar, N. L., Fay, G. C., & Liao, S. (1995). Recovery trends over three years following pediatric traumatic brain injury. *Archives of Physical Medicine Rehabilitation, 76,* 17–26.

Kolb, B., & Gibb, R. (2011). Brain plasticity and behaviour in the developing brain. *Journal of the Canadian Academy of Child and Adolescent Psychiatry, 20,* 265–276.

Marchman, V. A., Fernald, A., & Hurtado, N. (2009). How vocabulary size in two languages relates to efficiency in spoken word recognition by young Spanish-English bilinguals. *Journal of Child Language, 37,* 817–840.

Meyers, J., & Meyers, K. (1996). *Rey complex figure and the recognition trial: Professional manual. Supplemental norms for children.* Odessa: Psychological Resources Assessment.

Muscara, F., Catroppa, C., & Anderson, V. (2008). The impact of injury severity on executive function 7–10 years following pediatric traumatic brain injury. *Developmental Neuropsychology, 33*(5), 623–636.

Office for National Statistics. (2011). Census: Aggregate data (England and Wales). https://www.ons.giv.uk.

Oller, D. K., Pearson, B. Z., & Cobo-Lewis, A. B. (2007). Profile effects in early bilingual language and literacy. *Applied Psycholinguistics, 28,* 191–230.

Patterson, J., & Pearson, B. Z. (2004). Bilingual lexical development: Influences, contexts, and processes. In G. Goldstein (Ed.), *Bilingual language development and disorders in Spanish-English speakers.* Baltimore: Paul Brookes.

Poulin-Dubois, D., Bialystok, E., Blaye, A., Polonia, A., & Yott, J. (2012). Lexical access and vocabulary development in very young bilinguals. *International Journal of Bilingualism, 17,* 57–70.

Prifitera, A., Saklofske, D. H., Weiss, L. G., & Rolfhus, E. (2005). WISC–IV: Foundations of interpretation. In A. Prifitera, D. H. Saklofske, & L. G. Weiss (Eds.), *WISC-IV clinical use and interpretation.* London: Elsevier.

Taylor, H. G., & Schatschneider, C. (1992). Academic achievement following childhood brain disease: Implications for the concept of learning disabilities. *Journal of Learning Disabilities, 25,* 630–638.

Wechsler, D. (2004). *Wechsler intelligence scale for children* (4th ed.). New York: Harcourt Assessment.

Yeates, K. O. (2010). Traumatic brain injury. In K. O. Yeates, M. D. Ris, H. G. Taylor, & B. F. Pennington (Eds.), *Pediatric neuropsychology.* London: Guilford.

Yeates, K. O., Swift, E., Taylor, H. G., Wade, S. L., Drotar, D., Stancin, T., & Minich, N. (2004). Short- and long-term social outcomes following pediatric traumatic brain injury. *Journal of the International Neuropsychological Society, 10,* 412–426.

Yeates, K. O., Armstrong, K., Janusz, J., Taylor, G. H., Wade, S., Stancin, T., et al. (2005). Long-term attention problems in children with traumatic brain injury. *Journal of the American Academy of Child and Adolescent Psychiatry, 44,* 574–584.

Chapter 9
An Integrative Approach to Differential Diagnosis of Subarachnoid Haemorrhage and Korsakoff's Dementia

Martha Sorensen

In a case involving review of a gentleman following a quantifiable subarachnoid haemorrhage (SAH) and the cognitive impact on his life (Greebe et al. 2010; Becske et al. 2010; van Gijn et al. 2007; Feigin et al. 2005), the findings were actually not so obvious until a neuropsychological evaluation was completed and additional investigation took place. SAH with probable underlying and unidentified Korsakoff dementia (also known as Wernicke–Korsakoff syndrome; Ingram et al. (2003)) was indicated after careful review of findings, identification of inconsistencies, and a thorough interview with collateral sources. It greatly impacted the expected outcome, discharge planning, and longer term follow-up.

Work Setting/Introduction

The setting for this case was a large, public teaching hospital servicing some of the country's most diverse populations, spanning the lowest to highest socioeconomic levels. A multidisciplinary team approach with a clearly identified stroke pathway was used. For those who can participate in ongoing medical rehabilitation, the provision of services focuses on the relearning of activities versus compensation which is used when the patient lacks the ability to relearn a task. This begins in the hospital and is carried over into the community following discharge. The role of the team neuropsychologist was as a specialist taking on cases only after screens and functional evaluations by other team members were completed. If those screenings did not provide enough information to explain the patient's symptoms and behaviours, and act as a guide for treatment, a more in-depth review and further assessment would be completed by the neuropsychologist. The primary contributions would be in the clarification of diagnosis, identification of strengths and weaknesses in abili-

M. Sorensen (✉)
AT&R Unit, Middlemore Hospital, Neuropsychology and Rehabilitation, Colvin Complex, Reception B, Private Bag 93311, Otahuhu, Auckland 1640, New Zealand
e-mail: Martha.Sorensen@middlemore.co.nz

J. A. B. Macniven (ed.), *Neuropsychological Formulation*,
DOI 10.1007/978-3-319-18338-1_9

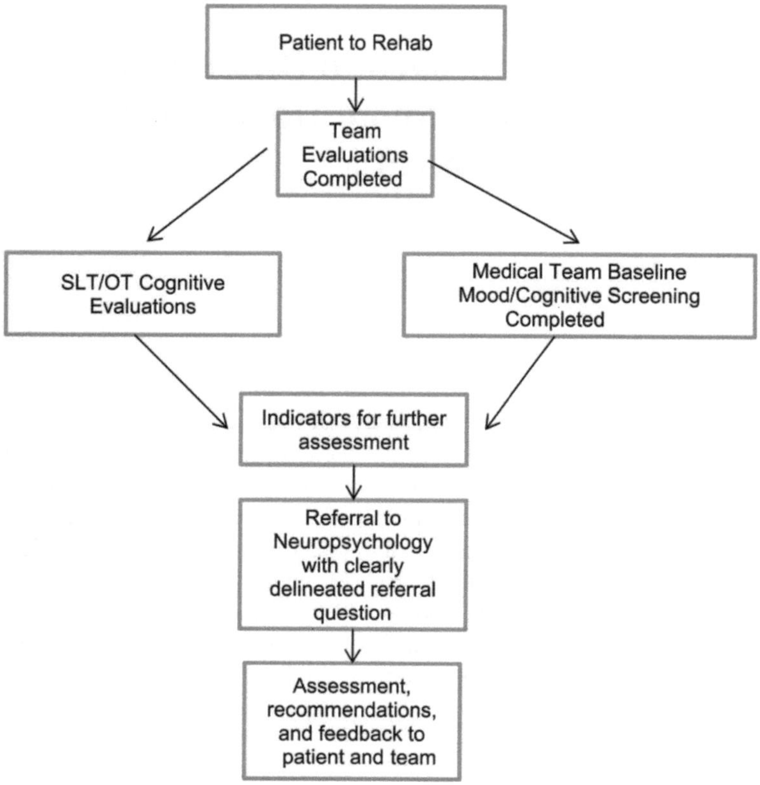

Fig. 9.1 Referral process

ties, recommendation of strategies for management of symptoms, and guidance of treatments in hospital. Additionally, findings would be incorporated into discharge planning for ongoing community rehabilitation efforts (Fig. 9.1).

The Process of Evaluation

Following a set process of evaluation allows more efficient use of services and clarity in evaluations. It guides the flow of work, the processing of findings, and the ability to provide clear, concise results for the referring party. While each evaluation is unique with unique requirements, the process remains relatively stable and is described above. This chapter describes a case, used to highlight the process with suggestions on how to create an approach to gathering and managing data (often large amounts), review and consolidation, and how to use results for presentation in a meaningful way.

Receipt and Review Referral

Upon receipt of a new referral, a determination of the purpose and focus of the assessment takes place. Clarifying the purpose of the assessment helps us to avoid unnecessary testing, clinician frustration, and saves time and resources. For example, is the referral focused on understanding abilities/deficits, looking at return to work, assessing complicating factors, reviewing safety, making a differential diagnosis, measuring overall cognitive functioning, educating a capacity evaluation, or evaluating if and what type of brain damage might be present?

Having a discussion with the referring clinician at the outset of the assessment helps us to assure clear understanding of the question to be answered. Knowing the referral question is important: without clarity, the focus of the assessment might go in the wrong direction. For example, if the referral asks for a diagnostic clarification and instead findings highlight strengths and weaknesses without the requested findings, this could leave the referring clinician frustrated once results are presented. With a focused referral question, assessment efforts will be more directed and the tendency to over-test can be avoided. Use of the additional information gleaned from discussions can guide and focus the assessment, interpretation, and feedback. This enables increased certainty the information gathered will be of use to both the patient and the clinician, make efficient use of resources, and decrease the chance of over-testing.

The tendency to fill the space between referral and the real question with too much testing is a common and easily managed problem. Over-testing puts off referrers as well as causes unnecessary patient stress and over exposure to testing measures.

It is a bit like answering a "why?" question without understanding what they really want to know. Rather than answering vague "why" questions (e.g. "please review cognition" or "assess mood and cognition"), it is useful to focus the process and answer by using a scientific method approach: asking questions of who (who is the patient/client, the referring party, audience the report goes to, etc.), what (what is the purpose of this evaluation, the intent of use for findings, what will this evaluation add to patient care, what agencies are involved-hospital, community teams, private clinicians, insurance carriers, disability/ACC/military, etc.), where (inpatient, outpatient, school, forensic, medical, mental health, etc.), when (when is it needed, when did the injury occur, when is the patient available for assessment, etc.), and how (how long in the hospital, how findings used, how in depth does this need to be, how will results be provided, etc.). This ultimately provides the answer to "why."

Meetings with patients and family members overseeing their care prior to testing are used to help build rapport, review role and purpose of testing, and receive consent; verbal consent is generally all that is required for in-patient evaluations as they have completed consent for treatment forms on admission. However, written consent is easy to collect and highly recommended regardless of the setting or purpose of the assessment. Reviewing consent allows a patient time to understand the purpose of assessment, the demands being requested of them, and allows the clinician to respond to questions while further assessing the willingness of the patient to fully participate. In addition, this is a good time to assess appropriateness of the referral and testing of this patient. Doing this prior to starting data collection (including records review) helps prevent unnecessary work; at this juncture, discovery of declined assessment might occur and all actions stopped until a plan is clearly identified. While most assessments continue after further discussion with patient and family, there are times when assessment is declined regardless of the treating team's requests.

Once consent is received and prior to actual testing, attendance at the multidisciplinary team meeting allows time to discuss the patient with team members. A review on their findings, concerns, needs for assessment, and coordinate testing time within the rehabilitation schedule is essential. Other activities to complete prior to assessment would include a full review of records, viewing of scans, seeking of additional written records (previous level of functioning, work-related information, etc.), previous testing/screens, review of capacity issues, and identification of holder for enduring power of attorney for those patients not considered capable of providing full consent at this stage. This serves as a preparation of the clinician's focus for the assessment.

Consideration of the use of the collected data is important. Keeping in mind questions such as, "How is this assessment impacting patient rehabilitation?" (or use of questions appropriate for the setting/situation) helps to keep the assessment focused on outcome and purpose. Reviewing issues of culture, language and verbal comprehension, patient ability to comply with testing demands, physical limitations, time of day and duration constraints, time from assessment to discharge time which results are required, and a practiced avoidance of over-testing helps us to guide choices and minimises patient stress.

Appointments and Follow-Up

Setting up appointment times to complete evaluations allows for patient certainty and mental preparation for the task ahead. It also allows for preparation to meet special needs in the assessment; if an interpreter is needed or special arrangements need to be made to accommodate communication, vision, hearing, or movement issues, these are addressed prior to evaluation and save valuable time.

Providing a quiet space for both the assessment and feedback sessions with patient/family after evaluation is completed allows for assessment and discussion without interruption or confusion as to where and when to meet. Including a table/desk, good lighting, good ventilation, and allowance for sufficient space to accommodate special needs (wheelchairs, extra seating, etc.) provides ease of assessment. Consideration of the location of assessment room helps to assure patient and family are comfortable and put at ease, thus decreasing the potential effects of anxiety.

Assessment

Patient reviews may need to be done over several shorter sessions to accommodate fatigue issues following illness/acquired brain injury (ABI)/traumatic brain injury (TBI), or fatigue related to age. The length of the testing session tolerated is clinically relevant in interpreting findings. Caution is advised in not fatiguing a patient beyond their capabilities for their best performance unless the goal of assessment includes determination of fatigue's part in the assessment. This is a common aspect of rehabilitation testing and is monitored carefully.

Interviews with patient, family, or collaborative sources (employer, teacher, and friends) for in-depth history and collaborative history taking would commence during the assessment phase. This can be abbreviated if a good history already exists but the use of interviews can help to confirm information already gathered highlighting unknown facts that would help to clarify findings, or inaccuracies found in the record that may skew findings. Setting a feedback session date puts forth a deadline for results; clinicians are less inclined to procrastinate in scoring and writing up results, puts a stop to chasing information, and prevents delayed feedback thus keeping the information fresh and useful (Fig. 9.2).

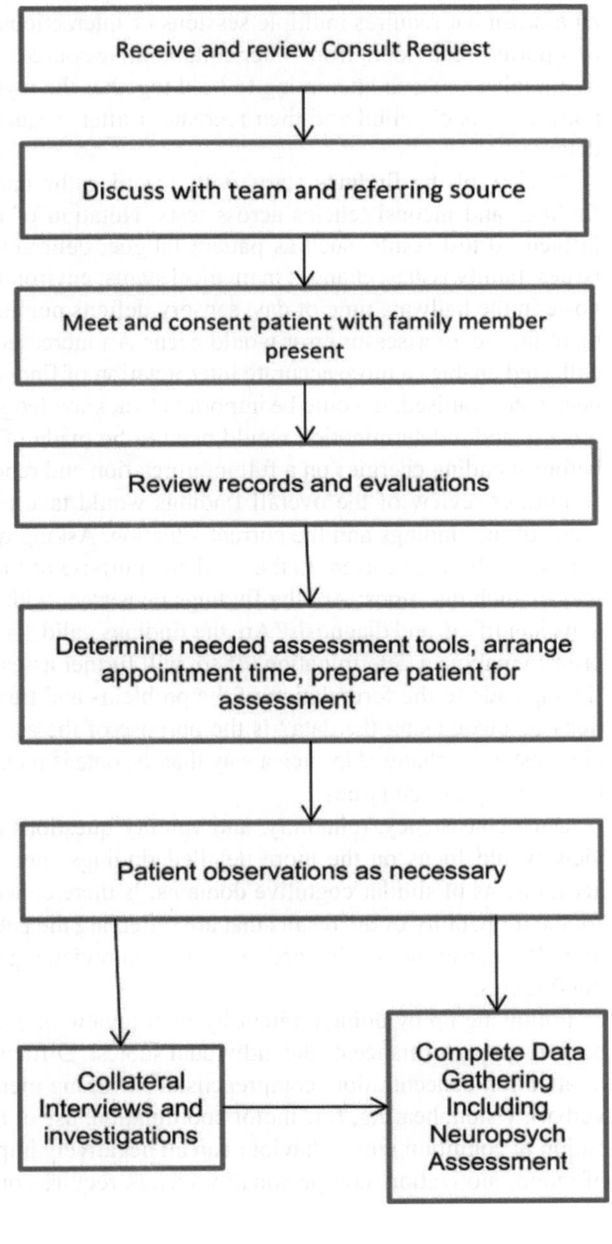

Fig. 9.2 Data gathering

Scoring and Review

Scoring results as soon as possible, making notations of observations, difficulties during the assessment, utterances by patient during testing, behavioural observations, and tracking a general sense of the assessment session allow for maintenance of the gleaned information. These types of observations can be lost or quickly forgotten when other patient issues come up between the actual assessment and times of scoring and interpretation. Process information impacts on the interpretation of the data collected and informs beyond the snapshot gained in the data collection time. These observations can be useful in making comparisons across times when an assessment requires multiple sessions or interactions, and used as comparisons to reported behaviours from other collaborative sources. It also decreases the levels of clinician stress in attempting to hold together the myriad of informational components in one's mind and then recreate it after frequent interruptions or lengthy delays.

Review of the findings starts with scanning the data collected for validity of findings and inconsistencies across tests. Notation of any factors that may have influenced test results such as patient fatigue, delirium, confusion, mental health issues, family issues, changes in medical status, environmental disturbances such as noise in the hallway, time of day, sensory deficits not noted prior to testing, equipment failure, or assessor error would occur. An increased understanding of the data collected enables a more accurate interpretation of findings. If the testing data have been compromised, it would be important to acknowledge early in the interpretation process and a determination would need to be made of the usefulness of the data before spending energies on a full interpretation and report.

Further review of the overall findings would take place looking for a general sense of the findings and the current situation. Asking questions during this phase keeps the clinician current to the need and purpose of the assessment. Some examples of such questions: Are the findings consistent with the reported illness, problems identified, and diagnosis? Are the findings valid? Is more information required prior to making a determination? If so, will further assessment be required? Do the findings add to the formulation of the problems and treatment? Can recommendations be made using the data? Is the purpose of the assessment still valid or have circumstances changed in such a way that the data is rendered useless or invalid due to externally driven issues?

Once consistency, reliability, and validity questions are considered, further review would focus on the more detailed findings specifically looking at patterns across items of similar cognitive domains. Is there consistency across domains? If so, the probability of the results that are reflecting the patient situation accurately is high. If not, caution would need to be taken in reviewing the results and in reporting the findings.

Following up by doing an item-by-item review of each test helps us to identify patterns in performance of the individual subtest. Difficulties in specific areas such as attention/concentration, comprehension, working memory, language (written or verbal), vision, hearing, fine motor coordination, use of manipulatives, and coordination of cognition with behaviour can all negatively impact findings. Examination of mood, motivation, and personality factors require consideration as well as they impact performance and outcomes significantly. Reviewing results for effects of education (e.g. illiteracy) could prove crucial as not all patients admit to being illiterate out of embarrassment and it is only in the assessment process this is identified.

Use of short, written summaries of each test administered provides a general summary of findings, a detailed look at the aforementioned items, and overall impression for analysis. Noting thoughts in this phase of how other test findings reviewed might collaborate or refute the individual test findings can be useful. Additionally, keeping notes regarding the findings in relation to the injury (in this case SAH: Are they consistent or inconsistent?) can be beneficial and point out discrepancies requiring follow-up or clarification.

In a medical setting, it would not be uncommon to run into findings or illnesses unfamiliar to the clinician. Literature searches focused on expected neuropsychological findings for the particular situation would illuminate expected patterns or breaks from the expected patterns. In this case, consultation with a colleague would be very acceptable and useful. Peer group discussions to help in the understanding and formulation of a case, and/or individual supervision to discuss the case in more depth would also be appropriate; remembering the goal is to help better understand the findings and use of them requires a good understanding by the clinician so dissemination of information educates and informs the patient, family and team.

Once the general reviews, the more detailed reviews and the initial impressions are formed, it is helpful to review the referral question again to determine if more information or assessment is needed to answer it clearly and concisely. If more information is needed, follow-up with patient and family, team members, or referring clinician may answer the questions easily. Or additional tests might need to be completed if any tests were considered invalid, the results are out of date (there have been significant changes in a patient's health status or cognition, delays in completion of the assessment, etc.), or there continues to be a lack of clarity between the findings and the patient behaviours.

The Report

Report writing can be the most difficult part of an assessment to complete. Using a fairly prescribed format, placed in template form, can ease the process significantly. Alterations can be made to reflect the type of case, the purpose of the evaluation, the referral question, and the audience's level of understanding of neuropsychological findings. The length of neuropsychological report and what is covered can change each time one's written. The formatting of the report is dependent on the setting, type of assessment (forensic, neuropsychology, rehabilitation, in-patient, out-patient and return to work/school), audience reviewing results, time frame allowed for completed assessment, and current reporting trends in neuropsychology (industry and legal standards). Again, many neuropsychologists find the written report the most anxiety provoking and labour intensive aspect of neuropsychological evaluations. Use of a template allows for the quick alteration of format without losing the overall gestalt of your findings across assessments and aids in the management of author anxiety.

Time constraints often require fitting report writing into a very full day and finding extended hours to complete this process in one sitting is rare. Beginning the write-up as soon as information becomes available across the entire evaluation helps to manage the data collected, the time available for write-up, and ease at determining gaps of information required to make an assessment. Turnaround time in the rehabilitation/hospital setting can be short for inpatient evaluations with longer time frames for outpatient evaluations; making use of short periods of time is very beneficial.

Demographics, known medical issues (illness/diagnosis, medications, known drug/alcohol/smoking/health factors that might impact on findings), social history a brief overview of early childhood, education, vocation, interests, recent activities, marital/relational issues that might impact on findings, etc., are usually available in the early stages and these sections can be completed prior to actual testing taking place. Additional information gleaned during the active process of the assessment can be input as work continues and throughout the assessment. These processes allow early identification of inconsistencies in information across the rehab situation and quick follow-up during the assessment. While some reports require brief histories, others benefit from detailed histories to put the findings into perspective and the report can be tailored to reflect specific requirements.

As testing is completed and the data is scored, checking for disqualifiers that portion of the assessment is important. Using the referral question as a guide, in determine if further testing is required in that domain to clarify findings. Disqualification of data can happen for a multitude of issues (medical issues, interruptions due to environmental issues, patient fatigue, patient frustration, etc.). If data are disqualified, making a clear statement and providing explanation for disqualification and potential implications for the assessment would be expected.

After completing the summary write-ups for the individual tests and pulling together the various findings, comparisons can be made across tests sharing similar cognitive domains. Watching for outliers and findings inconsistent with the majority of findings, a look for trends and patterns can begin. If there is not enough data to make comparisons (only one test within in this assessment was used or remains valid), a statement of understanding that the findings reflect only one element of measure within the domain and may not fully or accurately reflect the patient's abilities or difficulties would be appropriate.

Once all the data have been analysed at general, detailed, and cross-comparison levels, making summary statements about the various domains (e.g. attention measures = all finding divided attention difficulties in the mild–moderate ranges with some variability noted dependent on the length of time required to attend, complexity of task, etc.) can aid in the final written report. Each domain is addressed as a whole, not as an individual test: assimilated results are best received by most referral sources. In some evaluations, there needs to be much more detailed reporting of the scores, variations, individual findings, and how each of them impacted on the overall test findings; this is especially true in forensic evaluations or those with high impact on one's future. In general, the work of the neuropsychologist in the rehab setting involves both basic and very complex neuropsychological assessments. The type of report required is dependent on the age of the patient, the need to return to school or work, the question of capacity, the ability to retest in the future, and providing scores for comparison reasons in future evaluations. In these cases, keeping a separate page for actual test results would be appropriate and can be added to the end of the report for reference by those in need of the information. It is also acceptable to place this information in the body of the report but experience suggests most prefer it separated out to encourage reading of the report by referral sources.

Once the report has been written with assimilation of results, a review of the report with a summary of the results is completed. Placing a brief summary at the top of the report allows presentation of the salient findings for those who need a quick review. This is generally kept to less than half a page. There is always a note of encouragement to read the entire report in order to best understand the findings included. It is up to the individual reader to determine whether they require more information than the summary provides, would glean any further understanding of the patient, or if they only need to have a summary version in order to proceed with their treatment planning.

A full report is written, with discussion of issues of concern, additional findings, and recommendations for follow-up. Recommendations are directed to the referring clinician first (follow-up blood work, scans, testing of hearing, vision, movement, or medication review, etc.), to staff providing treatment (actions to take for rehab, discharge planning, and additional assessments to aid in patient care following discharge, etc.), and to the patient and family in general. The recommendations are meant to encourage the patient and family to continue on with their rehab once they return home. For some patients there is ongoing rehabilitation with staff after discharge, for others there is not. Making use of the report to make suggestions to enhance their recovery and life gives the report a stronger sense of purpose, aids clinicians attempting to help the patient after hospitalisation, provides a measurement of what the patient is willing and able to do for themselves, and guides other clinicians in their work (SLT, OT, PT, SW, Rehab specialists). It also provides the patient and family members with an understanding of the need to stay involved in their care following discharge.

The findings are reviewed with the patient and supportive family/friends that they want present. Discussion regarding the testing, findings, meaning and purpose of the findings, relevant concerns needing follow-up, and who they need to be in contact with for that follow-up is completed. Close review of the recommendations with provision of rationale behind them to enhance follow-up is completed. While recommendations are discussed with the medial and treatment team, the patient and family need to implement or follow-up on many items following discharge thus making it essential they understand them so they make best use of their efforts. This is the crux of the assessment for many patients and unfortunately one area that is often lacking.

A full copy of the report is placed in the medical chart with the patient's consent. Often personality testing is a part of the evaluation; when this occurs, a full discussion around the findings with the potential impact of releasing to a medical record is discussed. They have the right to determine whether this aspect of the assessment is included. If they opt to not include this portion, it is noted in the report that personality assessment was completed as part of the evaluation but not included secondary to confidentiality issues and on procurement of a signed release of information from the patient, it can be provided to the appropriate clinicians. However, a general statement is included regarding impact of personality on current rehabilitation (i.e. person showed high reliance on others prior to ABI and continues to need high levels of support). Should a patient not agree to releasing the full report to the medical record, a summary of findings (with patient knowledge) is released without full elaboration and a note informing the reader they can obtain a copy with full, written consent from the patient or family member in charge of their care. The complication of the hospital being the referring party, the need for the results to fully understand the patient's needs, and the benefits of releasing the information to the responsible clinicians would be discussed with both the patient and patient's family/caregiver should this situation arise.

Follow-up with the referring party and the team as needed is done immediately after the patient's feedback. Providing patient the information first allows them time to reflect and assimilate the news. Often they are faced with cognitive changes they may or may not fully understand or recognise within themself. It is also time to explain results, answer questions, and correct any misinformation. Inpatient follow-up with the patient during their hospitalisation is continued through individual meetings, team meetings, family meetings, and discharge meetings with outside entities. This is to encourage follow through, answer new questions, address treatment needs, and support the patient and family during the remainder of their rehabilitation.

Storage of both raw data and results is managed with regards to legal requirements for medical/psychological materials. It is imperative to maintain this for both the protection of patient confidentiality and copy right laws for assessment measures (Fig. 9.3)

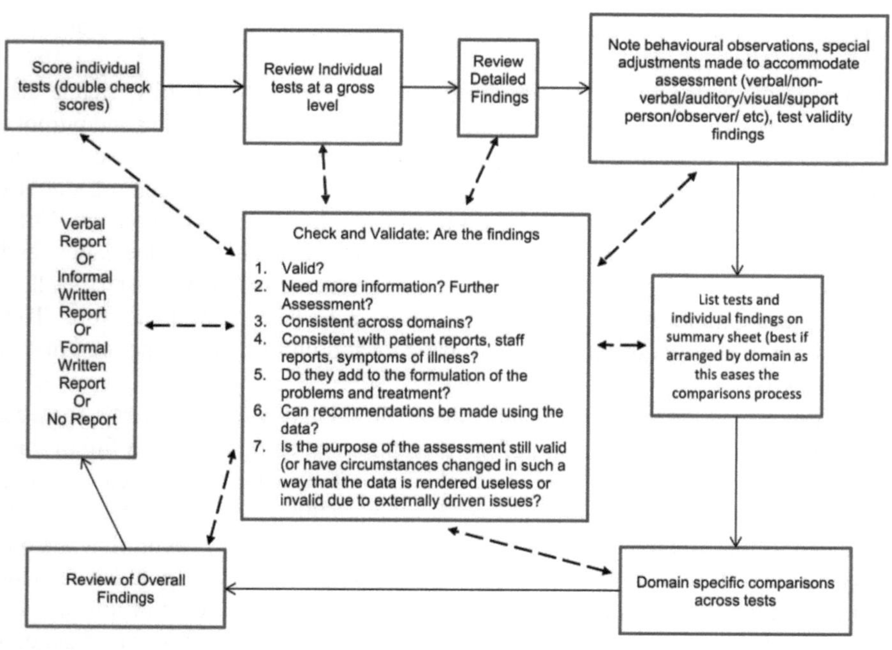

Fig. 9.3 Data analysis and write-up

Mr B

Background/Referral
After careful discussion and review of the purpose and limitations for the use of information gathered during evaluation and limitations and efforts to protect identity, both verbal and written consent were provided by patient and his wife who was acting on his behalf.

Initial Referral to Neuropsychologist
Mr B was a 67-year-old European male, usually fit and well with nil previous medical history with the exception of being a heavy, long-term smoker. He was status post surgery following a large SAH; blood was found in the lateral ventricles with hydrocephalus. His initial prognosis for recovery was poor but he showed marked improvement during his acute hospital stay.

His initial assessments (both functional and cognitive) were completed by various allied health staff. While he began his rehabilitation showing marked improvement in communication, alertness and interaction with others, he continued to be confused around issues of time, sit for long periods of time without activity or interest, and began behaving in ways that caused confusion amongst the staff in knowing how to handle his cares. A referral was sent with the following questions: "Please provide an overview of cognitive function and recommendations to enhance rehabilitation efforts. Discharge planning delayed due to need for this information and clarity of diagnosis. Please review behaviours that appear to be changing daily and not responding to the traditional responses by staff." He had progressed as one with SAH was expected but only to a point. His lack of continued progress and "odd" behaviour were the key concerns.

Relevant Medical History
This gentleman presented to Emergency Department via ambulance after being found by his wife with abnormal breathing early in the morning. He was intubated on arrival and transported to CT. Computer tomography angiogram (CTA) review identified a multilocular 8 mm anterior communicating artery aneurysm with rupture; blood extending into the ventricles including fourth ventricle with acute hydrocephalus. Primary diagnosis: sub-arachnoid hemorrhage (SAH), unspecified (SAH). He was stabilised and sent to neurosurgery for external ventricular drain (EVD) placement and supportive care. Over the next few days, he improved (GCS 10, E4, V1 and M5) and continued to improve up to about a week later when he required a second surgery to reinsert a permanent shunt. He also underwent coiling of the identified aneurysm rupture. At that time he showed moderate confusion and lower limb weakness but was alert and able to follow commands.

Diagnosis: primary: subarachnoid haemorrhage (SAH)
Secondary: anterior communicating artery (ACOM) aneurysm (coiled)
Hydrocephalus (ventricular peritoneal (VP) shunt inserted)

Sources of Information
Patient records and scans were reviewed carefully. Consultation with team members was held with discussions regarding previous test findings. A full clinical inter-

view with the patient and patient's wife was completed. The measures selected for the assessment included the Repeatable Battery for the Assessment of Neuropsychological Status-Form A (RBANS; Randolph 1998), Behavioral Dyscontrol Scale (BDS; Grigsby and Kaye 1996), Number and Writing Samples, Clock (Eknoyan et al. 2012).

Social History: Initial Evaluation Found the Following
On interview, Mr B was alert, maintained good eye contact, had a mild dysarthria, showed good verbal comprehension, reported difficulties with short-term memory (STM), and showed good humour. He was cooperative but fatigued easily.

He was born in England at the end of the World War II (WWII). He and his family moved to New Zealand when he was 5 years old (parents and two siblings). He is the middle child and only boy. He grew up in a very small beach community southeast of a large city. He liked his youth and growing up "care free." He was allowed freedom to wander around town, swim and play freely. He did chores at home but was not greatly overloaded or hindered. He denied any difficulties related to home life or trouble with authorities.

Schooling was limited. He declared himself "not academic" so he stopped formal schooling by age 14. He began working almost immediately in jobs with his father. At the age of 17, he took his first "adult" job. His overall employment focused primarily in sales, providing security and, later in life, consulting others on security systems. Any further education he attained took place on the job. He was reported as being successful in business in spite of educational limitations and opportunities.

Socially he spent his youth "running with the boys," "learning to drink a bit, smoke and meet girls." Once he began working, he spent even more of his spare time socialising with his peers. He never played sports and preferred just "hanging out with the boys" doing "boy things." He started using alcohol at a very early age (12) and drank socially for the majority of his life. He denied using drugs during his lifetime. He smoked most of his life, at times quite heavily. Physically he was fit and healthy rarely going to the doctor.

He met and married for the first time around age 19 but divorced after 10 years of what he described as "a stress filled life together due to too many differences." He remarried after an extended period of years and remains married to his life partner of more than 30 years. This relationship was described as a "good marriage" and "quite comfortable." Mr B's living situation prior to his stroke was middle-class living, working on a large property. While semiretired, he worked their large lifestyle block as well as working nights on a part-time basis, sleeping during the day while his wife worked days. This allowed them evenings together. He enjoyed his home projects, gardening, and being very involved with his wife and friends socially. His relationships with his siblings and two grown adult children were reported as being close. His marital relationship was reported as strong and supportive.

Initial reports of alcohol use were vague or nonexistent in history taking and in records. One report suggested he drank limited alcohol (two to three glasses of wine a few nights a week: social drinking only). Initially, Mr B's reports relating to alcohol use were "Never drank beer," "Never got drunk, only social drinker." No more information on alcohol use was available.

Team Review
Initial discussions started with the multidisciplinary team through multidisciplinary meetings or with individual clinicians reviewing their findings and assessments across the services. In this case, Mr B started on the restorative care ward due to the initial prognosis being poor. He settled into restorative care but remained confused. An initial contact with psychology requested cognitive assessment. This was attempted 2 months post surgery by the covering psychologist but was eventually declined due to the patient not being able to participate with evaluation (fell asleep during evaluation, confusion). He later was returned to surgery for increasing confusion. It was found he had bilateral subdural haematomas with midline shift.

Over a month's time, he showed good signs of recovery and was moved to the rehabilitation ward for a more intensive, active rehabilitation. A request for evaluation by psychology was received four and a half months following the SAH. Initial assessments had been completed by other staff members but were inconclusive and staff felt uncertain as to what to do with the patient on discharge. In order to direct discharge planning and management on the ward there needed to be an understanding of his general level of functioning.

Chart Review
An initial chart review was completed taking notes for relevant data. Medical diagnosis, initial evaluations, screening tests and issues related to psychological difficulties (mood, previous mental health issues, family issues, alcohol/drugs, legal issues) were all carefully screened for during this phase. Making use of a detailed interview format developed by the clinician for gathering information provided comprehensive information to educate the assessment. While the questionnaire has been tailored to fit the current setting and needs, it has gone through many format changes depending on the setting, purpose, and amount of detail needed to complete the requested evaluation. Since there were many parties involved in this patient's care, as much information possible was gleaned from the record, filling in as many portions of the form as possible prior to meeting with the patient. This information was used as collaborative data to compare against during the interview phase of evaluation with the patient and family members. The interview information provided was used to look for inconsistencies in reports, difficulties in completion of assessments, and making comparisons between evaluations where data was already collected. This formed the basis for the social history, test selection, and informed the interpretation and write-up of findings.

Records from earlier assessments such as the Montreal Cognitive Assessment *MOCA Version 7,* which measures short-term memory, visuospatial, executive functioning, attention/concentration, and working memory (Nasreddine et al. 2005), showed difficulties in orientation, attention/calculation, recall, repetition and sentence writing. He was unable to copy a design without significant distortion. His handwriting was reported to be "almost illegible, small in size and showing tremor." Clock-drawing attempts showed the ability to hold form with some distortion on left side. Numbers were placed correctly but repeated. The time indicated was incorrect. Insight into error was variable in that he recognised some errors but not others.

Later attempts at assessment by others found that he continued to have difficulties in orientation, visuospatial, executive functioning, attention, low verbal fluency, and delayed recall for verbal information.

Additional information was discovered during review of the records and in further discussions with patient and wife. In the notes, there were references by several staff stating that he made vague or subtle sexually suggestive comments. There were no overt actions or behaviours noted that caused distress but these subtle comments increased in frequency as he recovered and across a variety of staff and situations. When questioned about the thoughts behind this behaviour, he denied doing such things and did not recall any such events.

Further he was reported as having poor short-term memory, difficulties with time management, decreased attention/concentration, confusion regarding events, and often blending activities and time in "strange" ways, decreased insight into his behaviours and lacking in motivation. Staff reported he appeared to be lying to them regarding events as he told a variety of stories about his history, activities, and other people's actions. This created difficult staff interactions as well as made it difficult to gain an accurate history from him. On interview I noted his tendency to fill in information he could not fully recall, almost always on inquiry (probable confabulation). He did not appear to be confabulating without inquiry. He did not appear to be purposely misrepresenting himself or his actions. An obvious melding of ideas, memories, and stories with no clear temporal context was taking place (e.g. he gave a credible sounding work history but dates of employment were years off and tasks completed were not his jobs but those of his father's). He firmly believed what he was presenting and when querying his responses, he became somewhat distraught at not being believed. He would then withdraw from conversation, becoming quiet and disengaged. Confabulation is a memory disturbance and presents as fabricated, distorted, or misinterpreted memories about oneself or the world. This is without conscious effort or intention to deceive (Thomson and Marshall 2006; Sechi and Serra 2007; Kyoko 2009; Thomson et al. 2008; Kopelman et al.2009; Kessels et al. 2008). His lack of awareness about the falseness of the information, the fact that his responses held some truth to his history and daily activities, and observations that responses ranged from subtle alterations of the truth to strange combinations (e.g. "I worked in a morgue embalming dead bodies but as a security guard") all supported confabulation versus lying.

During initial interview, his wife identified changes starting approximately 2 years prior to the SAH. She noted he had become more withdrawn, less active, more forgetful, less engaging with her and family, and seemed to lack interest for he would loved to do before. Although previously he was interested and active in his gardens, on the property and with others, he now showed disinterest. He spent prolonged periods of time watching television or "just sitting." He rarely did the chores he normally took care of without prompt or "outright nagging." His sleep patterns were difficult to determine as he worked 2–3 nights per week while his wife was away during the days. His ability to provide an accurate history proved difficult due to short-term memory problems.

In light of the newer findings, a fuller alcohol history was taken. She noted he drank more in the evenings with her (prior to going to work). They used to have a glass or two of wine (large) but this was now at least 4–5 on his part. He often finished off an evening with gin or hard liquor. Both of them denied his drinking beer at initial interview. Ultimately it was identified that he drank as much as 2 L of wine, one bottle of spirits, and two–three six-packs of beer per day. He took to hiding the bottles or explaining them away. His social history had him drinking as early as 12 years old, throughout his adolescence and into adulthood. He reported that he decreased his drinking to the rare drink during the years following the divorce from his first wife (the divorce was negatively affected by his drinking). This information was collaborated. He began drinking again socially after remarrying, believing it was controlled. Over the next 15 years, he drank to excess leading to his current marriage being in jeopardy. Once confronted, he decreased his intake to "less than a glass of wine per night." His wife began suspecting he was drinking again when she smelled it on his breath. He began hiding his activities about that time. She never witnessed him drunk or out of control; however, at some point in the previous 2 years he started demonstrating more irritability and frustration with his wife. Their sexual life was sporadic and dependent on his mood. Both attributed the problems in their relationship to their different working schedules and feeling isolated from one another.

Direct Observations
When left alone Mr B would sit without moving. He made no attempts to move about the room, toilet himself, feed himself, join others in the day room, or interact with others. He had notable fatigue and could fall asleep while speaking with someone. This improved over the course of the evaluation but not as expected. His level of interaction continued to vacillate greatly; 1 min making good eye contact and answering direct questions, the next appearing detached and passive. His affect was relatively flat without emotional response to much of anything. On questioning about pain he would pause, consider the question and answer with "I guess so, not sure." He never complained of pain voluntarily. Since his physical balance was poor, he required a full watch be maintained for safety reasons. There was no marked impulsivity but there were times when attempting to go to the toilet or get into bed, he would fall. He failed to learn to use the call button for assistance. Since his test results showed osteoarthritis, there was concern regarding the risk of hip fracture.

Assessment
At the time of assessment he was 18 weeks post surgery with a variable recovery. He had been in intensive rehabilitation for about 4 weeks when the referral came through. The completed assessment required approximately 1 week to complete due to the difficulties in obtaining accurate information and following up on newly disclosed information.

Tests Administered
These were selected to enable a quick review of the issues identified, provide a baseline from which to work, and to keep testing to a minimum since cooperation was quite variable.

- *Repeatable Battery for the Assessment of Neuropsychological Status* (RBANS; Randolph 1998). This measure is found to be useful as a neuropsychological screening battery when it is impractical or difficult to use a longer, standardised battery. The tests provide a good overview of a patient's functioning without taxing them beyond their abilities to participate. This battery can be very useful in this type of situation where quick turnaround is needed for direction in services and the patient is not able to tolerate a lengthier process. The battery takes approximately 30 min to complete, and measures discreet neuropsychological domains including immediate memory, visuospatial/constructional, language, attention and delayed memory.
- *Clock drawing* (Eknoyan et al. 2012). This test assesses patient disinhibition and frontal pull. It uses errors to measure conceptualisation, disinhibition, executive functions including abstraction, planning, reasoning, problem solving, and behaviour response to command, stimulus-bound response, visual-spatial reasoning, fine motor control including graphical control, and perseveration. It also allowed for a direct comparison with previous efforts on clock drawing.
- *Behavioral Dyscontrol Scale* (BDS; Grigsby and Kaye 1996). It consists of measures of executive function using Luria principles and neurological responses. This is found to be a valid measure of functional autonomy in predominately geriatric population and found to be superior to mini-mental state exam (MMSE) (Folstein et al. 1975) and Functional Independence Measure (FIM; Keith and Granger 1987) in predicting living situation (independent versus assisted; Suchy et al. 1997). It is easy to administer and engage patient participation and takes under 15 min to administer.

Writing samples were attempted. He was asked to write his name, numbers, and letters. Careful review of his ability to attend to task, concentrate, organise and plan, orientation, fine motor control, and visual-spatial skills, short- and long-term memory was undertaken.

MRI (reviewed with NeuroRadiologist) reviewing structural changes within the brain as well as review report findings.

Findings

- Mr B was unable to write name, address, or phone number. He produced very small print with some form to letters. With great effort he was able to put together his name in a fashion but not legible for reading. Number writing was accurate 1–9 with pairing occurring between numbers (e.g. 123 space 45 space 67 space 89 space 9 space 1 space 11 space 0212 space 3). Written serialisation of letters was illegible.
- Clock drawing efforts were quite impaired. He drew an oversized, misshapen circle, placed anchor numbers at quarter hour segments with incorrect and repetitive numbers. When asked to place the hands at 10 past 11, he wrote a nonsensical number off to the side. He could place the centre point but did not successfully place hands or actually set the time. On confrontation to time telling using an actual clock, he was unable to give time, understand what the clock was used

RBANS Age 60-69	Index Scores	Percentiles	Classification
Immediate Memory	44	<0.1	Extremely Low
Visuospatial/Constructional	50	<0.1	Extremely Low
Language	74	4	Borderline
Attention	60	0.4	Extremely Low
Delayed Memory	48	<0.1	Extremely Low
Total Score	49	<0.1	Extremely Low

Fig. 9.4 RBANS results

for, or explain the number/hands on the clock. In fact, he asked if the clock was a mirror. Using the Sutherland scoring criteria (Eknoyan et al. 2012), he scored 1 for circle. He lacked insight into his performance.

- Behavioral Dyscontrol Scale (BDS) (6/19) was severely impaired. He showed difficulties in new learning, understanding directions, following directions, poor initiation, poor attention/concentration, failure to learn with verbal, visual, or demonstration prompts, he made echopraxic error, could recite the alphabet a–e then became confused and was unable to restart even with prompts and he showed poor insight into his difficulties.
- *Repeatable Battery for the Assessment of Neuropsychological Status* (RBANS) results showed extremely low performance in immediate memory/visuospatial/constructional/attention and delayed memory. His strongest performance was in language but remained in the borderline range. Overall score was extremely low. Word listing performance fell off rather than build up over trials. Story memory showed lack of presented details but rather elaborate story of a similar nature with confabulation and melding of materials previously presented and out of context. Figure copy held the gestalt but lost details. He was unable to grasp the line of orientation task regardless of extreme prompting. He found even simple line drawings difficult to determine direction or spacing. Performance on picture naming remained quite good with remaining subtest performance being poor: semantic fluency, digit span, coding, list recall, list recognition, and story recall (found the story "suspicious; don't recall a story"). There was no memory for figure copy (Fig. 9.4).

Formulation

The preferred method of approach in this case was a short, fixed battery with additional measures of short duration to help quantify the predicted ability to manage activities of daily living (ADLs) independently on discharge. Due to his difficulties in participating in activities for prolonged amounts of time, the investigation was limited in scope, focusing on his ability to use information, manage behaviour, and then make a determination where he might best receive the care and oversight he would need on discharge.

Selection of the RBANS-Form A came about as it was short in duration, simple to score, quickly interpreted, and could be used to determine if there was a dementia-type pattern underlying the SAH effects. Augmentation with the BDS reviewing behavioural response to commands, new motoric learning, mental control, and insight awareness provided a fuller picture of his capabilities and limitations. Clock drawing was selected to help make comparison over time with previous given clock, to better understand his abilities to understand and use time, review overall organisational skills, abstraction, spatial management and look more closely at the temporal difficulties uncovered during the assessment process. The results highlighted his difficulties reading a clock face or alternatives (digital clocks) and use numbers to schedule or organise his time (unable to use timetables or plan for therapies). His difficulties making temporal relationships and accurately place events, people, and manage situations that required flexibility placed him in a situation where being alone for long stretches of time (as he would need to be to return home) unsafe and impractical.

While initially, staff thought his deficits were directly related to his SAH injury, his failure to recover in the expected pattern (cleared orientation, ability to schedule and use time, follow through on instructions, increased cognitive response to therapies, use of strategies to overcome some hurdles, etc.) and his propensity to "make up stories", it became evident very quickly there were other factors in play.

After the initial neuropsychology review, a repeat MRI with blood work to rule out thiamine deficiency was requested. This became even more important after uncovering his extensive alcohol history. MRI results supported small vessel disease both cortical and subcortical in addition to the damage associated with his SAH. There was remaining evidence of a receding subdural haematoma.

Additionally, blood work found a significant thiamine deficiency. These findings further supported the theory of a possible Wernicke–Korsakoff syndrome (or Wernicke's encephalopathy) with underlying Korsakoff dementia. Wernicke–Korsakoff syndrome is a neurological disorder typically characterised by years of chronic alcohol abuse and a nutritional thiamine deficiency (Todd et al. 1999). Additional records review was required to determine if he showed symptoms of such on coming into the hospital. These were located and reviewed in depth, finding a diagnosis of Wernicke's encephalopathy at the time of SAH. Verbal feedback was given to the medical team immediately on this information and thiamine replacement therapy was started.

The identification of confabulation within his communications was relevant. While confabulation is one salient symptom of this syndrome, it can also be found in subarachnoid haemorrhage and encephalitis. In his case, the confabulation occurred predominately when providing autobiographical information. This is indicative of a complicated and intricate process that can be led astray at any point during encoding, storage, or recall of a memory. This type of confabulation is commonly seen in Korsakoff syndrome. Someone with Korsakoff would most likely be provoked to confabulate when they are prompted with questions pertaining to episodic memory, not semantic memory, and when they are prompted with questions where the appropriate response would be "I don't know." In SAH, the amount and duration of confabulation would be expected to clear or improve over time, as opposed to Mr B's presentation; as he improved, he confabulated more and all on inquiry of episodic content.

When taking into consideration the findings from the neuropsychological testing, his drinking history, his propensity to confabulate, the Wernicke's encephalopathy diagnosis at time of admission, his low nutritional thiamine levels, and his lack of recovery in the expected manner, it became clearer that more than one process was taking place and the prognosis for recovery to independence was very poor.

A formal write-up was produced with review of findings and recommendations to both staff and patient/family. The path to rehabilitation efforts changed with a stronger focus on preparing the patient to manage many of his self-cares, make safe transfers, identify a safe and supportive environment at discharge, educate patient and family regarding needs and concerns, and provide emotional support to the family as a whole while they adjusted to the diagnosis and prognosis.

Recommendations Made

- B-12 plus thiamine (long-term alcohol user)
- Discharge to supervised environment
- Notify family of need to invoke power of attorney to manage his affairs
- Reposition therapy focus to enhance areas of strength and accommodate areas of weakness.
- Retest in 6 months to 1 year if notable changes in cognitive status

After a delay of 1 month limited retesting took place to measure the effects of treatments. While some improvements had been noted in his rehab after thiamine therapy started, he continued to suffer from temporal difficulties, confabulation, and orientation to time/place but was now fully oriented to self. He continued to exhibit symptoms of a dementia process with a failure to learn new information, decreased comprehension, poor sequencing, significantly impaired problem solving, poor STM and decreased concept formation (National Institute on Alcohol Abuse and Alcoholism 2003). Review of self-management found him to be significantly impaired. Clock drawing highlighted his difficulties reading a clock face and use numbers to schedule or organise his time. His deficits in mental flexibility, poor temporal relationships, inaccurate placement of events and people, and difficulty in self-management of ADLs'. Placed him in a situation where being alone for long stretches of time (as he would need to be to return home) both impractical and unsafe.

Outcome

This patient required full-time supervision due to the dementia and added difficulties resulting from SAH. He was placed in rest home with supervision and full-time care support. His family remains quite involved in his everyday management but is able to continue in their work and social lives without concern for his safety. Of note, after discharge this gentleman managed to leave the rest home, got lost, spent a night out on the streets and was found under a bush in the early morning hours, unconscious. He'd been drinking which he denied. He now resides in a secured section of a private hospital due to continued cognitive decline and progressive dementia.

Reflection/Discussion

What initially appeared to be SAH recovery proved much more complicated and required an open mind to other contributing factors. It was remarkable that this gen-

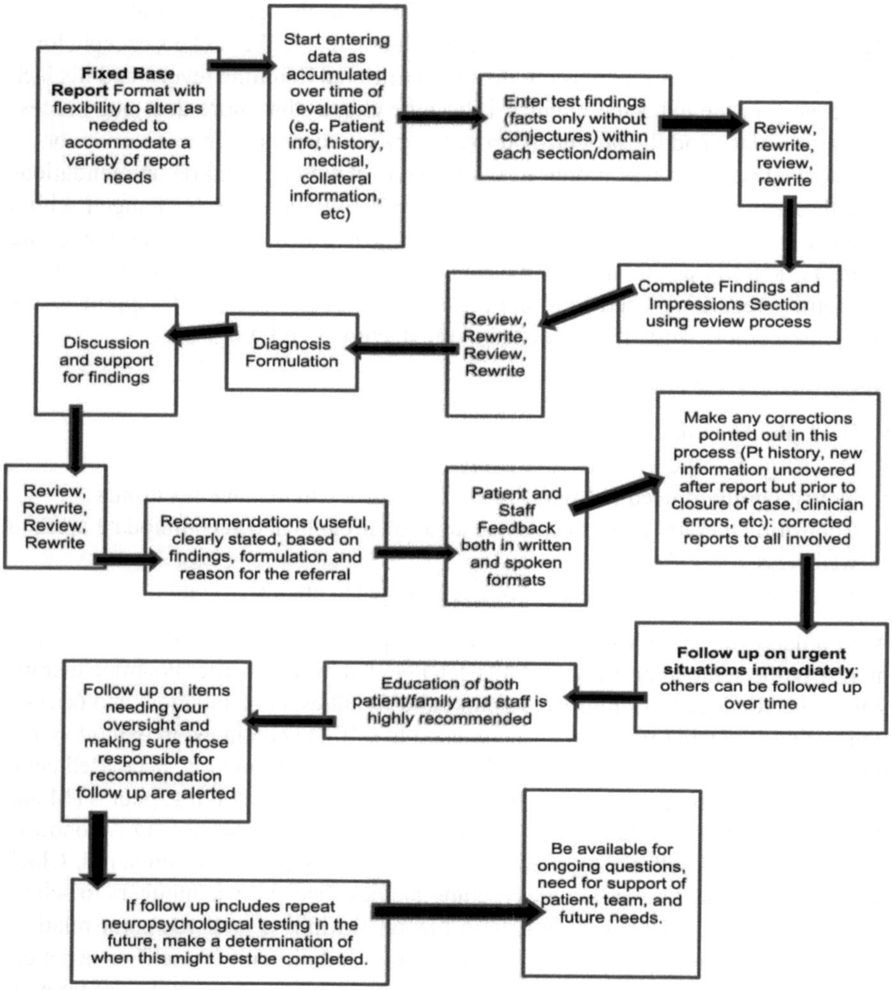

Fig. 9.5 The process

tleman went through two hospitals, multiple treatment specialists and staff without anyone identifying his significant alcohol history and use. It was the investigative stance that neuropsychologists take, looking under rocks and behind doors, that helped clearly identify what other factors were contributing to the ongoing difficulties. The process of understanding findings from a neuropsychological evaluation is not straightforward; it requires both fixed processes to guide the evaluation and flexibility to adapt as things change, new information emerges, and outcome requirements change (treatment adjustment, informational feedback, recommendations, etc.) (Fig. 9.5).

Of note, it was not the testing per se in this case that made the difference; it was the investigation into other potential causes. The testing was quite limited in nature and more testing would not have been extremely helpful. While the preference for full neuropsychological evaluation (in-depth and detailed) remains, the use of neuropsychological tools must reflect the purpose, the use of the results, consider the cost/benefits, and information necessity must support the process.

A solid approach to selecting, gathering, reviewing, and integrating neuropsychological data will inform diagnosis and recommendations for treatment. Use of an investigative approach (asking who, what, where, when, and how questions) enables answers to why-type questions. Consultation with others remains imperative as does continual updating of knowledge regarding ailments and expected findings. It is in the close investigation and integration of the details that neuropsychologists stand out and can contribute.

References

National Institute on Alcohol Abuse and Alcoholism. (2003). Alcohol's damaging effects on the brain. *Alcohol research & health. 27*(2).

Becske, T., et al. (2010). Subarachnoid haemorrhage, eMedicine (Dec).

Eknoyan, D., Hurley, R., & Tabor, K. (2012). The clock drawing task: Common errors and functional neuroanatomy. *The Journal of Neuropsychiatry and Clinical Neurosciences, 24,* 260–265.

Feigin, V. L., Rinkel, G. J., Lawes, C. M., et al. (2005). Risk factors for subarachnoid haemorrhage: An updated systematic review of epidemiological studies. *Stroke, 35*(12), 2773–2780.

Folstein, M. F., Folstein, S. E., & McHugh, P. R. (1975). Mini-mental state. A practical method for grading the cognitive state of patients for the clinician. *Journal of psychiatric research, 12*(3), 189–198. doi:10.1016/0022-3956(75)90026-6. http://dx.doi.org/10.1016%2F0022-3956%2875%2990026-6. PMID 1202204. http://www.ncbi.nlm.nih.gov/pubmed/1202204.

Greebe, P., Rinkel, G. J., Hop, J. W., et al. (2010). Functional outcome and quality of life 5 and 12.5 years after aneurismal. *Journal of Neurology, 257*(12), 2059–2064.

Grigsby, J., & Kaye, K. (1996). The behavioral dyscontrol scale manual (2nd Ed.). Colorado: Authors.

Ingram, V., Kelly, M., & Grammar, G. (2003). Abstracts presented at the thirty-first annual international neuropsychological society conference. *Journal of the International Neuropsychological Society, 9,* 135–330.

Keith, R. A., & Granger, C. V. (1987). The functional independence measure: A new tool for rehabilitation. *Adv Clin Rehabil, 1*(3503663), 6–18.

Kessels, R. P. C., Kortrijk, H. E., Wester, A. J., & Gudrun, M. S. (2008). Confabulation behaviour and false memorises in Korsakoff's syndrome: Role of source memory and executive functioning. *Psychiatry and Clinical Neurosciences, 62,* 220–225.

Kopelman, M. D., Thomson, A. D., Guerrini, I., & Marshall. E. J. (2009). The Korsakoff syndrome: Clinical aspects, psychology, and treatment. *Alcohol & Alcoholism, 44*(2), 148–154.

Kyoko, K. (2009). The cognitive profile of elderly korsakoff's syndrome patients. *Master's thesis presented to department of neurological science*. Montreal Canada: McGill University.

Nasreddine, Z. S., Phillips, N. A., Bedirian, V., Charbonneau, S., Whitehead, V., Colline, I., Cummings, J. L., & Chertkow, H. (2005). The Montreal cognitive assessment, MoCA: A brief screening tool for mild cognitive impairment. *Journal of the American Geriatrics Society, 53,* 695–699.

Randolph, C. (1998). *Repeatable Battery for the Assessment of Neuropsychological Status (RBANS)—Form A*. Bloomington: Pearson, Inc.

Sechi, G., & Serra, A. (2007). Wernicke's encephalopathy: New clinical settings and recent advances in diagnosis and management. *Lancet Neurology, 6,* 442–455.
Suchy, Y., Blint, A., & Osman, D. C. (1997). Behavioral dyscontrol scale: Criterion and predictive validity in an inpatient rehabilitation unit population. *The Clinical Neuropsychologist, 11*(3), 258–265.
Thomson, A. D., & Marshall, E. J. (2006). The natural history and pathophysiology of Wernicke's encephalopathy and Korsakoff's psychosis. *Alcohol and Alcoholism, 41*(2), 151–158.
Thomson, A. D., Cook, C. C. H., Guerrini, I., Sheedy, D., Harper, C., & Marshall, E. J. (2008). Wernicke's encephalopathy revisited. *Alcohol and Alcoholism, 43*(2), 174–179.
Todd, K. G., Hazell, A. S., & Butterworth, R. F. (1999). Alcohol thiamine interactions: An update on the pathogenesis of Wernicke encephalopathy. *Addiction Biology, 4,* 261–272.
Van Gijn, J, Kerr, R. S., & Rinkel, G. J. (2007). Subarachnoid haemorrhage. *Lancet, 369*(9558), 306–318.

Chapter 10
Themes in the Formulation of Repeat Assessments

Patrick Vesey and Robert D. Stephens

In this chapter, two patients are presented that were each seen several times for neuropsychological assessment and opinion, over a period of months and years. This chapter illustrates and discusses issues related to serial assessment, the progression of symptoms and increasing familiarity with the cases. The first patient presented with subtle subjective cognitive change and underwent subsequent serial assessment over several years to help clarify the nature of her condition and monitor change in the context of other neurological investigations. Issues are discussed concerning the role of the patient's account in understanding her condition and the utility of increased familiarity with the patient over time. The second patient underwent neurosurgery as a treatment for intractable epilepsy. The assessments addressed questions about risk to his cognition, the cognitive outcome of surgery, and the role of psychological and behavioural disturbance. Issues of test selection and the psychometric evaluation of change are discussed.

Case 1. JK—A Case of Multidomain Cognitive Impairment

Background of JK

A 55-year-old woman was seen in the neurology clinic in the context of concerns about subtle changes in numerous aspects of functioning. She gave a 2-year history of gradually worsening confusion, speech difficulties and unsteadiness. She had

P. Vesey (✉)
Department of Clinical Psychology and Neuropsychology, Nottingham University Hospitals NHS Trust, QMC Campus, Derby Road, Nottingham NG7 2UH, UK
e-mail: Patrick.vesey@nuh.nhs.uk

R. D. Stephens
Department of Clinical Psychology and Neuropsychology, Nottingham University Hospitals NHS Trust, QMC Campus, Derby Road, Nottingham NG7 2UH, UK
e-mail: robertd.stephens@nuh.nhs.uk

J. A. B. Macniven (ed.), *Neuropsychological Formulation*,
DOI 10.1007/978-3-319-18338-1_10

become more aggressive and less tolerant. She had developed a new liking for chocolate. She retained the same hobbies and interests and, if anything, her mood had improved of late. She slept well and had a good appetite. Her dressing sequencing had been normal. In recent weeks, she had intermittent symptoms of unsteadiness when walking, with swaying and bumping into items. She had long-standing left-foot numbness in relation to previous lumbar spinal problems, worse on exertion. She had occasional attacks of slurred speech but normal comprehension. She was a retired healthcare assistant who lived with her husband. She had a spinal fusion in the 1970s and also suffers from hypertension. She smokes ten cigarettes a day but did not drink alcohol. Her father was said to have developed dementia in his late 30s. Mini Mental State Examination was normal at 28/30. Fundoscopy was normal but there was no visualisation of venous pulsations. The rest of the neurological examination was entirely normal. There were no extrapyramidal features and finger nose testing was accurate. There was no obvious myoclonus or other movement disorder on examination. Speech was normal. She was to be referred for blood tests and magnetic resonance imaging (MRI) brain imaging. In subsequent weeks, MRI revealed a small area of atrophy on the left side of the brain and an ill-defined area of high signal in the left frontal lobe. It was felt that both of these may be coincidental to the memory problems but repeat imaging was recommended after an interval.

The patient was reviewed in the neurology clinic 12 months later. She reported worsening of her memory difficulties, stammering, normal face recognition and geographical orientation. There was thought to be possible worsening of her writing even despite a history of dyslexia. She had on-going dizziness without headaches. There was said to be no evidence of dementia but she understandably remained concerned about the family history of such. Repeat MRI showed areas of confluent high signal within the pericallosal white matter, as before, and unchanged focal atrophy in the left parietal lobe. There were no areas of abnormal enhancement post contrast. The appearances seemed to be long standing and unchanged.

She was referred for neuropsychological assessment with a view to refining the nature of her subjective cognitive changes and monitoring progress.

Neuropsychological Contact with JK

Clinical Interview She was seen in the neuropsychology clinic 8 weeks later (assessment point A1). She repeated her history, comprising a 3-year history of mild slurring, being unable to articulate sentences formed in her mind, and memory disturbance comprising forgetting of intended activities and information she had been told. She felt her memory had worsened but her speech had possibly improved, although possibly because she was being more deliberate in speaking and had been speaking less to avoid embarrassing mistakes. In recent weeks, she had noticed upper limb jerks a few times a week. She had fallen several times although without hurting herself. She revealed that 25 years previously she drank heavily and had contact with mental health services. She smoked cigarettes and denied illicit drug use. Current medication was codeine for back pain, an antihypertensive and amitriptyline. She was right handed. She passed the time now by reading and had not noticed any change in her reading ability.

Assessment On examination, pre-morbidly she was indicated to have functioned in the low average range for the population. Linguistically, confrontational naming was consistent with the expected level. There were no gross difficulties with comprehension. Her reading of a newspaper passage was reasonable as was single-word reading, number reading, number copying, single-word repetition and phrase repetition. Basic attention, as assessed by digit span, was broadly consistent with the expected level at five digits forwards and three digits in reverse. The memory results were variable. Immediate recall of a word list over repeat trials was low but there was reasonable learning from first to last trials and there was good retention after both short and long delay. Recognition was poor, however. Immediate and delayed recall of a complex geometric figure was low, but copy of the figure was itself poor. On further exploration, clock drawing was equivocal. Line bisection was reasonable but performance on numerous other visuospatial tests was below the expected level. Block Design was reasonable but Picture Completion was poor. There was no agnosia or apraxia. On frontal-executive tests, there were variable results. Similarities, BADS Key Search and Temporal Judgement were reasonable but letter fluency was low, as was performance on the Brixton test. Qualitatively, despite being somewhat anxious initially she became more relaxed and a substantial interference from mood or anxiety disturbance was felt unlikely. She was well engaged with the tests and performed well on a formal test of performance validity.

Formulation JK gave a frank and straightforward account. A number of low results were obtained in the assessment, compared to the estimated pre-morbid level. Mood and anxiety were felt likely to compromise day-to-day activities but not to have significantly contributed to the test results.

Overall the presentation was felt to be clinically authentic, with a clear neurological correlate for the reported subjective cognitive changes albeit that a somewhat unusual pattern of results had been obtained. There were prominent difficulties in visuoperceptual performance, aspects of memory, and frontal-executive functioning. The results were felt to be consistent with the imaging findings, severe in places and unlikely to be long standing, although the history of dyslexia and possible non-uniform abilities pre-morbidly complicated interpretation of the current results.

Subsequent Assessment and Clarification of Initial Formulation Despite JK's cognitive difficulties having a suspected primary neuropsychological basis, lack of clarity existed regarding whether the deficits formed part of a syndrome that was long standing, acquired and static, or progressive and deteriorating. It was, therefore, felt advisable to keep her under neuropsychological review, and indeed she also remained under neurological review.

JK was reassessed 12 months later (A1 + 12 months). She felt her memory had continued to worsen. She reported difficulty in operating certain objects such as the remote control, difficulty in dealing with change when shopping. She felt her jerks had worsened. Of note, 2 months previously she had been admitted to hospital with an unprovoked generalised seizure. MRI at the time had shown no interval change from the previous one, and no evidence of bleeding, ischemia, tumour or hydrocephalus. On examination, her neuropsychological functions continued to involve multidomain impairment. Qualitatively, phrase repetition was impaired, as was basic calculation. Left–right orientation was hesitant but eventually reasonably well demonstrated. Alternating hand movements were impaired as were the Luria three-stage hand movements bilaterally. Conversely, single-word repetition was reasonable, as was spelling (of regular and irregular words), praxis (buccofacial, mime and symbolic gestures), reading of a newspaper passage, converse tapping, name and novel sentence writing. Quantitatively, copy of a complex figure was poor as was clock drawing. There were impairments in expressive and receptive language, basic attention and working memory, memory for verbal and nonverbal information. There was patchy frontal-executive impairment. Close analysis of deficit severity was complicated by the marked visuospatial impairment which predominated the profile and which impinged on many of the nonverbal functions formally examined.

There were felt to be subtle qualitative changes compared to the previous assessment. There was a tendency to line-bisect to the left of centre that was not evident previously. Figure copy was poorer. Visuospatial impairment was more pronounced, evident on more tests than the previous one (five of nine tests compared with one of nine previously). There was equivocally lower performance on some of the auditory anterograde memory tests. Overall, the changes were evident mainly on qualitative assessment, and tended to be less evident quantitatively.

She was assessed on two subsequent occasions: A1+24 months and A1+60 months, and she remains under review. Over that period, she felt that her memory had perhaps worsened. She noticed more problems with dizziness and also some continued jerks, but no further seizures.

At A1+24 months, there were no neuropsychometric changes from previous one, including on tests of memory, basic attention and working memory, visuospatial function, and numerous frontal executive functions (fluency, rule formation, problem solving and estimates). Clock drawing was good and line bisections no more impaired than the previous one. The results were regarded as providing no indication of further deterioration in the previously evident impairments.

At A1+60 months, she reported increased confusion and difficulty with some day-to-day tasks including using remote controls or calculating change. She felt there had been no further speech changes. She tried to remain active with family and friends. Her medication continued to be Epilim and she had not had a seizure for over 3 years. She does continue to have fairly constant pain associated with her spondylitis. On qualitative assessment, single-word repetition was good but phrase repetition was impaired. Spelling and calculations were slightly poor. Alternating hand movements were impaired. Clock drawing, name and sentence writing were reasonable. Her reading of passages and long number strings was impaired. Quantitatively, many results were unchanged from previously but there were some slightly lower results. Specifically, no change was evident on forward and reverse digit span, verbal list learning and recall, letter fluency and category switching, estimates, novel problem solving and reasoning (verbal and nonverbal). Naming of drawn objects was unchanged with no obvious semantic or perceptual errors. Line bisections were similarly impaired. Conversely, construction of blocks to match a given design was poorer than the previous one. Copy of a complex figure was also poorer than the previous one (and subsequent recall, perhaps as a result of poor copy; Table 10.1).

Table 10.1 JK data across assessments

	A1 (assessment 1)			A1 + 12 months			A1 + 24 months				A1 + 60 months		
Test	Raw	*z*	Comment	Raw	*z*	Comment	Raw	*z*	Percentile	Comment	Raw	*z*	Comment
WTAR estimated pFSIQ		−1.5			−1.3			−1.3				−1.5	
Graded naming test	11			9			9				12		
Wechsler-III SS													
Vocabulary													
Similarities		−0.8			−2			−0.3					
Digit span		−1.2			−1.6			−1				−0.3	
Picture completion		−2.7			−2.3			−2				−2.3	
Block design		−0.8			−2			−1				−2	
Matrix reasoning		−1.2			−1.6			−1				−1.7	
Information		−1.6			−1.6			−1.3					
Arithmetic		−2.3			−2							−1.3	
Picture arrangement		−2.3			−2.3								
Word list I RTS		−2.3			−3.5			−2				−2.3	
Word list II RTS		0			−0.8			−0.3				−0.3	
Word list I learning slope		−1.2			−1.2			−1				−1.3	
Word list I short delay ret		−0.5			1			−0.3				0	
Word list II long delay ret		0.3			0			0				0.3	
Word list II recognition		−2.7			−2.3			−2				−2.3	
Rey figure													
Rey figure copy		−2.7			−2.7			−2.7				−2.7	
Immediate recall		−2.2			−2.2			−2.3				−2.2	
Delayed recall		−2.2			−2.2			−2.7				−2.2	

Table 10.1 (continued)

Test	A1 (assessment 1)			A1 + 12 months			A1 + 24 months				A1 + 60 months		
	Raw	*z*	Comment	Raw	*z*	Comment	Raw	*z*	Percentile	Comment	Raw	*z*	Comment
Frontal-executive tests													
Brixton test		−2.2			−2.7			−2.2				Not repeated	
Letter fluency		−3.1			−2.3			−2.3				−2.3	
Category switching total CR												−1.7	
BADS temporal judgement		0	Normal			Normal							Normal
BADS key search						Impaired							Abnormal
Other (qualitative)													
Line bisections			Normal			Abnormal				Abnormal			Abnormal
Clock drawing			Equivocal			Equivocal				Normal			Normal
Number reading			Impaired										Abnormal
Paragraph reading			Normal										Impaired
VOSP (items correct)													
Screening test	20		Pass	18			18					14	
Incomplete letters	20			18			18					12	
Silhouettes	19			14			14						
Object decision	16			12			12						
Progressive silhouettes	8			10			10						
Dot counting	8			10			10					2	
Position discrimination	19			11			11						
Number location	4			6			6						
Cube analysis	8			3			3						

Table 10.1 (continued)

Test	A1 (assessment 1)			A1 + 12 months			A1 + 24 months				A1 + 60 months		
	Raw	*z*	Comment	Raw	*z*	Comment	Raw	*z*	Percentile	Comment	Raw	*z*	Comment
Illustrations													
Rey figure copy	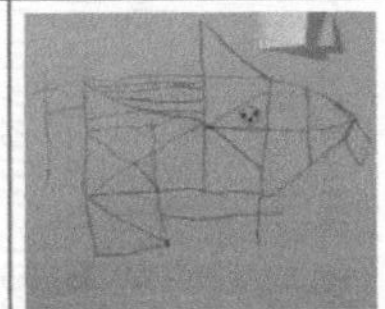			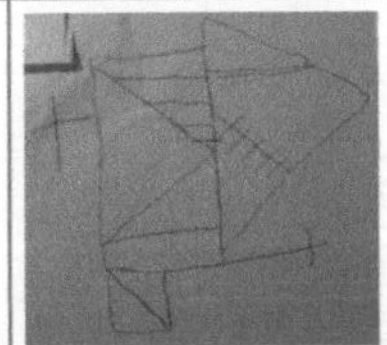			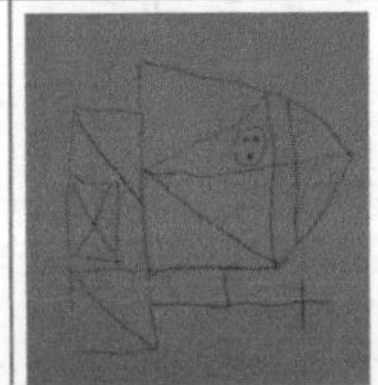				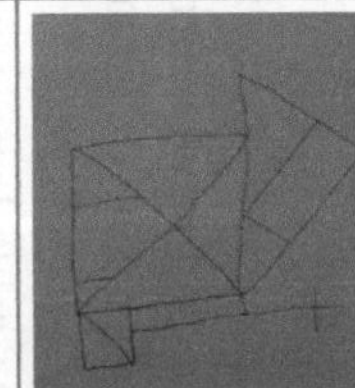		
Line bisections				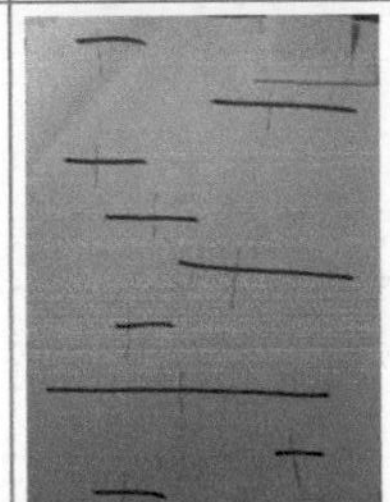			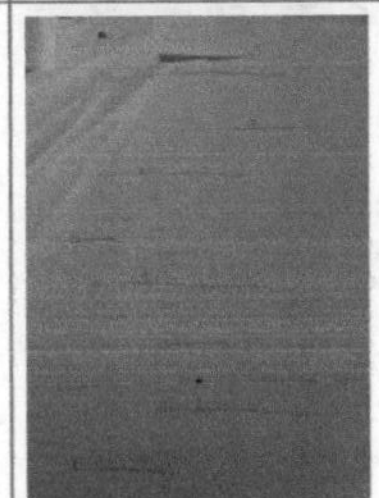						
Clock drawing	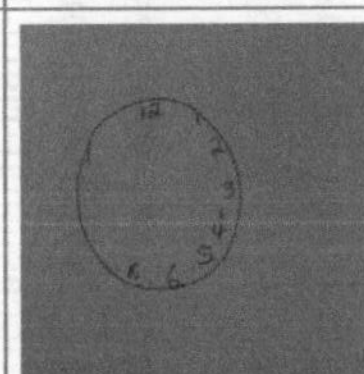 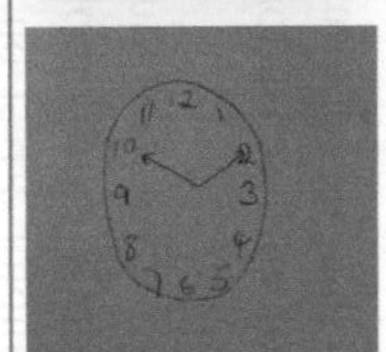			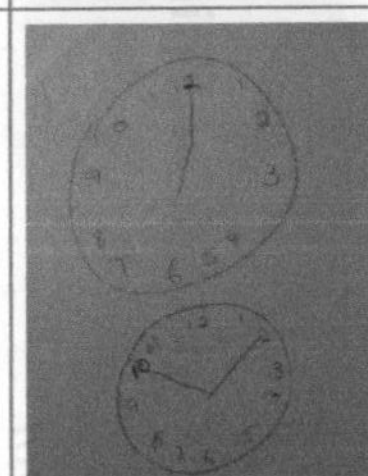			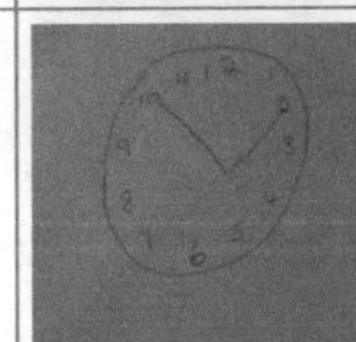				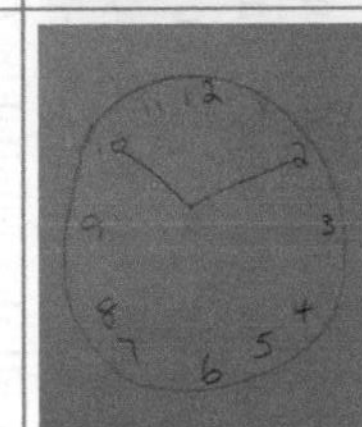		

Outcome and Overall Formulation of JK

The patient's general condition is contributed by various factors including her psychological and psychosocial wellbeing (including mood and anxiety factors), her underlying neurological status, and the impingement of her neurological status on her neuropsychological functioning. It is likely in this case that her psychological wellbeing affects her subjective cognitive wellbeing, and her understanding and account of her cognitive and functional condition.

Understanding of the case is based on the quality and accuracy of her own account and that of her family, her engagement and performance on formal neuropsychological tests, and information deriving from other specialist sources including neurology consultations and associated investigations.

Considering all the available factors, there are felt-to-be multidomain neuropsychological impairments compared to the estimated pre-morbid level, with some evidence of increased neuropsychological impairment over the course of the assessments, A1 to A+60 months. Over time, this impression has been conveyed to the patient and she has come to the understanding that she does indeed have an underlying neurological condition substantively accounting for the changes she has experienced in aspects of her cognitive and functional abilities. She has been given advice at various stages regarding strategies to minimise the impact of the cognitive impairments on her quality of life, although it was recognised that the impact of the cognitive impairments was increasingly significant and less amenable to such approaches.

Case 2. AH—A Case of Epilepsy Surgery

Background

AH Medical History Right-handed AH experienced meningitis as a child and then epileptic seizures until age 10. Seizures returned as a 46-year old (mostly episodes of aura sensations or blank spells). Radiological investigations at that time were unremarkable.

Over subsequent years, seizures increased in frequency up to 4 per day, developed into complex–partial then more frequently, tonic–clonic in type (involving motor arrest but occasional right-hand movement and no speech; afterwards, he was able to speak but did not seem to comprehend speech). Throughout this time, antiepileptic medications of Carbamazepine, Keppra and Clobazam were ineffective, although treatment compliance was questioned.

At 66 years old, video telemetry electroencephalogram detected slow waves from the left temporal region.The MRI found increased signal on fluid-attenuated inversion recovery (FLAIR) from both mesial temporal lobes; the right showed no volume loss, whereas the left exhibited greater signal intensity and volume loss consistent with hippocampal sclerosis. In addition to this, the radiologist commented on a background of mild cerebral atrophy and multifocal white matter ischemia of undetermined significance. His records noted a history of excessive alcohol intake, although when assessed age 67 his intake was well within recommended limits. His consultant neurologist requested neuropsychological opinion about AH's suitability for surgery.

AH Psychosocial History AH left school at 15 years with no qualifications, then trained as an electrician, which he worked as until early retirement due to a shoulder injury. He was married and had children, however leading up to the age of 67 years he experienced a series of bereavements of immediate family, including the trauma of discovering his son's suicide. He reported symptoms consistent with mild depression on the Beck Depression Inventory Fast screen for medical patients; raw score of 8 where range 4–8 is categorised as mild (Beck et al. 2000). He also described a worsening daily problem with verbally aggressive behaviour. He attributed some of his frustration to the activity limitations associated with the risk of seizure; he tended to take risks by going running or cycling alone and indeed, sustained numerous injuries from these activities. Around this time he contemplated suicide. When assessed at 68 years, symptoms of depression had worsened; his BDI-fast screen raw score was 17 (range 13–21 is categorised as severe); and he described his mood as "bumping along the bottom."

AH Cognitive Complaints AH reported that he frequently repeated himself during conversation or within an hour, and that he would quickly forget the content of recent conversations. He reported word finding difficulty more than once per day. He reported frequently losing objects and getting lost. Overall, he believed that these cognitive problems had worsened.

AH Timeline AH completed three neuropsychological assessment in all, although only the second and third are the focus of this report. The findings of the previous assessment are summarised below. Eleven months later, surgery to treat his epilepsy was reconsidered and so he was re-referred for assessment (T1). Six months after assessment T1, AH underwent surgical resection of his left temporal lobe. Unfortunately surgery did not go well, and was complicated by the development of haematoma at the site (which required evacuation), along with evidence of localised oedema and ischemia on CT scan. In addition, tonic–clonic seizures returned. Follow-up neuropsychological evaluation was completed 8 months post surgery, which equates to a retest interval of 14 months between T1 and T2.

AH Previous Neuropsychological Assessment AH completed neuropsychological evaluation prior to assessment T1. In summary, his pre-morbid general intellect was estimated to be high average; his general intellect at the time of assessment was estimated to be average, and judged to represent a borderline significant decline in ability. There was evidence of impaired verbal fluency and some evidence of impaired verbal learning (although it was concluded that his performance may have been affected by attention difficulties). Performance on other tests of verbal and visual memory was within normal limits, and no problems were evident relating to visuoconstruction, space perception, visual naming and executive ability (using the Brixton Spatial Anticipation Test).

Referral Questions for AH

1. *Laterality.* Prior to surgery, the multidisciplinary team requested opinion about the concordance between neuropsychological and other sources of evidence, i.e. the presence of left-sided brain abnormality and absence of right-sided brain abnormality. If AH's right hemisphere was a seizure focus then surgery to the left would be less likely to offer an effective treatment.
2. *Predicted cognitive outcome.* The team requested opinion about the risks of post-surgical cognitive decline, of which language and verbal memory were of particular concern due to the surgery being proposed for the (presumed) language dominant hemisphere (Schramm 2008).
3. *Actual cognitive outcome.* The third question was whether there was evidence of cognitive decline in neuropsychological functioning following surgery.

Assessment Data

Table 10.2 Case AH, table of psychometric results collected presurgery (T1) and postsurgery (T2) expressed as a raw score and point estimate percentile, based upon published normative data. For information, the *predicted* raw score at T2 derived from regression formula is also shown. The difference between predicted and obtained score at T2 is expressed as a percentile, representing the percentage of people expected to show the same or greater change at retest

	T1		$T2_{pred}$	$T2_{obt}$		Difference
	Raw	Percentile	Raw	Raw	Percentile	Percentile
Visual perception						
WMS-IV Visual Reproduction II Copy	41.0	26–50		42.0	26–50	
Language						
Graded Naming Test	15.0			3.0		
DKEFS Verbal Fluency Letter	17.0	2	18–20	20.0	5	↓49
DKEFS Verbal Fluency Category	17.0	1	22–23	10.0	<1	↓04
DKEFS Verbal Fluency Switching	4.0	<1	8	3.0	<1	↓11
Processing speed						
DKEFS Towers time per move	5.4	25		4.2	50	
DKEFS Towers move accuracy	1.6	37		1.2	63	
Attention						
WAIS-IV Digit Span forwards	8.0	25	8.0	5.0	2	↓<1
WAIS-IV Digit Span backwards	5.0	9	6.0	6.0	25	↑41
WAIS-IV Digit Span sequencing	3.0	5	5.0	4.0	9	↓27

Table 10.2 (continued)

	T1		$T2_{pred}$	$T2_{obt}$		Difference
Reasoning						
DKEFS Towers achievement	12.0	25	17	22.0	95	↑06
Visual memory						
WMS-IV Visual Reproduction I	29.0	37	34–35	26.0	16	↓02
WMS-IV Visual Reproduction II	22.0	50	29–31	10.0	16	↓<1
WMS-IV Visual Reproduction recognition		26–50			3–9	
Verbal memory						
WMS-IV Logical Memory I	23.0	37	26–28	8.0	<1	↓<1
WMS-IV Logical Memory II	14.0	16	20–21	2.0	<1	↓<1
WMS-IV Logical Memory recognition		17–25			10–16	
WMS-IV Verbal Paired Associates I	4.0	1	16–18	2.0	<1	↓03
WMS-IV Verbal Paired Associates II	2.0	2	5.0	0.0	<1	↓<1
WMS-IV Verbal Paired Associates II recognition		3–9			3–9	
Mental health						
Beck depression inventory—fast screen for medical patients	8/21			17/21		

Interpretation of Results AH

1. *AH laterality.* Qualitatively AH's copy of the WMS-IV figures contained few omissions to one side or the other (attention to space), and his construction of the figures exhibited no gross errors of size, orientation, relation and so forth (Stern et al. 1994). His recollection of details of the drawings after 30 min was statistically average compared to his age peers. AH was able to recognise and name pictures of objects. Overall, assessment in this domain revealed no evidence of impairment for the processing, storage and retrieval of visual information. In which case there was no sign that the functioning his right hemisphere had been affected by seizure activity, assuming left hemisphere dominance for language.

During conversation, AH's expressive language was fluent and unremarkable in terms of articulation, rate and overall quantity; there was no evidence of word finding, paraphasia or errors/omission of grammatical construction. According to normative data, his performance during visual object naming would be expected of someone of average general intelligence and vocabulary. He exhibited no difficulty in understanding conversational speech or test instructions (Table 10.2).

AH was able to focus his attention and hold in mind an average amount of information presented verbally. However, when required to manipulate or perform calculations on the information, his performance in the low average range suggested that this was an area of weakness, but not necessarily impairment.

AH struggled with semantic and phonemic versions of the verbal fluency task. In the literature, various cognitive processes have been proposed to be especially important when performing this task, including, for example energising and selection. Performing the task has been associated with activation or integrity of the prefrontal cortex (Andrewes 2001, pp. 260–266) particularly in the left lateral region (Robinson 2012). Regarding the pattern of performance between the tasks, patients with temporal lobe damage tend to exhibit relatively worse semantic fluency (Henry and Crawford 2004; Costafreda 2006), but this was not evident for AH. Therefore, AH's known left temporal lobe abnormality did not offer a good fit for his poor performance on these tasks, in addition to which, he exhibited no other language problems. Two alternative hypotheses could be proposed. First, seizure activity from the temporal lobe is thought to spread to the frontal lobe, inhibiting processes reliant on those regions (case report by Campo 2011). Second, the use of multiple antiepileptic medications (and specifically Carbamazepine) is known to impair cognition, of which processes of mental control appear to be especially vulnerable (Eddy 2011).

AH's results on tests of verbal memory were varied, and posed a challenge to interpret. His memory for word-pairs was consistently poor during learning, retrieval and recognition, suggesting that he failed to consolidate the words effectively. However, his memory for stories was generally better. His immediate recall performance in the average range suggested effective learning, whereas after a delay of 30 min his recall and recognition performance were both low average compared to peers. Whilst a little below expectations, this low average delayed recall was within normal limits and it would be reasonable to take this (being his best score) as a more accurate reflection of ability. However, this seemed to be premature. We know that AH has TLE and that the base rate of verbal memory problems is higher for this population, in addition to which, he had reported everyday memory problems. Without attempting to quantify this using Bayes' theorem, it was deemed appropriate to explore possible reasons for AH performance on these memory tests.

If AH's low test score on Verbal Paired Associates (VPA) II was retained for interpretation, then it is possible that his true verbal memory ability might fall somewhere between VPA-II and Logical Memory (LM) II. Using a confidence interval of 95 %, then the range estimate of two of the scores were LM-II 2–37 %ile and VPA-II 0.1−9 %ile; there is an area of overlap between the second and ninth percentiles. Despite this overlap, the discrepancy between LM-II and VPA-II seemed quite large. This can be quantified by using the known correlation between the two tests; from which it was estimated that about 10 % of the healthy population have a discrepancy of this magnitude or greater. This is quite uncommon; so might there be a neuropsychological explanation for it?

Stories offer the learner an inherent meaning and structure that aids learning and retrieval (Lezak 2004, p. 444). Patients with a problem organising new material, such as following mild traumatic brain injury, are less disadvantaged when structure is provided, compared to a task like word-pair learning (Guilmette and Rasile 1995). We would not expect the same difference with temporal lobe damage, and indeed no difference has been found between stories and word lists for people with TLE (Wilde et al. 2003; Doss et al. 2004). However perhaps counter to this, Helmstaedter et al. found that for people with TLE, story recall performance correlated with performance on executive tests such as verbal fluency (Helmstaedter et al. 2009). This brief consideration of neuropsychological evidence did not yield a satisfactory rationale to link AH's known left TLE pathology to his worse performance on VPA. Consideration of AH's worsening depression might offer a better fit to this pattern of results (Veiel 1997; Elliott et al. 1996; Diana et al. 1995).

In view of the above considerations, the possibility of memory impairment was retained and would be consistent with his left hippocampal sclerosis, but the amount of decline was judged to be relatively minor. Certainly, the severity of reported everyday problems seemed beyond that suggested by his psychometrics. Considering the wider context of worsening mood and intolerance towards condition-related problems, it was formulated that his everyday difficulties were exacerbated by psychological factors, along with other cognitive problems associated with medication and seizure activity.

2. *Predicted cognitive outcome.* Evidence suggests that memory functioning undergoes a decline over time without surgery, for example ~29% of one sample exhibited a reliable decline in verbal memory over ~5 years (Helmstaedter 2003). From the same study, ~47% experienced a decline in verbal memory after surgery to the left temporal lobe. Since presurgical decline in AH's verbal memory was minor if at all, then we assume that the brain tissue supporting this function was largely intact. As a consequence, if that tissue was removed or damaged by surgery then the impact on memory function was likely to be greater than otherwise (a "more to lose" principle; Schwarz 2005). There is also evidence to suggest that surgery later in life confers a greater risk to memory (Baxendale et al. 2006).

AH's profile of results was consistent with his known left-sided pathology and there was no reason to suspect other than left hemisphere dominance for language; therefore, language-based functions were more at risk from surgery to this hemisphere. Language problems are relatively common following surgery to the dominant hemisphere; estimates of the incidence of naming problems vary in the region of 34% (e.g. Ives-Deliperi and Butler 2012). For AH the risk is reduced somewhat because his seizures began in childhood, when brain function has more opportunity to adapt (Schwarz et al. 2005), although arguably AH had already acquired language before the onset of seizures. The presence of hippocampal sclerosis is a factor that reduces the likely severity of language problems should there be any (Davies et al. 1998).

It was formulated that processes relating to mental control and verbal fluency were inhibited by seizure activity and medication side effects, both of which might be "released" depending on the seizure outcome of surgery (the idea of "double winners"; Helmstaedter et al. 2003).

3. *Actual cognitive outcome and reformulation.* Because AH experienced complications during surgery, the likelihood of cognitive impairment unfortunately increased what might have been expected otherwise. On testing, no change was evident in his perceptual ability in terms of visuoconstruction, space perception

> or object recognition. His speed of performance during a nonverbal test of planning and reasoning was unremarkable. In fact, his success at this task exhibited an uncommonly large improvement, now performing in the superior range.

Whereas previously AH's retrieval of figural material (Visual Reproduction II) had a point estimate at the 50th %ile, 14 months later and after surgery the point estimate on this test was 16th %ile (in terms of standard score points this was a drop from 10 down to 7). Change analysis adopted a regression-based approach (Crawford and Garthwaite 2007) and was based upon data published in the test manual, which has a retest interval of 23 days. This normative sample revealed quite a large practice effect on this test, of near 3 standard points. Against this data, the magnitude of AH's decline was quite unusual, estimated to occur in less than 1 % of the healthy population (the upper confidence limit around this estimate being 1.3 %; not really changing the impression of rarity). However, it would be reasonable to question the equivalence of 23 days versus 14 months retest interval, and to suppose that improvement due to practice would decline over time; however, pending a more appropriate data set, there was no basis on which to quantify this. A decline in figural memory after *left* temporal lobe surgery is not uncommon (Helmstaedter et al. 2003) and so AH's decline to the low average range was interpreted as abnormal even though not large.

Whereas AH's picture naming ability was average prior to surgery, afterwards he exhibited a marked dysnomia during assessment. The onset or worsening of dysnomia has already been noted as a risk factor of temporal lobe surgery to the dominant hemisphere, and the complication of a bleed in this brain region offered an addition mechanism of damage.

Prior to surgery AH's performance on word fluency was near the floor of the test, and remained so after surgery. This was again attributed to seizure activity and/or medication. For information, his letter fluency score at T2 was slightly higher than at T1, but less than the mean increase of the normative sample, and so AH was in the direction of decline (albeit nonsignificant).

AH's performance on tests relating to attention and mental control was somewhat mixed. His recitation of digits forwards reduced to yield percentile point estimates from 25 % down to 2 %; a magnitude of change that occurs in less than 1 % of the healthy population. However, his recitation of digits backwards improved, from 9 % up to 25 %; a magnitude of change that occurs in up to 41 % of the healthy population. The longest number string he reversed was still less than that recited forwards, but after standardisation this pattern of results (forwards versus backwards) is difficult to make sense of under the well-known working memory model (Baddeley 2012). Specifically, any impairment of the phonological loop should limit more complex mental operations performed on information held therein. There are many possible reasons why AH did not perform at his best during digits forwards, whereas he might have found reverse digits more of a challenge and motivating. AH's seemingly uncommon decline in digits forwards was discarded because it did not make neuropsychological sense.

Prior to surgery, AH's performance on tests of verbal memory were quite mixed; he clearly struggled to learn word-pairs, whilst his story learning was only a little below expectations. After surgery he performed near the floor of both tests, LMII, for example dropped from a scaled score of 7 down to 1. Change analysis was not really required to support the conclusion that this magnitude of decline was clinically significant; analysis confirmed that less than 1 % of the healthy population exhibit such change. This finding was consistent with the known damage to his left cerebral hemisphere, and reported everyday memory problems that now required marked dependence on his wife in all activities of daily living.

AH's mood had declined progressively over time, which in itself might have contributed to worsening test performance. Whilst memory functioning has been implicated (Burt et al. 1995), it was observed that AH improved on cognitively effortful tasks (such as reverse digits and towers) which argued against mood playing a major role (Porter et al. 2007). For information, his psychological needs were prioritised clinically, and to date, he and his wife have engaged well with a specialist community service for neurological conditions.

Reflection and Discussion: Themes Associated with Serial Assessment of Cases over Longer Periods

Theme 1: The Role of the Patients' Account in Understanding the Processes Involved in Their Condition and Reaching a Formulation

The role of the patients' account in reaching a formulation is of key importance especially when there is equivocal evidence otherwise of whether or not impairment exists. Patients' accounts are one of several primary sources of information regarding the presenting or updated history. They can provide valuable information on the neuropsychological condition, narrowly, or on the patients' broader psychological wellbeing. They can corroborate or diverge from other aspects of the clinical picture.

In Case 1, at the time of JK's initial presentation to neurological services, uncertainty existed about the nature of her complaints; there was uncertainty about the significance of the left parietal lobe findings evident on MRI. However, JK gave a clear account at A1 of distinct neuropsychological changes that neatly matched the subsequent evidence from imaging and lent additional weight to the recent-onset nature of the difficulties. At A2, there was only patchy and inconsistent evidence from the neuropsychological assessments of further cognitive change: perhaps most evident in some of the perceptual tests and, most markedly of all, in line bisections. However, JK was clear that she had experienced further cognitive decline since the first assessment and this added important corroboration to the neuropsychometric evidence even in the absence of further changes on imaging.

For Case 2, AH was able to valuably identify the contribution of numerous life stressors to his general adverse condition, these including bereavements, psychological traumas, and frustration deriving from the impact of epilepsy on his activities and quality of life. At the same time, his insightful account of the nature and severity of his cognitive difficulties persuasively implicated a neurological basis to the cognitive changes rather than a basis from factors such as pain, fatigue, or stress despite there being no shortage of the latter.

As often in neuropsychological formulation, the account offered by both patients provided a vital and unique complement to the neuropsychological test data regarding the nature of the underlying difficulties and of cognitive change too subtle to be detected by formal tests.

Theme 2: Familiarity with the Patient and Their Family over Time—How This Can Make Formulation Both Easier and Harder

Time brings an additional quality to the neuropsychological clinical environment, namely of increased familiarity between patient and clinician. It is well accepted in other areas of psychological practice, such as psychological therapy, that familiarity is an important contributor to clinical outcome as it facilitates relationship building, increased trust, refinement of the information exchanged between patient and psychologist, and better exploration of the basis and meaning of the patient's experiences. Similarly in neuropsychological practice, increased familiarity is often an inevitable property of repeat assessments and can be key to securing the best information from the patient about their condition and it's impingement on their function. Increased familiarity over a longer period of contact can allow patients to reflect more safely and accurately on the nature of their difficulties. As such, it can help to clarify the nature and presence of neuropsychological changes and better characterise their resulting disabilities.

Conversely, familiarity can also complicate clinical progress, perhaps more so than in other areas of psychological practice where narrative development is more explicitly a goal of clinical contact and more intrinsically favourable to clinical outcomes. In neuropsychological formulation, the accuracy of patients' perceptions, including about neuropsychological change, can be central to accurate formulation and therefore clinical progress. Increased familiarity over time can potentially work against this, providing an inadvertent opportunity for patients to speculate beyond what is necessarily helpful about the nature of their difficulties.

For Case 1, JK, there were numerous occasions throughout the clinical contact when both factors were relevant. Increased familiarity facilitated the clinical relationship but, particularly during earlier periods of contact, JK speculated more than was warranted that her subjective cognitive difficulties were singularly associated with non-neurological factors such as low mood and stress (although it is accepted that a partial contribution from these at the time was likely). This meant that when neuropsychometric evidence emerged of a distinct neuropsychological basis for some of her subjective difficulties, she in turn experienced increased distress about the nature of the difficulties.

However, in Case 2, familiarity enabled a valuable additional perspective to be gained on AH's postsurgical progress. In addition to the neuropsychometric evidence of a favourable postsurgery neuropsychological state, familiarity that had built up over numerous contacts with the neuropsychologist enabled AH to give a clear, more rounded, and more honest account of his postsurgical condition including areas in which he had responded well and those in which he had not.

Theme 3: Test Selection

The above report of AH focused on the pre- and postsurgery assessment, however he had been assessed previously by another clinician. They had evaluated a broad range of cognitive domains beyond the mental processes of most interest. Given that no wider problems were found, there was no clinical reason to revisit them a second time around, hence a more targeted approach to testing could be adopted. On reflection, one could argue in favour of further testing of language and visual memory in this case, because these domains had the greatest clinical implications. A residual doubt from the case is whether the recurrence of seizures after surgery derived from a right-sided focus or not. However, there is often a case for further testing and a limit needs to be drawn somewhere. In addition to which his presurgery performance on the figural memory test was not equivocal. Another factor that drove towards a narrow test selection was concern about the overall number of analyses and attendant risk of spurious results (Binder 2009). Aside from the number of individual tests, the planned evaluation of change over time multiplied the number of analyses yet further.

Theme 4: Statistical Evaluation in Serial Assessment

To support the evaluation of change in AH's psychometrics, regression-based analysis was used, drawing largely on the work of Crawford and Garthwaite. The arguments for this approach are compelling and well described in their publications, such as Crawford (2013). Regression formulae have the potential to accommodate multiple factors, such as the polynomial solution used in the Test of Premorbid Functioning UK (Crawford et al. 2012; Wechsler 2009, p. 23). However, sample data are not readily available for many clinically useful factors and this raised two issues for the assessment of AH. First, one might suppose that someone with impaired memory at first testing is going to benefit less from the practice than someone with a good memory. Second, practice effect is likely to decay somewhat over time. As reported earlier, the only available data with which to evaluate performance change across AH's 14 month interval used a 23-day interval (Wechsler et al. 2009, p. 51). So in this instance, did regression analysis improve interpretation by correcting common biases (Crawford et al. 1998), or did the analysis give a frankly incorrect impression? On reflection it seemed better to have the information from the analysis, but reduce the weight of it within the wider interpretive context. It is relevant to note that the uncommon change in AH's digits forward score was rejected, because it did not make sense with his other results. A risk is that this interpretive approach becomes ad hoc and biased towards confirmatory evidence. However, the counter risk is to become data driven away from formulation that makes clinical sense. These issues go beyond the scope of this discussion, but they were considered when formulating AH's case.

Conclusions

The cases in this chapter have served to illustrate a number of themes important to formulating neuropsychological cases that are seen for repeat assessments over longer episodes of care. Four themes have been explored: the role of the patients' account in reaching a formulation; the role of increasing familiarity with patients over time; the selection and introduction of new tests; and the evaluation of serial data. Numerous issues within these themes are important in navigating the complex process of neuropsychological formulation which itself is key to the value of neuropsychology to patients, within the broader multidisciplinary care process.

References

Andrewes, D. G. (2001). *Neuropsychology: From theory to practice*. Taylor & Francis: New York

Baddeley, A. (2012). Working memory: Theories, models, and controversies. *Annual Review of Psychology, 63*, 12.1–12.29

Baxendale, S., Thompson, P., Harkness, W., & Duncan, J. (2006). Predicting memory decline following epilepsy surgery: A multivariate approach. *Epilepsia, 47*(11), 1887–1894.

Beck, A., Steer, R., & Brown, G. (2000). *Beck depression inventory fast screen for medical patients manual*. San Antonio: The Psychological Corporation.

Binder, L., Iverson, G., & Brooks, B. (2009). To err is human: "Abnormal" neuropsychological scores and variability are common in healthy adults. *Archives of Clinical Neuropsychology, 24*(1), 31–46.

Burt, D., Zembar, M., & Niederehe, G. (1995). Depression and memory impairment: A meta-analysis of the association, its pattern, and specificity. *Psychological Bulletin, 117*(2), 285–305.

Campo, P., Garrido, M., Moran, R., Maestu, F., Garcı´a-Morales, I., Gil-Nagel, A., Pozo, F., Dolan, R., & Friston, K. (2011). Remote effects of hippocampal sclerosis on effective connectivity during working memory encoding: A case of connectional diaschisis? *Cerebral Cortex, 22*(6), 1225–1236.

Costafreda, S., Fu, C., Lee, L., Everitt, B., Brammer, M., & David, A. (2006). A systematic review and quantitative appraisal of fMRI studies of verbal fluency: Role of the left inferior frontal gyrus. *Human Brain Mapping, 27*, 799–810.

Crawford, J. (2013). Quantitative aspects of neuropsychological assessment. In L. H. Goldstein & J. E. McNeil (Eds.), *Clinical neuropsychology: A practical guide to assessment and management for clinicians* (2nd ed.). West Sussex: Wiley-Blackwell.

Crawford, J., & Garthwaite, P. (2007). Using regression equations built from summary data in the neuropsychological assessment of the individual case. *Neuropsychology, 21*(5), 611–620.

Crawford, J., O'Carroll, R., & Venneri, A. (1998). Neuropsychological assessment of the elderly. In A. S. Bellack & M. Hersen (Eds.), *Comprehensive clinical psychology, volume 7: Clinical geropsychology*. Oxford: Pergamon.

Crawford, J., Garthwaite, P., Denham, A., & Chelune, G. (2012). Using regression equations built from summary data in the psychological assessment of the individual case: Extension to multiple regression. *Psychological Assessment, 24*(4), 801–814.

Davies, K., Bell, B., Bush, A., Hermann, B., Dohan, F., & Jaap, A. (1998). Naming decline after left anterior temporal lobectomy correlates with pathological status of resected hippocampus. *Epilepsia, 39*(4), 407–419.

Diana, B., Mary, Z., & Niederehe, J. (1995). Depression and memory impairment: A meta-analysis of the association, its pattern, and specificity. *Psychological Bulletin, 117*(2), 285–305.

Doss, R., Chelune, G., & Naugle, R. (2004). WMS-III performance in epilepsy patients following temporal lobectomy. *Journal of the International Neuropsychological Society, 10*(2), 173–179.

Eddy, C., Rickards, H., & Cavanna, A. (2011). The cognitive impact of antiepileptic drugs. *Therapeutic Advances in Neurological Disorders, 4*(6), 385–407.

Elliott, R., Sahakian, B., McKay, A., Herrod, J., Robbins, T., & Paykel, E. (1996). Neuropsychological impairments in unipolar depression: The influence of perceived failure on subsequent performance. *Psychological Medicine, 26*(5), 975–990.

Guilmette, T., & Rasile, D. (1995). Sensitivity, specificity, and diagnostic accuracy of three verbal memory measures in the assessment of mild brain injury. *Neuropsychology, 9*(3), 338–344.

Helmstaedter, C., Kurthen, M., Lux, S., Reuber, M., & Elger, C. (2003). Chronic epilepsy and cognition: A longitudinal study in temporal lobe epilepsy. *Annals of Neurology, 54,* 425–432.

Helmstaedter, C., Wietzke, J., & Lutz, M. (2009). Unique and shared validity of the "Wechsler logical memory test", the "California verbal learning test", and the "verbal learning and memory test" in patients with epilepsy. *Epilepsy Research, 87*(2–3), 203–212.

Henry, J., & Crawford, J. (2004). A meta-analytic review of verbal fluency performance following focal cortical lesions. *Neuropsychology, 18*(2), 284–295.

Ives-Deliperi, V., & Butler, J. (2012). Naming outcomes of anterior temporal lobectomy in epilepsy patients: A systematic review of the literature. *Epilepsy & Behavior, 24*(2), 194–198.

Lezak, M., Howieson, D., & Loring, D. (2004). *Neuropsychological assessment* (4th ed.). New York: Oxford University Press.

Porter, R., Bourke, C. & Gallagher, P. (2007). Neuropsychological impairment in major depression: Its nature, origin and clinical significance. *Australian & New Zealand Journal of Psychiatry, 41,* 115.

Robinson, G., Shallice, T., Bozzali, M., & Cipolotti, L. (2012). The differing roles of the frontal cortex in fluency tests. *Brain, 135,* 2202–2214.

Schramm, J. (2008). Temporal lobe epilepsy surgery and the quest for optimal extent of resection: A review. *Epilepsia, 49*(8), 1296–1307.

Schwarz, M., Pauli, E., & Stefan, H. (2005). Model based prognosis of postoperative object naming in left temporal lobe epilepsy. *Seizure, 14*(8), 562–568.

Stern, R., Singer, E., Duke, L., Singer, N., Morey, C., Daughtrey, E., & Kaplan, E. (1994). The Boston qualitative scoring system for the Rey-Osterrieth complex figure: Description and interrater reliability. *The Clinical Neuropsychologist, 8*(3), 309–322.

Veiel, H. (1997). A preliminary profile of neuropsychological deficits associated with major depression. *Journal of Clinical and Experimental Neuropsychology, 19*(4), 587–603

Wechsler, D. (2009). *Wechsler test of premorbid functioning—UK edition; administration, scoring and technical manual.* UK: The Psychological Corporation, Pearson.

Wechsler, D., Holdnack, J., & Drozdick. (2009). *Wechsler memory scale–Fourth edition: Technical and interpretive manual.* UK: Pearson.

Wilde, N., Strauss, E., Chelune, G., Hermann, B., Hunter, M., Loring, D., Martin, R., & Sherman, E. (2003). Confirmatory factor analysis of the WMS-III in patients with temporal lobe epilepsy. *Psychological Assessment, 15*(1), 56–63.

Chapter 11
Decisional Capacity in the Traumatically Injured

Christina Weyer Jamora and Ron Ruff

Introduction

Loss of capacity in patients with moderate to severe traumatic brain injuries (TBIs) is a common issue that clinicians face. In the adult inpatient setting, upwards to 75% of neuropsychological referrals relate to decisional capacity (Moberg and Kniele 2006).

Decisional capacity can be defined as the ability to (1) appreciate one's circumstances and the inherent consequences of one's actions, (2) understand relevant information, (3) communicate a consistent choice in treatment or lack thereof, and (4) reason rationally (Applebaum and Grisso 1988; Marson 2005). Additionally, (5) individuals must be able to retain information over time in order to make use of all of the above constructs. The primary aim of this chapter is to present a TBI case that highlights the neuropsychological formulation approach for determining capacity. We also aim to provide a framework by which neuropsychologists can think through clinical questions, and provide practical suggestions by which to implement this suggested framework.

C. W. Jamora (✉)
San Francisco General Hospital & University of California-San Francisco,
909 Hyde St #620, 94109 San Francisco, CA 94109, USA
e-mail: Christina.Weyerjamora@UCSF.edu

R. Ruff
University of California-San Francisco, c/o 909 Hyde Street #620,
San Francisco, CA 94109, USA
e-mail: ronruff@mindspring.com

J. A. B. Macniven (ed.), *Neuropsychological Formulation*,
DOI 10.1007/978-3-319-18338-1_11

Case

The patient that we will describe was seen for an inpatient neuropsychological assessment as part of the neurosurgical service at a large urban metropolitan, level I trauma centre. This is a high-volume neurosurgical service that has been approved by the Joint Commission as a TBI specialty program in the USA. In particular, the neurosurgical service focuses on TBI-specific multidisciplinary treatment planning and research, as well as inpatient and outpatient clinic follow-up care and support. The following patient was seen and followed in the context of the aforementioned program.

TN (fictitious initials) is a 36-year-old bilingual English and Vietnamese speaking, right-handed man who suffered a moderate TBI after being assaulted. After the assault, his friends brought him into the emergency room where staff noted that he was quite confused and repeating himself. His last memory prior to his injury was dropping his girlfriend off at home. While on the medical unit, he was quite confused and his posttraumatic amnesia lasted for 5 days. For example, he attempted to leave the hospital to "go back to work" despite not knowing where he lived nor where he worked. Serial CT imaging revealed multifocal damage, including bi-frontal subdural haematomas (left worse than right), left temporal subdural haematoma, cerebellar subarachnoid haemorrhage, and facial fractures.

As his thinking became clearer, he was able to remember where he was and the reason for his hospitalisation. However, the nursing staff noticed that TN struggled to remember information he was told. For example, he had difficulties recalling what medications he was given, and who had visited him. After 2 weeks, the neurosurgical team was considering discharging TN from the hospital; however, the team was unsure what kind of help TN would require once he left the hospital.

The patient's girlfriend, who lived in another town, agreed to help TN; however, her ability to do so was limited. She agreed to help him in the evenings and on weekends, but she was unavailable for most of the day. She tearfully described wanting to help him even more, but explained that she needed to work during the day. Thus, for much of the day and night, we understood that he would be unsupervised. This available level of supervision was concerning, and therefore prompted the neurosurgical team to refer TN for a neuropsychological assessment, to determine whether he possessed the capacity to independently make his own medical decisions and the level of supervision he would need upon discharge.

Neuropsychological Evaluation

At the time of the neuropsychological evaluation, TN was alert and oriented to person, place, and date. He presented as a fit man who looked approximately his stated age. When asked, he stated that he felt equally or even more comfortable with the evaluation being conducted in English, as he was educated in the USA from the age of 7.

TN was observed by the staff to be quite sensitive to environmental stimulation such as bright light and loud sounds. Moreover, when there was increased light and noise in his room, he became restless or even irritable. Thus from the outset of the examination, the clinician drew the window curtains and closed the door, which allowed the patient to remain fully engaged.

Clinical Interview

During the clinical interview, he was able to appropriately answer questions regarding his medical care and the ways in which he would go about taking care of himself. He correctly stated why he was in the hospital ("I had a brain injury"). He was also able to articulate the risks of various aspects of his medical care (risks of reinjury, how to contact his primary care physician, risks of alcohol use, and side effects of his medications, etc.). In a more general way, he was able to state the purpose for his medications ("To keep me from having seizures"); however, he struggled to remember which pills he had taken that day. Reminders from the nurses about his medication regimen were helpful in this regard. He acknowledged that once he returned home, he would need help with managing aspects of his life such as his medications, medical appointments, and bill paying.

Similarly, he was able to recall hypothetical medical information, weigh risks and benefits of proposed treatments, articulate a choice in treatments, and recall his treatment choice 2 h later. As part of this exercise, the patient was also told to pretend that the doctor had told him that he had a heart condition and to treat this condition he could either undergo surgery (which would cure the condition) or medication (which would help the condition, but not cure it). In this vignette, he was given various risks and benefits about the proposed treatments. When he was asked what he would do under these circumstances, he stated, "I would have surgery. I would want it cured since the procedure sounds pretty safe; I think it would be worth it".

In terms of cognitive issues, TN reported minimal cognitive sequelae from his injury. He acknowledged some "mild forgetfulness" since his injury, but minimised the significance of his memory deficits. That said, he did report having difficulty thinking quickly and becoming more easily distracted.

Prior to his injury, much of TN's life revolved around his work as a real-estate agent. He began working as a real-estate agent shortly after he graduated from college with an Associate degree. He proudly described, "loving to help Vietnamese families find homes, which is my professional niche". Therefore, much of his personal and professional time was spent speaking Vietnamese.

Financially, he stated that he would live off savings until he was able to return to work. He also explained that with the help of the Social Work staff, he was going to apply for short-term disability. He acknowledged feeling frustrated that he could not return to work, but overall he felt grateful for his girlfriend's support. When he was asked whether any of his family (who lived near him) could help him, he lamented that he had been estranged from his family for years and tearfully described fear-ing that he could not rely on their support. Finally, he reported no history of prior psychiatric, addiction issues, or major medical illness.

Neuropsychological Test Results

A summary of the neuropsychological test scores is provided in Table 11.1.

Overall, the neuropsychological screening battery captured diminished cognitive functioning across all assessed domains. However, his test performances were particularly compromised in verbal learning, memory, and word-finding tasks. In light of his prior education and occupational attainment, these scores were clearly lower than expected.

Despite of these impaired test scores, TN understood the nature and implications of his injury, and was able to articulate the implications of not following up with medical care, as well as the risks of reinjury. When asked during the clinical interview how he would care for himself upon discharge, he said, "my girlfriend will help me".

Despite TN's ability to articulate a plan of care when prompted in the clinical interview, his neuropsychological test performance raised concerns about his ability to independently recall taking his medications and practice good judgment. This was particularly worrisome, since upon returning to his home he was going to spend the great majority of his time alone and thus unsupervised. Moreover, when he would leave his home to run errands, the concern was raised whether he could find his way around. In this regard, the formal testing was less instructive and helpful in guiding the supervisory recommendations.

Table 11.1 Neuropsychological test scores

Tests	Scores
Galveston orientation and amnesia score (Levin et al. 1979)	95/100
WAIS-III digit span (Wechsler, 1997), (5 forward, 4 back)	16th percentile
RBANS list learning (Randolph 1998) (4, 4, 4, 4)	< 1st percentile for immediate delay
	< 1st percentile, long delay (no words)
	Recalled 80 % of the list with cues
RBANS story memory (Randolph 1998)	< 1st percentile for immediate delay
	16th percentile, long delay
RBANS naming (Randolph 1998)	< 1st percentile
RBANS figure copy (Randolph 1998)	4th percentile
Trail making A (Reitan and Wolfson 1993)	16th percentile
Trail making B (Reitan and Wolfson 1993)	10th percentile
Beck depression inventory-II (Beck 1996)	21, moderate depression
Endorsed moderate levels of anxiety, depression, and increased anger and irritability	

RBANS repeatable battery for the assessment of neuropsychological status

Functional Assessment

Functional tasks were added to the assessment to help clarify the patient's abilities and needs for supervision upon discharge. To assess his need for supervision while finding his way around in the community, he was asked to do a path finding task whereby he used the signs in the hospital to find his way to the hospital cafeteria, the clinic he would receive his follow-up care, the gift shop to purchase items, and then back to his room. On this task, he did well navigating in a new and novel environment with no cueing. Additionally, he avoided bumping into oncoming people and environmental hazards such as spills on the floor. His social graces were also normal in that he opened doors for others and engaged in typical social repartee.

Since the patient was likely to need to shop for food occasionally, the medical team was concerned about TN's ability to perform this task also independently. To assess his ability to make purchases, he was asked to remove $20 from the hospital ATM, and thereafter purchase a number of items from the hospital's gift shop. He was told the items shortly prior to leaving for the path-finding task and he was expected to remember the items on the list with no written reminders. TN completed all these tasks without errors. However, on a subsequent prospective memory task where he was asked to take three pills out of a mock pill bottle in 2 h after the instructions were given, he was able to recall/remember to take the pills in 2 h, but forgot how many pills he needed to retrieve. With multiple-choice cueing his recall improved and he was able to recall how much medication to take.

Formulation of Capacity

Historically, there has been a shift in the discipline of neuropsychology from a focus on localising brain damage towards establishing the nature and extent of impaired cognition, as well as the implications of these impairments on a person's activities of daily living. Increasingly referral sources are not only interested in whether a patient has decisional capacity but also need us to determine the level of supervision that is needed for the patient function in a safe manner.

Capacity to make one's own decisions generally requires clinicians to assess an individual's ability to articulate the nature of their difficulties, weigh risks and benefits of their various decisions, articulate a choice in care, and retain this information over time (Marson 2005). In this process, neuropsychological testing can be instructive; however, generalising from one's test performance to functioning in the real world is fraught with difficulties.

The neuropsychological tests indicated that TN's verbal memory was significantly impaired, consistent with the left fronto-temporal damage confirmed by neuroimaging. Thus, based on this information alone, we may have concluded that he was unable to function independently. However, in the clinical interview, TN was clearly able to articulate the nature of his medical issues and his need for help upon discharge. TN understood the reason for his hospitalisation and the implications of not following up with medical care, and could identify symptoms that would necessitate emergent medical intervention. He also acknowledged that he would need help with managing his medications, medical appointments, and bills and he was willing to accept help.

In terms of weighing risks and benefits, TN was able to adequately articulate the risks of reinjury, not following up with medical care, and failing to take his antiseizure medication. Similarly, on a medical decision-making vignette he was able to weigh the risks and benefits of various hypothetical treatments and articulate a consistent treatment choice. This suggests that he not only is able to recall and critically process previously learned information but also incorporate new information. This is contrary to his neuropsychological test scores, which would suggest that his ability to do this is quite limited. Therefore, it is unlikely that the test scores accurately reflected his abilities. The reason for the discrepancy is unclear; however, factors such as issues with ecological generalisability, premature assessment in the post-acute phase, and possible patient factors (headaches and bilingual status) may have played a role. Unfortunately, the demands and realities of busy inpatient services necessitate early assessment, which is often under suboptimal conditions.

Further, TN was able to recall information germane to his medical care and discharge planning over extended periods of time. This ability to hold on to pertinent information is a particularly important aspect of capacity assessment that should not be overlooked. He initially was only able to recall basic information and those who visited him; however, this became less problematic as his recovery progressed. Even when the examiner returned 2 days later, he was able to recall much of our conversation, the choices he had made about where he would live, the fact that his girlfriend was to support him on discharge, and the risks of reinjury and not taking his medications.

Finally, TN's ability to both articulate his plan of care and to demonstrate successful completion of complex functional tasks was promising. His performance on functional tasks such as path finding, purchasing food, and using an ATM suggested that he could implement his intentions for caring for himself. His need for cueing on medication management informed the patient's after-care plan and allowed for the team to address this in the care planning conference. His girlfriend agreed to fill his medication box and to call him to remind him to take his medications. These findings gave the neurosurgical team confidence that he could live a more autonomous life, and clarified areas that he would need additional help.

Ethical Concerns

Ethically, clinicians are bound to hold principles such as veracity, autonomy, and beneficence even when the patients themselves cannot do so (Larkin et al. 2001). Veracity may be thought of as articulating a truthful narrative about the patient (Larkin et al. 2001). At its core, veracity mandates accuracy in both score reporting and clinical observations. Beyond this, grappling with veracity may take on a subtler form. For example, a clinician may unknowingly be imprinted with early compelling information about a case. Without an a priori framework upon which to guide the assessment, the hypothesis testing becomes problematically circular.

Autonomy and beneficence are connected, but disparate constructs central to our role as providers and evaluators (Berg et al. 2001). The principle of autonomy maintains that a clinician should avoid unnecessary impingement upon the patient's decision-making, even if the decision is not fully in the patient's best interests (Larkin et al. 2001). In TN's case, the team supported the patient's preference to return home with his girlfriend's support in accord with preserving his autonomy, but not at the cost of causing undue harm.

In contrast, it may not always be ethically appropriate to champion a patient's autonomy. For example, the concept of justified paternalism (intervening on the patient's behalf with life-saving interventions) has been argued as being ethically appropriate in some circumstances, particularly in a medical crisis (Buchanan 2008).

Interestingly, it is the magnitude of damage and not the likelihood that the patient will be debilitated that has been argued as being of utmost importance (Brown 1985). In the face of little information about the patient's premorbid wishes, it assumes treatment should be aggressive and lifesaving, but the ethical viability of this expires once the emergency passes (Andy Bruenner, Esq., personal communication, 2012). For example, in the subacute setting, if an emergency can be anticipated, (i.e. an intractable seizure disorder) the reasoning for justified paternalism becomes less robust. Often consulting with a hospital's medical ethics board for risk management and/or colleagues with ethics expertise can be immensely helpful in thinking through these thorny ethical dilemmas.

Beneficence insists that a provider acts in the best interest of a patient, even if this means not fully complying with the patient's wishes. Given the nature of decisional capacity, there is a natural tension that can arise between maintaining a balance between autonomy and beneficence (Pantilat 2008). Such as in the case of TN, the team ethically addressed issues of beneficence through a supervised transition to home, close outpatient follow up, and engaging his girlfriend as a caregiver.

Outcome

The neurosurgical team decided that (1) TN was capable to make decisions on his own behalf, yet (2) he did need help with his daily affairs to ensure his safety, and (3) his girlfriend was the appropriate person to provide the needed help in this regard. A supervision plan was devised in conjunction with the patient and his girlfriend. The neurosurgical team allowed him to continue his recovery at home, while taking into account his unique limitations.

TN and his girlfriend were relieved that he would be able to return home; however, they were apprehensive about his discharge. TN, his girlfriend, and the neurosurgical team agreed that the initial post-discharge period was crucial for his understanding how he would adjust and work around his difficulties. To ease this transition, the patient's girlfriend agreed to stay with him for the first 2 weeks. In this interim phase, she agreed to observe his abilities with independent activities of daily living such as food shopping, laundry, navigating in the community, and medication management. Additionally, the patient was scheduled for an outpatient clinic visit 1 week after he was discharged to evaluate how the transition to home was progressing and to refer him to additional services as needed.

TN expressed concern about managing his finances (e.g. tracking bills that had been paid, balancing his check book, making sure his bills were paid on time). The patient discussed that while he was open to his girlfriend helping him, he preferred to largely manage his own finances. The team suggested that he work with his bank to set up automatic bill paying, online budgeting, and tracking his expenses. The patient agreed to do this and at the time of discharge he had already began working with his local banker to set this plan in motion.

When TN and his girlfriend presented for their follow-up clinic visit 1 week after discharge, they reported that he was doing well. As predicted, he was able to food shop, do laundry, and navigate in the community to familiar places such as his favourite coffee shop and grocery store. He was also working successfully with an outpatient social worker and his banker to manage his financial issues. His girlfriend reported that he had some difficulty remembering to take his medications, despite his medication box, and thus reminder phone calls were needed in the foreseeable future. At this point, it was determined that he did not require any additional supervision and the patient agreed to follow up in the clinic in 1 month and for every 3 months thereafter for the first year.

Over the course of that year, TN's post-concussive headaches and fatigue became less prominent. By 6 months post-injury he had returned to work on a part-time basis doing administrative tasks in his real-estate office. As the 1-year anniversary of his injury drew near he had returned to work as a real-estate agent on a part-time basis. His fatigue was the primary barrier to his returning to work on a more full-time basis.

Discussion

Overall, TN's case contained many of the typical elements often seen in busy metropolitan neurosurgical services. Providing an accurate assessment of the patient's functioning in a timely manner is often challenging. Neuropsychologists in this setting are often under pressure to render decisions about clinical care based on little information and suboptimal circumstances. In this context, one often must undertake a thoughtful and reasoned approach that not only takes into account the patient's unique needs but also the available resources and the limitations therein. While inpatient evaluations are often suboptimal, they provide crucial information to assist in discharge planning.

TN's case taught us much in terms of the importance of critically thinking through a case using multiple informational sources. In particular, this case highlighted the importance of not overvaluing the neuropsychological testing when functional information is potentially contradictory. Additionally, utilising Marson's capacity framework allowed the assessment to be focused on the components needed to answer important issues such as the ability to make one's medical decisions (Marson 2005). Further, the functional testing clarified the patient's post-discharge supervision needs.

In this case, it would have been beneficial to have additional information regarding TN's premorbid functioning to better understand his unique strengths and limitations. Upon reflecting back, it would have also been helpful to explore the patient's cultural resources in greater detail before he was discharged. In subsequent clinic visits, the team learned that the Vietnamese culture was an important part of his identity. Despite the rift with his family, TN and his girlfriend benefited from the help and emotional support that they received from their Vietnamese community. Exploring this early on may have allowed us to provide recommendations that could have incorporated the support that was available by their Vietnamese community.

Beyond addressing the issue of decisional capacity, this case also highlights the importance of carefully implementing supervision recommendations and monitoring post-discharge needs. As a rule, providers are well served to involve potential caregivers early on and throughout the discharge process. This allows for enhanced continuity of care and support for the patient and helps caregivers to be more informed and realistic in their expectations. Additionally, pacing supervision that fades as the patient becomes more capable allows the patient to enjoy additional autonomy. That said, caregivers might need some guidance in this regard. Repeated outpatient follow up to track progress and provide support can facilitate this process and allow caregivers and patients to feel more confident and grounded in their transition through the various recovery phases.

References

Applebaum, P. S., & Grisso, T. (1988). Assessing patients' capacities to consent to treatment. *The New England Journal of Medicine, 319*(25), 1635–1638.

Beck, A. T., Steer, R. A., & Brown, G. K. (1996). *Manual for the beck depression inventory-II*. San Antonio: Psychological Corporation.

Berg, J. W., Appelbaum, P. S., Lidz, C. W., & Parker, L. S. (2001). *Informed consent: Legal theory and clinical practice*. New York: Oxford University Press

Brown, K. (1985). Can medical paternalism be justified? *Canadian Medical Association Journal, 133*(7), 678–680.

Buchanan, D. R. (2008). Autonomy, paternalism, and justice: Ethical priorities in public health. *American Journal of Public Health, 98*(1), 15–21.

Larkin, G., Marco, C. A., & Abbott, J. T. (2001). Emergency determination of decision-making capacity: Balancing autonomy and beneficence in the emergency department. *Academic Emergency Medicine, 8*(3), 282–284

Levin, H., O'Donnell, V., & Grossman, R. (1979). The Galveston Orientation and Amnesia Test: A practical scale to assess cognition after head injury. *Journal of Nervous and Mental Disorders, 20,* 694–705

Marson, D. C., Dreer, L. E., Krzywanski, S., Huthwaite, J. S., DeVivo, M. J., & Novack, T. A. (2005). Impairment and partial recovery of medical decision-making capacity in traumatic brain injury: A 6-month longitudinal study. *Archives of Physical Medicine and Rehabilitation, 86*(5), 889–895.

Moberg, P. J., & Kniele, K. (2006). Evaluation of competency: Ethical considerations for neuropsychologists. *Applied Neuropsychology, 13*(2), 101–114

Pantilat, S. (2008). *Decision making capacity*. San Francisco: UCSF School of Medicine.

Randolph C. (1998). *Repeatable battery for the assessment of neuropsychological status*. San Antonio: The Psychological Corporation.

Reitan, R. M., & Wolfson, D. (1993). *The Halstead Reitan neuropsychological test battery: Theory and clinical interpretation* (2nd ed.). Tucson: Neuropsychology Press.

Wechsler, D. (1997). *Wechsler adult intelligence scale III*. San Antonio: The Psychological Corporation.

Chapter 12
Educational Disengagement Following Mild Traumatic Brain Injury in Childhood

Ingram Wright

Work Setting

Bristol is a city of 400,000 people in the southwest of England. Our specialist services include a regional paediatric neurosciences service based at Bristol Royal Hospital for Children and serving the southwest region with a population of 6.5 million. Our neurosciences centre has 20 beds and an additional 5 neurorehabilitation beds. Our neuropsychology service is principally assessment-focused and designed to meet the needs of children following acquired brain injury. We offer over 190 outpatient appointments per year comprising an initial consultation, brief focused assessment and subsequent feedback session to discuss written reports. Opportunities for extensive treatment are limited, but we make good use of links with educational psychology and child mental health services.

Background/Referral Details

Katie was referred to our service by a community paediatrician specialising in chronic fatigue syndrome (CFS) who had concerns about the likely relationship between Katie's head injury and her presentation with fatigue and cognitive problems. The principal concerns were memory and concentration difficulties thought to be affecting Katie's schooling. Prior to our service receiving the referral, Katie had been referred to the community paediatrician by her general practitioner (GP) who had expressed concern regarding her presentation with debilitating fatigue and withdrawal from school attendance.

I. Wright (✉)
Department of Experimental Psychology, University of Bristol, The Priory Road Complex, Priory Road, Clifton BS8 1TU, Bristol, UK
e-mail: ingram.wright@bristol.ac.uk

J. A. B. Macniven (ed.), *Neuropsychological Formulation*,
DOI 10.1007/978-3-319-18338-1_12

Katie had suffered a head injury 2 years prior to the referral. She had tripped on a step and hit her head on a pipe protruding from a wall. The accident was witnessed by her friends who had managed her sympathetically but had not sought to attract medical attention. Katie was reported to have lost consciousness briefly and had retrograde amnesia for several hours prior to the injury.

Katie completed her school day and on returning home appeared pale, and complained of a headache. She was puzzled that her phone was broken and could not recall how this had happened. On enquiring via her friends, her parents heard details of the accident and also noted bruising and tenderness at the top of her head. Katie was not taken to the Emergency Department at this stage but was monitored by her parents and visited her GP the following day for advice. Katie was absent from school for 2 weeks initially but experienced worsening of her symptoms on return to school when she had engaged in a sports session. She was then advised to take a further 4 weeks off school.

Since the time of her injury, and up to the point of her referral to neuropsychology, Katie had suffered persistent dizzy spells and headaches. Her GP had initially referred her to a general community paediatrician 12 months after the injury. This referral was initiated given her complaints of memory and concentration difficulties at school with accompanying poor attendance. Initial investigations undertaken by the paediatrician included routine blood tests and screening specifically for possible medical causes of her fatigue and headaches. All investigations had returned negative results. At 18 months post head injury, a follow-up appointment documents normal neurological examination but with Katie's parents reporting that her symptoms were worsening and particularly problematic when she was stressed or anxious. A referral was subsequently made to a paediatric specialist in chronic fatigue.

Since the initial injury, Katie had experienced numerous additional ailments, including recurrent infections of her chest, throat and urinary tract. She was also experiencing gradually more debilitating fatigue with frequent headaches alongside memory and concentration problems. She had found these issues so problematic that she had experienced symptoms of significant low mood and anxiety about her schoolwork.

Katie attended her local state secondary school but had not been able to keep up with her academic work. She had planned to attend school every day but only achieved average attendance of 60 %. Her school had been unable to get any additional finance to support her inclusion in school or to provide any additional support in classroom learning. Despite poor school attendance, Katie had continued to maintain contact with her friends on a regular basis using social media and arranging social activities outside school.

Sleeping remained a significant problem, and Katie tended to go to bed at 10 p.m. but then read or listened to music and was typically awake until around 4 a.m. Katie described the mental aspect of her fatigue as the most debilitating. In terms of physical and social activities, she was not reporting any significant limitations, although often chose to engage in more sedentary activities with her friends. Katie had not reported any other restrictions relative to her previous level of physical activity. However, she reported some fatigue when engaged in sustained activity and, for example, was able to go shopping for no more than an hour before needing to rest. One year after the injury, she had reported some improvement in her concentration, although she experienced persistent memory problems.

The specialist paediatrician considered the onset of symptoms as too specific to the head injury to warrant a diagnosis of CFS. This conclusion precipitated the referral to neuropsychology approximately 2 years after the initial injury.

Clinical Interview

Katie attended an appointment accompanied by her parents. She was smartly but casually dressed and appeared initially rather nervous. She became increasingly confident during the consultation and addressed questions fluently. She appeared socially oriented and articulate.

Katie lives at home with her parents and two sisters. Her sister Megan is 18 years old and was diagnosed with ME/CFS (Myalgic Encephalomyelitis) at 15 years of age following a viral illness at the age of 11. Katie also has a much older sister who is 31 years old, who has complex partial seizures following a diagnosis of epilepsy as an infant. Katie's parents are self-employed and run a small business in the computing sector. Both parents were educated to university level and reported no further history of learning or neurological problems in the family.

Katie was born following an uneventful pregnancy and delivery, and there were no reported early developmental concerns. Prior to Katie's injury she had no reported history of learning difficulties or educational concerns. There was no history of any previous accidents or injuries. She integrated well into initial primary school, enjoyed school, and generally made good educational progress. Some concerns regarding possible mild dyslexia were highlighted by her teacher but were not formally investigated. She obtained average level attainments on completion of her primary education. Katie had some subsequent difficulties settling into secondary school but this improved and, immediately prior to the injury, she was performing well both academically and socially. She had been predicted above average A–C grades in all subjects with the exception of mathematics.

Katie was in year 9 at the time of the injury, 2 years prior to school examinations and the completion of her secondary education.

Katie described the accident as reported above. She was described by a friend as having lost consciousness for a few seconds but returned to the classroom looking pale and unwell. She did not mention the injury to her parents on returning home, but on noticing her broken mobile phone, failed to remember what had happened during the day. Her friend subsequently volunteered information regarding the accident.

Katie went to see her GP who suggested that some of her symptoms might be secondary to a urinary infection for which she had tested positive. She was advised to take 2 weeks off school.

In the days following her injury, Katie reported not feeling her normal self and described feeling “on edge and frustrated”. Katie continued to experience symptoms of dizziness and headaches and her GP apparently advised her to undertake rest and she had 4 weeks absence from school at this point. On return to school she was again apparently advised to refrain from undertaking physical education (P.E.) for a further couple of weeks. However, her P.E. teacher advised her to jog around the field and to do star jumps. This apparently made her feel sick and her headache returned. Following these events, Katie’s GP apparently advised a further 2 weeks off school, with concern about ongoing bad headaches and dizzy spells. Katie eventually returned to school after 8–9 weeks but became significantly frustrated in the class. She experienced several recurrent illnesses and often became tearful, frustrated and unable to concentrate, finding it difficult to tolerate how far she was falling behind with her work.

Katie was initially diagnosed as having post-concussion syndrome (PCS) and subsequently ME/CFS. She experienced significant anxiety and reported loss of social confidence following the injury. During her period of convalescence she had done no schoolwork for 9 weeks.

Katie reported the onset of symptoms of significant fatigue around 3 months after the accident with prominent dizzy spells and headaches. A referral to neuropsychology was made by a specialist paediatrician who felt that Katie’s symptoms did not entirely fit with CFS, the onset of her symptoms being too specific to the head injury.

Katie continued to suffer problems including recurrent infections and illnesses and increasingly debilitating fatigue with associated headache, memory and concentration problems. At the time of our appointment, Katie was 2 years post-injury and was attending the final year of secondary/high school. She experienced ongoing difficulties keeping up with academic work, with reduced school attendance, despite no apparent physical or social limitations.

At the time of our appointment, Katie had returned to school part-time, but her attendance remained poor and she had supplementary home tuition for 5 hours per week split over 4 days. She had reduced her number of academic subjects at school from nine to six.

Following her head injury, Katie reported some hearing problems, memory loss, poor concentration and working memory. Her parents expressed a specific concern regarding her apparent poor hearing, with a need for her to keep music and television at high volume, although referral to an audiology specialist revealed no apparent problems.

Katie maintained contact with three good friends and reported no ongoing social difficulties. There had been some previous bullying in primary school and Katie found it difficult to discuss this in our consultation and became tearful when it was raised. Parental accounts indicate that Katie had lost confidence while at primary school but did not receive counselling at this point.

Katie’s sleep was reported to be very poor. She would often not fall asleep when going to bed around 10:30 p.m. and would either watch television or engage in artwork and often be worried about not sleeping. She had tried some medication but had not found this effective. She also tended to sleep during the day as a consequence of her poor sleep.

There were some concerns regarding memory functioning. Katie reported having a limited capacity for verbal instructions, preferring these to be kept short and simple. She reported similar difficulties at home and school, although experienced more prominent problems in the classroom environment. She was noted to have reasonable attentional skills and, for example, was able to read very lengthy novels and could subsequently recall the narrative without difficulty. She described a reasonable memory for details of recent past events. Katie also commented that her prospective memory was intact. There were no concerns regarding her language, communication or adaptive functioning. Katie reported taking good care of herself in terms of activities of daily living and eating a varied diet but taking exercise only infrequently. She remained organised and relatively independent despite her other disabling symptoms.

On talking to Katie on her own she was open about her future plans to take school examination in English, Maths and Art, with a goal to take a photography course at college. She was open about her lack of confidence and felt that she had not been offered support, although it would have been helpful to her in the past. Her friends have currently been very supportive and encouraged her to be positive and to socialise with them. Katie told me that she occasionally avoided social interaction and had persistently struggled with confidence in social situations, although had never received any formal support with this. Katie told me that she would like some help with her education once at college. When I asked Katie to elaborate on this she told me that meeting new people would be the hardest thing and that if she could manage this, then things would be a lot easier. Katie expressed optimism that many of her symptoms would improve on leaving school, and she compared herself to her sister for whom things improved when she left school. Katie felt that she may need help with some of her education when she goes to college as she finds meeting new people one of the hardest things she has to do. She reported her ambition to be a music photographer and talked enthusiastically about attending a recent music festival with this in mind.

Assessment

Katie generally engaged well with the formal assessment process but lacked confidence and was somewhat inhibited. She appeared to be very hesitant when providing answers to the verbal reasoning subtests of the Wechsler Intelligence Scale for Children-Fourth Edition (WISC-IV), often responding by saying "I don't know". If prompted, Katie would occasionally try to expand on answers, but her apparent lack of confidence seemed to inhibit her responses. She did respond well to praise and encouragement. When completing the picture concepts task Katie required instructions to be repeated several times. Following this she worked well. Katie appeared easily distracted during the presentation of some stimuli, particularly on memory tasks, and reported fatigue towards the end of the assessment session. For example, when completing the family pictures task from the Children's Memory Scale, Katie would look out of the window while being presented with the stimulus and was quite easily distracted by people walking past. Katie completed the Conner's Continuous Performance Test-Second Edition (CPT-II), on occasion she would rest her head on her arm but seemed to remain focussed.

A summary of formal assessment results and parental and self-reported symptoms is shown in Tables 12.1 and 12.2.

Assessment of Katie's intellectual abilities was undertaken using a short form of WISC-IV intelligence scale for children (Wechsler 2003). This assessment revealed verbal comprehension and perceptual reasoning within the average to low average range (19th–30th percentile). There was no marked discrepancy between verbal and nonverbal reasoning.

Katie's performance on memory tests was consistent with her intellectual abilities with no material-specific deficits. On a broad-based test of attentional functioning (CPT-II; Conners 1994), she produced relatively fast responses with a consequent high frequency of commission errors, suggesting poor impulse control. The overall pattern was of mild inattention and impulsivity, with no evidence of significant problems with vigilance. A discriminant function analysis of the pattern of results suggested a relatively low likelihood of a clinically significant attention problem.

As an adjunct to the above formal assessment of Katie's cognitive abilities, we asked both parents and Katie to complete the Strengths and Difficulties Questionnaire (SDQ; Goodman 1997), a self-report assessment of a child's emotional and behavioural functioning. Both parents and Katie highlighted significant emotional

Table 12.1 Formal cognitive assessment results

	Percentile rank	Classification
Wechsler Intelligence Scale for Children-Fourth Edition (WISC-IV)		
Verbal Comprehension Index	19	Low average
Perceptual Reasoning Index	27	Average
Memory (Children's Memory Scale)		
Verbal memory	12	Low average
Visual memory	30	Average
Conner's Continuous Performance Test-Second Edition (CPT-II)		
Omissions	37	Inattention
Commissions	91	Impulsive
HIT reaction time (RT)	30	Fast
HIT reaction time (RT) block change	55	Typical
HIT standard error (SE) block change	67	Typical

Table 12.2 Parental Report of Childhood Cognitive Abilities (PRECCA; Williams et al. 1991) and Strengths and Difficulties Questionnaire (parental and self-reported problems). Table shows classification of parental and self-rated concerns relative to clinical threshold

Domain	Classification	
PRECCA	Parental concerns	Self-reported concerns
Memory and learning	Elevated	–
Language	No concerns	–
Orientation	No concerns	–
Higher cognitive abilities	Elevated	–
Apraxia	No concerns	–
Hyperactivity/impulse control	Highly elevated	–
Learning behaviour	No concerns	–
Skills	No concerns	–
Cognitive problems	No concerns	–
SDQ		
Prosocial	No concerns	No concerns
Peer problems	No concerns	Borderline elevated
Innatention—hyperactivity	Borderline elevated	Borderline elevated
Conduct problems	No concerns	No concerns
Emotional symptoms	Highly elevated	Elevated
Total difficulties	Borderline elevated	Borderline elevated
Impact score	Highly elevated	Highly elevated

symptoms and attentional problems having a significant impact on her life. In a broad-based questionnaire assessing everyday cognitive and academic abilities, a high level of concern was expressed regarding attentional symptoms.

Overall, on the basis of self-report, parental report and formal cognitive assessment, there did not appear to be any significant decrement in Katie's general level of reasoning compared to her pre-existing level of functioning and her academic history. However, her IQ scores were somewhat lower than expectations on the basis of her previous educational attainment.

Despite reported memory and learning problems, Katie performed relatively well on formal assessment of episodic memory and obtained scores within a range consistent with her general reasoning ability. As is consistent with her reported attention problems, she exhibited some difficulties on attention tests with elevated omission and commission (impulsive) errors.

Reported data from the questionnaires including the SDQ and parental reported evaluation of childhood cognitive abilities (PRECCA) suggest a high level of concern regarding memory, learning problems and attention/executive difficulties alongside endorsement of symptoms indicative of probable emotional/psychiatric disorder.

The dominant concerns initially following the head injury were dizziness, nausea, headache, fatigue alongside attentional symptoms and poor school attendance.

Formulation

Evidence on Symptomatology Following Paediatric Mild TBI

The trajectory of Katie's symptomatology is broadly consistent with the literature on PCS (King 2003) and specifically the trajectory observed in paediatric samples (Eisenberg 2014). Common early reported symptoms include headache, fatigue, dizziness and nausea. Such symptoms are reported by over 50 % of children and lead to forgetfulness, poor concentration and slow processing in those whose symptoms persist beyond 28 days. Persistence of symptoms up to 28 days occurs in only 15 % of the cases reported by Eisenberg, with no more than 5 % reporting continued symptoms at 90 days post-injury. These longer term symptoms are correspondingly unpredictable on the basis of injury features. Some sensitive imaging techniques have revealed organic brain injury in patients with persistent post-concussive symptoms 1 year after injury. The incidence of minor head injury is highest in young adults with an increased prevalence of PCS in females (King 2003; Eisenberg 2014).

Mismanagement of return to education is common following mild TBI (mTBI). Teachers may not be aware of or fully understand the implications of the mTBI and are often unaware of a child's mTBI. Twenty percent of the children have difficulties with schoolwork and 18 % are disciplined for problem behaviour after mTBI (Hawley 2004).

While injury factors are highly predictive of symptoms in the first 3 months following injury, pre-existing psychological risk factors and ongoing psychological reactions are most predictive of persistent symptomatology (Butler 2013). King (2003) highlights unhelpful premorbid cognitive schemas, concerns regarding potential permanence of symptoms, and unhelpful strategies for coping as risk factors in those with continued symptoms. Those with persistence over 6 months may have misperception of having suffered a severe brain injury coupled with a lack of understanding from others.

Evidence for treatment efficacy is largely focused on prevention of PCS via early provision of education and advice or targeting of high-risk groups. Such evidence supports early intervention, leading to significantly reduced PCS prevalence in mTBI (King et al. 1999). Information provided to parents at discharge from the Emergency Department leads to reduced levels of parental stress, childhood anxiety and PCS symptoms (Kenardy et al. 2008; Ponsford et al. 2002). Evidence for the treatment of persistent symptoms leading to a diagnosis of PCS is extremely sparse; there is no randomised controlled trial (RCT) evidence to support the effectiveness of symptom-specific interventions and to demonstrate enhanced recovery from PCS in response to intervention with children (Pangilinan et al. 2010). However, in adults at "high risk" for PCS following mTBI, those who received cognitive behavioural therapy (CBT) intervention delivered shortly after the injury reported a faster and more complete recovery (Mittenberg et al. 1996; Silverberg et al. 2013).

Katie's performance on tests of general reasoning is slightly below expectations, given reports of her previous educational progress. However, it is likely that her pre-existing social and educational vulnerability had contributed to a high level of anxiety and corresponding hypervigilance on returning to school. Her symptoms of fatigue and nausea, particularly in response to exertion, are consistent with prevalent symptoms reported after mTBI. The initial failed attempts to return to school full time followed by retreating into nonattendance and sedentary behaviour are likely to have reinforced her beliefs about organic damage in the absence of any clear guidance on the likely trajectory of her recovery.

The combination of Katie's previous vulnerability and an extended period of convalescence from school had left Katie feeling further behind in her studies and frustrated with her inability to keep up with her peers. Although we did not think there was any strong evidence for any ongoing cognitive deficits, Katie had clearly developed a pattern of poor sleep, which was having an additional adverse effect on her school attendance, social and educational functioning.

Intervention/Feedback/Reformulation

Despite the considerable time that had passed since Katie's head injury, we believed it would be helpful to address the likely origin of her early cognitive and somatic symptoms at the time of her initial return to school. Katie and her family accepted the likely interaction between pre-existing vulnerability, short-lived cognitive symptoms following her injury and longer-term symptoms mediated by psychological factors and based on a mismanaged return to school. Reassurance was provided regarding the general integrity of her reasoning and episodic memory on the basis of positive test scores. Her educational difficulties on returning to school were reframed as a likely combination of subtle pre-existing problems, several weeks of missed school, relatively mild attention problems and excessive vigilance regarding cognitive symptoms.

A number of suggestions were made regarding treatment and intervention. We suggested the need to target her sleep pattern and provide support to promote her gradual re-engagement with education. Reduced expectations were set regarding her likely achievement given the months of school absence, and we highlighted the need for interim educational support. We also supported a referral to child mental health services for emotional support and to provide additional support with regard to a school reintegration programme.

Outcome

At the time of our follow-up appointment, Katie had returned to college to complete her exams and had obtained average results but in only three of the original nine academic subjects that she had started prior to her injury. She had enrolled at a further education college on a full-time course and was undertaking a vocational qualification in business administration. Initial communication with the college had served to set reasonable expectations regarding her attendance and a plan for her to build up to full-time attendance. Despite modest initial expectations, her college attendance had been 100 % and she had successfully completed all of her coursework.

Symptoms of fatigue continued but were much reduced, occurring approximately once a week. Katie remained relatively inactive outside college attendance but had successfully maintained her social relationships within college and via social media. Her sleep remained disrupted, with sleep onset difficulties being most prominent.

Katie had maintained her long-standing aspirations to pursue a career in photography but had been unable to enrol on her chosen course due to her poor examination results and attendance record. Her future educational opportunities had, therefore, been severely constrained but options remain to address this. Katie was also concerned that she may have to fund her studies having spent more than 2 years at college and therefore exhausted the usual government funding. We have therefore undertaken to make strong representation regarding recognition of the impact of her head injury and the need for discretion in extending her funding for further education.

Reflection/Discussion

Katie's symptoms are consistent with diagnosis of PCS and possibly CFS. The initial referral to a specialist paediatrician was indeed made on the basis of her likely having CFS. The onset of fatigue symptoms shortly following a mTBI is sufficient to exclude CFS as a diagnosis. However, some effort should be made to clearly distinguish the conditions on the basis of presenting symptoms, formulation and recommended treatment.

The most commonly used diagnostic criteria and definition of CFS for research and clinical purposes were published by the United States Centers for Disease Control and Prevention. The fatigue causes a significant reduction of previous activity levels. The presence of persistent symptoms of impaired memory or concentration, post-exertion malaise, poor sleep and headaches is sufficient for a diagnosis of chronic fatigue where there are no other specific medical causes (Afari and Buchwald 2003). CFS was reasonably excluded as a diagnosis on the basis that a minor head injury provides a potential medical cause of the subsequent symptoms.

A minor head injury is classified as a blow to the head with a brief period of loss of consciousness, posttraumatic amnesia or disorientation. Although the terms concussion and mTBI are used interchangeably, the term concussion would explicitly exclude evidence of any abnormality on imaging.

Although no universally accepted definition of PCS exists, most of the literature defines the syndrome as the development of at least three of the following symptoms: headache, dizziness, fatigue, irritability, impaired memory and concentration, insomnia, and lowered tolerance for noise and light. DSM-IV would include symptoms of affective disturbance, personality change or apathy in addition to the above. Symptom onset must occur soon after the injury and persist for several months.

The early symptoms such as headache and dizziness were reasonably believed to reflect underlying organic factors and are largely predictable on the basis of injury characteristics, whereas most of the symptoms that persist beyond 3 months, typically fatigue, mood disturbance and impaired concentration/memory, were likely to have a psychological basis.

Formal assessment in this case was deliberately brief as our practice is to only undertake formal assessment where there is either clear risk of likely deficits given known underlying pathology or where there are convincing parental or self-reported difficulties. Assessment of specific domains in the absence of such evidence is more likely to yield false-positive results and may simultaneously reinforce maladaptive illness beliefs or behaviour.

Neuropsychological consultation had highlighted potential cognitive deficits in memory and attention, with evidence of impaired educational progress but no suggestion of any change in underlying intellectual ability. Corresponding formal assessment revealed only mild attention problems in the context of intact memory and general reasoning ability. Anxiety and misattribution of symptoms to severe and permanent cognitive change is regarded as an important predictor of the evolution of symptoms in PCS (Dischinger et al. 2009).

The intervention in this case, although based on a characterisation of PCS consistent with the literature, utilised an approach with proven efficacy only as a preventative measure in the acute stage of recovery. Despite limited evidence for direct application to PCS symptomatology in children, more direct targeting of specific persistent symptoms such as fatigue and attention problems may have been helpful in this case. Consideration of further diagnostic investigations for attention problems is unlikely to have been fruitful, but some form of remediation could nonetheless have been considered. Furthermore, definitive management of fatigue and sleep disturbance was not undertaken and the evidence base for this is reasonably well developed in the paediatric population (Lloyd et al. 2012).

References

Afari, N., & Buchwald, D. (2003). Chronic fatigue syndrome: A review. *The American Journal of Psychiatry, 160*(2), 221–236. doi:10.1176/appi.ajp.160.2.221. (PMID 12562565).

Butler, I. J. (2013). Postconcussion syndrome after mild traumatic brain injury in children and adolescents requires further detailed study. *Journal of the American Medical Association Neurology, 25,* 1–2.

Conners, C. K. (1994). *The conners continuous performance test.* Toronto: Multi-Health Systems.

Dischinger, P. C., Ryb, G. E., Kufera, J. A., & Auman, K. M. (2009). Early predictors of postconcussive syndrome in a population of trauma patients with mild traumatic brain injury. *The Journal of Trauma, 66*(2), 289–296, (discussion 296–7).

Eisenberg, M. A., et al. (2014). Duration and course of post-concussive symptoms. *Pediatrics, 133*(6), 999–1006

Goodman, R. (1997). The strengths and difficulties questionnaire: A research note. *Journal of Child Psychology and Psychiatry, 38,* 581–586. (Normative data from 9 European countries and the US. Meltzer, H., Gatward, R., Goodman, R., and Ford, F. (2000) *Mental health of children and adolescents in Great Britain.* Data from the UK includes over 10,000 school age children).

Hawley, C. A. (2004). Outcomes following childhood head injury: A population study. *Journal of Neurology, Neurosurgery, and Psychiatry, 75*(5), 737–742.

Kenardy, J., Thompson, K., Le Brocque, R., & Olsson, K. (2008). Information-provision intervention for children and their parents following pediatric accidental injury. *European Child and Adolescent Psychiatry, 17*(5), 316–325.

King, N. S. (2003). Post-concussion syndrome: Clarity amid the controversy? *The British Journal of Psychiatry: The Journal of Mental Science, 183,* 276–278.

King, N. S., Crawford, S., Wenden, F. J., Caldwell, F. E., & Wade, D. T. (1999). Early prediction of persisting post-concussion symptoms following mild and moderate head injuries. *The British Journal of Clinical Psychology/The British Psychological Society, 38*(Pt 1), 15–25.

Lloyd, S., CHalder, T., & Rimes, K. (2012). Family-focused cognitive behaviour therapy versus psycho-education for adolescents with chronic fatigue syndrome: Long-term follow-up of an RCT. *Behaviour Research and Therapy, 50*(11), 719–725.

Mittenberg, W., Tremont, G., Zielinski, R. E., Fichera, S., & Rayls, K. R. (1996). Cognitivebehavioral prevention of postconcussion syndrome. *Archives of Clinical Neuropsychology, 11*(2), 139–145.

Pangilinan, P. H., Giacoletti-Argento, A., Shellhaas, R., Hurvitz, E. A., & Hornyak, J. E. (2010). Neuropharmacology in pediatric brain injury: A review. *PM & R, 2*(12), 1127–1140.

Ponsford, J., Willmott, C., Rothwell, A., Cameron, P., Kelly, A., Nelms, R., et al. (2002). Impact of early intervention on outcome following mild head injury in adults. *Journal of Neurology, Neurosurgery, and Psychiatry, 73*(3), 330–332.

Silverberg, N. D., Hallam, B. J., Rose, A., Underwood, H., Whitfield, K., Thornton, A. E., & Whittal, M. L. (2013). Cognitive-behavioral prevention of postconcussion syndrome in at-risk patients: A pilot randomized controlled trial. *Journal of Head Trauma Rehabilitation, 28*(4), 313–322.

Wechsler, D. (2003). *Wechsler intelligence scale for children-fourth edition (WISC-IV)*. San Antonio: The Psychological Corporation.

Williams, K. S., Ochs, J., Williams, J. M., & Mulhern, R. K. (1991). Parental report of everyday cognitive abilities among children treated for acute lymphoblastic leukemia. *Journal of Pediatric Psychology, 16,* 13–26.

Chapter 13
Cognitive Neuropsychological Formulation

Greg Savage

The term *neuropsychological formulation* does not occupy a prominent position in the clinical neuropsychological literature. Not yet, anyway. It is a prominent concept in clinical psychology and psychiatry, however, providing a framework for understanding the nature of a person's disturbed mind, what factors played a role in causing and maintaining the disturbance, and importantly, how treatment might be planned. In light of this treatment focus, the notion of formulation may be more likely to be appealed to by neuropsychologists practising in rehabilitation settings, but with much general neuropsychological work focusing on assessment, formulation does not headline as a core construct. This chapter briefly outlines three perspectives on neuropsychological assessment, and will propose that formulation is central, in one way or another, to the tenets of practice across the board; what seems to vary across perspectives is how explicitly formulation plays a role. This chapter tells an Australian version of a story—not *the* Australian version, but one reflecting my own Australian experience starting out as a humble trainee. In particular, it reflects my initial training as a researcher, turning to a clinical career after completing a PhD and postdoctoral fellowship in experimental psychology.

I first learned about clinical formulation in my first year of the coursework masters degree in clinical neuropsychology at The University of Melbourne in the early 1990s. The clinical training programs had recently been restructured, teaching a common first year of coursework to both trainees in clinical neuropsychology and clinical psychology. At the time I considered some of the clinical psychology content ephemeral, suspecting that much of the knowledge I accumulated would never be accessed (the "empty chair technique" does linger vaguely in my memory, but only as a model example of something I doubt I will ever use). But the idea of formulation was appealing. It was taught only briefly, with readings from the Oxford

---

G. Savage (✉)
ARC Centre of Excellence in Cognition and its Disorders (CCD),
and Department of Psychology, Macquarie University, Australian Hearing Hub,
Level 3, 16 University Avenue, Sydney, NSW 2109, Australia
e-mail: greg.savage@mq.edu.au

J. A. B. Macniven (ed.), *Neuropsychological Formulation*,
DOI 10.1007/978-3-319-18338-1_13

Textbook of Psychiatry and a class exercise, but the idea of constructing an argument about differential diagnosis, citing evidence for and against plausible ranked contenders, resonated with my research experience in evaluating experimental hypotheses. Formulation involved consideration of predisposing, precipitating and maintaining factors in order to gain *understanding* of the case. This academic exercise soon translated into clinical reality: all first year students experienced a 30-day introductory placement in an acute psychiatric setting, and the glimpses I had into the cracks (and crevasses) of fractured minds while at Dandenong Hospital were extremely fascinating. I did wonder, though, if I would ever find myself drawing on insights I had gained, once working as a neuropsychologist. As for formulation, I appreciated no more about it at the time than how it was used in the psychiatric context in which it was being taught.

Ironically, it turned out that my first job was a newly created clinical neuropsychology position in acute psychiatry at St Vincent's Hospital in Melbourne. And it also turned out that my experiences there, following on from sharing a common first year of training with clinical psychologists, shaped views about neuropsychological assessment which I still hold 20 years later, and form the focus of this chapter.

Approaches to Neuropsychological Assessment

Placements in a variety of neuropsychological settings around Melbourne commenced in the second year of training, and the remaining coursework became neuro-specific. Presentation of patients seen on placement in the weekly case conference meeting back at the university opened my eyes to an issue which had received coverage in lectures but was not really appreciated until actively engaged in clinical work. That issue centred on the role of clinical/qualitative information in the assessment process, as opposed to (and I mean polemically opposed to) actuarial/psychometric data. Back-to-back case presentations might feature a hypothesis-driven assessment performed with minimal testing to aid diagnosis of corticobasal syndrome, followed by reporting of a comprehensive fixed battery comprising the Wechsler tests plus the MMPI-2 in support of a presurgical epilepsy evaluation.

Variety in approaches taken around Melbourne's hospitals were championed on the teaching course, represented by what appeared to be polar opposite views. Michael Saling followed the hypothesis-testing methodology of the influential Russian neuropsychologist Aleksandr Luria, articulated more recently and locally by the "grandfather" of Australian neuropsychology, Kevin Walsh (see Walsh 1992). The broad perspective shared by Walsh and Saling pegged out one end of a spectrum of approaches to neuropsychological assessment practised in Australia and internationally (Walsh 1991, 1992). It shared a kindred spirit with the Boston Process Approach advocated by Edith Kaplan and colleagues such as Harold Goodglass, Norman Geschwind and, more recently, Dean Delis. Stephen Bowden, on the other hand, took a strong psychometric position. Bowden's perspective has a North American heritage shaped by fixed-battery advocates such as Halstead and

Reitan, which places confidence about cognitive characterisation in a statistically reliable normative profile. For a sampling of local views on this zeitgeist issue at the time of my training, see a series of papers published in *The Australian Psychologist* (Bowden 1995; Caine 1995; Saling 1995). For another Australian's account of this spectrum of approaches, outlining some strengths and weaknesses of the methods used, see the more recent book by Simon Crowe (2010). I do perceive that the polemic tone has mellowed more recently, and a rapprochement between the process and actuarial perspectives may be nigh. As a sign of the times, perhaps, the process-badged California Verbal Learning Test-Second Edition (CVLT-II; Delis et al. 2000) is endorsed as a substitute for the Verbal Paired Associates subtest of the Wechsler Memory Scale-Fourth edition (WMS-IV; Wechsler 2009). In a similar acknowledgment, subtests from the Delis–Kaplan Executive Function System (D–KEFS; Delis et al. 2001) feature in actuarial computations within the Wechsler-oriented Advanced Clinical Solutions (ACS; Pearson 2009) software. The bottom line here seems to be that hypothesis-testing is endorsed when the hypotheses are framed and tested using reliable psychometric data.

Formulation in the Hypothesis-Testing Approach

My first neuropsychological placement was formative in acute neurology at the Austin Hospital under the supervision of Michael Saling. In that setting I began to appreciate what I later recognised as an extreme version of neuropsychological formulation. The approach to testing was minimalist, with Saling seeking to test specific hypotheses suggested by the clinical history. A report was written as a direct communication to the referring doctor, and I was tutored in streamlining the content, pruning unnecessary detail to ensure that the critical findings evidently supported the "impression" offered. The impression section was essentially a formulation, *arguing the case* for a diagnosis, or statement about recovery or decline, or return to work, and so forth, built on *understanding* the patient's neuropsychological state. Crucially, Saling impressed on his interns that the impression had to *make neuropsychological sense*.

On placement at the Austin I also learned about the inception of an Australian brand of neuropsychology, by virtue of the symbiotic collaboration between Kevin Walsh and his Austin Hospital colleague, neurologist Peter Bladin. Their collaboration was close but not close enough, realised Walsh: a hybrid kind of specialised clinician needed to be trained "from the ground up" with the expertise of the neurologist and psychologist "in the same head". Walsh started training clinical neuropsychology students at The Austin in 1973, and so began a uniquely Australian masters level qualification which became highly regarded in the international scene.

Walsh (2001) recounts an early referral from Bladin about a presurgical candidate with temporal lobe epilepsy which is poignantly relevant to the theme of this book. Bladin simply asked: "Does this patient have deficits to which he is not entitled?" That is, taking into account the relevant context of the case (an identified unilateral lesion, with some likely consequences on memory performance), are there deficits which might suggest other pathology (e.g. an unidentified lesion compromising the contralateral temporal lobe's ability to support adequate memory functioning following surgical removal of its diseased counterpart)? The referral question was subtle in its framing but fundamentally about formulation.

Formulation in the Psychometric Approach

In the early years of my first job I had the opportunity for engaging in discussions with Stephen Bowden at St Vincent's Hospital: Bowden was based in neurosciences, while I was in psychiatry. I came to appreciate that his position was not only grounded by a cornerstone of psychology's virtues—empirical metric strength—but the whole story was told in metric terms. Interpretation was conveyed by reference to statistical and clinically meaningful differences among test scores, which might suggest no room for formulation. It might be proposed that there is a *sense* of formulation, however, if spoken in a different dialect. Here, the data are *themselves* modulated in a context provided by normatively estimable effects of demographic factors such as age, sex and education, and base rates of abnormality. And ultimately, a formulation must be expressed outside the terms of reference provided by the data—that is, in the terminology of diagnosis and management. This formulation is garnered taking into account features of the patient's history as highlighted in the section on "The intelligent testing philosophy" in the psychometrically irreproachable text by Alan Kaufman (1990). Interestingly, quotes from Kaufman's text on this point feature in both Saling's and Bowden's contributions to the debate published in *The Australian Psychologist* in 1995, acknowledging a patch of common ground between contrasting assessment methods at the level of formulating the case.

Formulation from a Cognitive Perspective

As a fledgling clinical neuropsychologist with a research background I was continually struck by what appeared to be a chasm between the clinical characterisation of abnormal cognition and the theoretical characterisation of normal cognition developed over many decades of work in experimental cognitive psychology. This gap was also apparent in the labelling of cognitive constructs such as "performance IQ" and "freedom from distractibility"; these terms did not speak about models of perception or of working memory.

A bridge of sorts had been formed across the chasm by the more recent emergence of the research discipline named *cognitive neuropsychology,* which sought to understand normal cognition by testing hypotheses using data from patients with brain dysfunction. But that bridge had a one-way flow of traffic—cognitive neuropsychology did not set out to understand *the patient's* cognition. The discipline was evolving, though, and in the 1990s a flagship collection of work applying insights from cognitive neuropsychology to rehabilitation was edited by Jane Riddoch and Glyn Humphreys (Riddoch and Humphreys 1994). Around this time, tests began to appear which were based on theoretical models of cognition, themselves now informed by neuropsychological data. The Thames Valley Test Company in particular championed the cause with tests such as Doors and People (Baddeley et al. 1994) structured to assess encoding and retrieval memory processes, and the Test of Everyday Attention (Robertson et al. 1994) which assesses performance in theoretically motivated domains such as selective attention, sustained attention and attentional switching.

A few years into my clinical working life I happened upon a book edited by Robert Mapou and Jack Spector whose introductory chapter resonated with the views I had formed about the "theoretical agnosia" that seemed to exist in neuropsychological practice (Mapou 1995b). The book contained an excellent selection of chapters, each addressing a cognitive domain and outlining an approach to testing which was reconciled with models of cognition. Mapou's overarching chapter, entitled *A Cognitive Framework for Neuropsychological Assessment*, particularly influenced my outlook (Mapou 1995a). It outlines principles which consider layers of context provided by global intellectual functioning and academic achievement, foundation skills such as attention and executive abilities, modality-specific skills such as language and visuospatial functions, and at the top of the pile, potentially affected by all these subordinate abilities, learning and memory. This kind of schema for thinking about cognitive dependencies shaped my approach to conducting an assessment, with early testing of attention, working memory and speed of processing, setting the stage for what is likely to be achievable with a patient. Plans to administer a potentially overwhelming test such as the Rey Auditory Verbal Learning Test (Rey 1958) might be reconsidered in a patient who cannot repeat back three digits in reverse order or who cannot focus well enough to understand the simple instructions of the Coding subtest of the Wechsler Adult Intelligence Scale-Fourth edition (Wechsler 2008). This game plan was crucial to providing effective neuropsychological assessment in acute psychiatry, where patients were frequently agitated, or withdrawn, or suspicious about the process. Strategic assessment based on a cognitive approach frequently allowed essential tests to be done early in case the session needed to be truncated.

Importantly for the theme of this chapter, cognitively focused assessments afford cognitively framed formulations. They reveal opportunities for deductive inference about underpinning roles of processes: of verbal memory difficulties being secondary to semantic degradation or working memory impairment, of constructional problems mirroring underlying visuoperceptual deficiencies, or of reduced verbal fluency stemming from lifelong phonological processing deficits and associated poor literacy. Accounting for dependencies among cognitive processes allows for parsimonious formulation—applying the scientific tool of Occam's razor to cut through redundancies and find the simplest and most plausible account. It also allows for articulation of that formulation in cognitive terminology. I have found that formulations which talk in terms such as "…having difficulties retrieving information which has been taken in, but stored inefficiently…", are readily understood by patients, their families, the referrer and other clinicians.

This cognitive approach fundamentally involves hypothesis-testing but endorses use of the best psychometric tools to achieve its goal. As such, cognitive neuropsychological formulation resolves what appear to be differences between historically opposing views and also adds a new dimension in terms of the way that the findings of neuropsychological assessment are communicated.

Cases Illustrating Aspects of Cognitive Neuropsychological Formulation

The first case to be outlined had existing clinical features which provided challenges to the process of assessment, limiting options for testing. Formulation relied heavily on deductive inference and provided a "best guess" opinion about the diagnosis. The diagnosis is less contentious in the second case, which is described mainly to highlight the importance of considering the bedrock foundation level of Mapou's hierarchical framework, where the context provided by global intellectual level and academic achievement is pivotal.

The Case of Mr K: A Formulation About Dementia in a Hearing-Impaired Patient

Referral Details and Background

Mr K was a 79-year-old right-handed retired industrial designer who immigrated to Australia from an Eastern European country as a teenager after the Second World War. He had a history of a right hemisphere stroke almost a decade prior to the assessment, significant deafness and a recent fall. His family believed that his cognitive abilities appeared to be declining, and Mr K's general practitioner referred him to a neurologist in private practice for an opinion about the likelihood he had early Alzheimer's disease. The neurologist reviewed his recent history and referred him for a "full neuropsychological assessment".

Clinical Interview

Mr K was seen as a private practice outpatient. He attended with his wife, who provided essential input to the interview given Mr K's difficulty responding to questions due to his deafness. When asked if he had any problems with his thinking skills, Mr K denied any cognitive difficulties. On direct questioning about forgetfulness, problems with paying attention or language skills, he again denied any problems. He agreed his hearing was profoundly poor, however, and had been deteriorating over the preceding 7 years or so.

Mrs K provided a different perspective—and quite frankly, with Mr K not able to hear much of the conversation. She had noticed emerging problems with him interacting with new technology and navigating websites (activities he would normally have no difficulty with), forgetting passwords, and problems buying and selling shares. He was absent-minded, and once paid someone with a blank cheque. Mrs K believed these kinds of problems emerged after he suffered a right-hemisphere stroke affecting most of the left side of his body about 9 years previously but that the problems had been worsening over the preceding 2 years or so. He had recovered some physical functionality since the stroke: He could use his left hand but he walked with a cane and had difficulty using his left leg (this was evident as he sat down in his chair at the start of the assessment). At this point I asked Mr K about his stroke, and he described the physical consequences but denied any cognitive impact; Mrs K added he had difficulty reading for a few months after the stroke.

Two years after the stroke he had a subdural haemorrhage (I was unable to ascertain how this happened), and he had fallen a few times in the preceding few years, most recently only 3 months prior to seeing me. This latest fall required admission to hospital for a few days where a CT of the brain revealed no evidence of a recent stroke. He subsequently underwent physiotherapy as an inpatient at a specialist rehabilitation hospital.

His deafness had developed over the preceding 7 years and was worsening and quite debilitating, but he was reluctant to use his hearing aid (and therefore was not familiar with having it on when he did use it). He had diabetes and related hypertension, both of which were well managed. He had bowel cancer 15 years earlier which required removal of his sigmoid colon, and he had also had his gallbladder removed. He was a nonsmoker and drank only the occasional beer. His mother died aged 75 of diabetes-related complications, and his father aged 68 of septicaemia related to kidney stones.

Mr K settled in Australia in his late teens and learned English sufficiently well to complete both a bachelors and masters degree in industrial design. He worked in industry and later taught design at a technical college. Since retirement he has run a small business unrelated to his past vocation.

His social skills had deteriorated and he appeared indifferent to what was happening in his family life; his interests had narrowed, and he tended to read old European history books (ones he had read before and liked). He still played bridge three times a week and had no difficulty remembering the rules, but Mrs K said he was not playing as well as he used to and his friends "humoured him". He spent a lot of time reading the newspaper; on questioning, however, he could not provide adequate details of recent news items and tended to make general (but true) remarks about "trouble in the Middle East and Africa" (although he correctly remembered there had recently been "protests in Bangkok").

Mr K was a polite man who attempted his tasks with diligence. His speech was laboured but clearly articulated. His facial expression was largely impassive, but he was capable of expressing emotion (becoming animated when correctly naming an abacus on a language test and describing its adept use by merchants in various cultures). His mood appeared passive and affect was restricted (possibly reflecting his detachment due to deafness). His writing was well formed; he could write a grammatical sentence on command, he could copy intersecting pentagons and a "wire cube", and he could draw a clock and place hands to show a specified time. He was well oriented and could name current and recent political figures.

Formal Assessment

The scope of the assessment was compromised significantly by Mr K's deafness, and many routine tests relying on verbal administration were not able to be given. Specifically, in a typical assessment I would administer tests of auditory attention and working memory (WAIS-IV Digit Span), verbal learning and retention (CVLT-II), reasoning about verbally provided concepts (WAIS-IV Similarities) and inhibition of prepotent responses on a sentence completion task (The Hayling Test; Burgess and Shallice 1997). For Mr K, inferences about these cognitive domains needed to be based primarily on nonauditory tests, and occasionally I resorted to using written aids to help explain the task (e.g. to demonstrate switching in the last item of Mental Control from the Wechsler Memory Scale-Third edition (WMS-III; Wechsler 1997b)) and in the D–KEFS Trail Making Test. The scope was also impacted upon by reduced dexterity in his left hand (e.g. WAIS-IV Block Design was not administered as performance would have been marred by manual and not necessarily cognitive issues) and by the cultural and linguistic influences of immigrating to Australia in his late teens and only subsequently learning English. Nevertheless, I will suggest in the formulation that an adequate range of tests was given and responded to.

Mr K's premorbid level of intellect was informally estimated to lie in at least the high average range, based on his academic and vocational achievements. Against this background, some aspects of cognition appeared preserved (see Table 13.1). His copy of the Rey-Osterrieth Complex Figure (Meyers and Meyers 1995) was intact, and his approach was well organised, and memory for the figure after a short delay was adequate.

A test of language requiring naming of line drawings of objects (the Boston Naming Test; Kaplan et al. 2001) produced an equivocal finding: the test is culturally biased, and on debriefing he said he had never known the names of some of the items (e.g. *stilts, muzzle*). Moreover, I could not reliably provide phonemic cues when he failed to name the object spontaneously as he could not hear such minimal utterances adequately. I did attempt a "band-aid" solution by writing orthographic cues instead (e.g. pro… for *protractor*), with occasional success. Some neuropsychologists might challenge this approach, even to the extent of suggesting that this deviation from standardised administration is unethical. However, if one considers the purpose of the assessment in the context of significant sensory impairment, the qualitative data derived from the approach arguably justifies this method. Thus despite the challenges provided by Mr K's deafness, he had the opportunity

Table 13.1 Raw and metric test scores for Mr K

Test name	Raw score	Metric score	Interpretation
Rey-Osterrieth Complex Figure	Copy: 32/36	>16 %ile	Preserved
	3' delay: 14/36	69 %ile (T=55)	
Boston Naming Test	38/52≈43/60 (spontaneous)	<10 %ile	Mildly impaired
Coding[a]	36	25 %ile (SS=8)	
Mental Control[b]	16	16 %ile (SS=7)	
Spatial Span[b]	Total: 11	25 %ile (SS=8)	
	Forward: 7	50 %ile (SS=10)	
	Backward: 4	16 %ile (SS=7)	
Trail Making Test[c]	Numbers: 76 s	16 %ile (SS=7)	
	Letters: 79 s	16 %ile (SS=7)	
	Motor speed: 70 s	16 %ile (SS=7)	
Category Fluency	Animals: 10	5 %ile (SS=5)	Markedly impaired
Faces I[b]	22	5 %ile (SS=5)	
Picture Completion[a]	4	<1 %ile (SS=2)	
Trail Making Test[c]	Number–letter switching: 225 s	<1 %ile (SS=2)	

[a] Denotes subtest of the Wechsler Adult Intelligence Scale-Fourth edition *(WAIS-IV)*
[b] Denotes subtest of the Wechsler Memory Scale-Third edition *(WMS-III)*
[c] Denotes subtest of the Delis–Kaplan Executive Function System *(D–KEFS)*

to demonstrate that any naming difficulty he had was cueable. In any case, he produced a patchy pattern of hits and misses across the range of difficulty, and at worst his performance might be interpreted as showing mild impairment.

Most of the remaining test findings suggested more clearly some degree of decline from premorbid levels. He was moderately slowed on simple graphomotor tasks (sequencing numbers or letters on the D–KEFS Trail Making Test, or transcribing symbols according to a key with WAIS-IV Coding) and reduced speed also penalised his scores on the mental manipulation tasks in Mental Control from the WMS-III (e.g. reciting the months in order and then in reverse order). Errors in mental manipulation were also prominent for the backwards phase of WMS-III Spatial Span (briefly holding in mind a sequence of random locations and tapping them in reverse order).

Mr K's performances on some tests usually considered to tap into executive functioning were well below expected levels. A switching version of the psychomotor sequencing task (alternating between letters and numbers on the Trail Making Test) was extremely laboured and slowed, but notably he made no errors. Generation of words under time pressure given a theme (animals) was also quite impaired.

Low performances on two other tests stood out as potentially anomalous, and might be explained by failure to appreciate the instructions due to his deafness or withdrawal of effort. Specifically, he had great difficulty remembering a series of photographs of faces when tested immediately afterwards (WMS-III Faces I). His total score of 22/48 in making yes/no decisions about whether he had just seen a face or not suggests chance responding and profound amnesia. But inspection of the pattern of responses suggests Mr K was not performing the task as intended. He began with a tendency for a positive response bias (endorsing 12 of the first 17 items, in an otherwise variable pattern), but after that point he appeared to change his criterion, responding "no" to 25/31 remaining items with long runs of consecutive "no" responses. Similar concerns arose about appreciating task instructions when he failed five of the initial seven (extremely easy) items in the WAIS-IV Picture Completion subtest, where he was required to identify structural or logical missing elements from pictures.

Formulation

Mr K is a 79-year-old retired industrial designer with profound deafness who experienced a severe right-hemisphere stroke a decade ago. Cognitive difficulties were noticed after the stroke and appear to have worsened in recent years; hearing loss also developed since the stroke and has worsened steadily. Concerns were raised that recent cognitive decline might represent neurodegenerative changes in the form of Alzheimer's disease.

In terms of predisposing factors for cognitive change, the stroke and associated vascular risk factors (hypertension, diabetes) may be relevant. Emerging deafness may represent a precipitating factor; a relationship between hearing loss and dementia has been recently identified (Lin et al. 2011), but the nature of the relationship is not yet understood and may implicate mediating variables such as social withdrawal. Deafness likely represents a maintaining factor in terms of forming barriers to improving cognitive function via environmental stimulation. Note that these factors do not necessarily relate to the question of neurodegenerative change.

The typical course of Alzheimer's disease involves early forgetfulness and repetitive questioning, together with word-finding difficulty, progressing to loss of temporal orientation ahead of more generalised cognitive decline. Mr K does not fit the mould. He was said to be forgetful, but he did well on an incidental test of visuospatial memory, his naming difficulty was mild at worst, and he was not disoriented. There was evidence of cognitive decline apparently affecting disparate domains of thinking (executive functioning, working memory and processing speed), which could possibly be taken to represent Alzheimer's disease presenting in an atypical manner. A more parsimonious interpretation is that Mr K fared poorly in the tests normally representing these domains primarily due to reduced speed of mentation. The lowest common denominator across these tests was his slow and effortful processing; even his speech was laboured.

If his cognitive profile does not fit with an Alzheimer's differential, what is the most plausible account of his reported decline and his poor test performances? Given his history of cerebrovascular events and risk factors, prominent small vessel disease could explain his mental slowness, and plausibly many of the cognitive errors noted by Mr K's family (an MRI of the brain was recommended in order to throw light on this possibility). The role of Mr K's worsening deafness could also be significant. He had become progressively withdrawn and his interests had narrowed; mood disturbance is frequently present and undiagnosed in the context of deafness and also associated with slowed thinking, and a formal assessment of his mood by a clinical psychologist or psychiatrist was recommended. It remains possible that fluctuations in engagement due to deafness, dysphoria or their combined impact might be entirely responsible for his apparently reduced cognitive abilities. While no formal measures of effort were administered, neither was their inclusion particularly suggested as any point in the assessment. Mr K performed well on incidental recall of the Rey Figure. Confronted with this unexpected memory test, many patients prone to withdrawing effort will show signs of disengagement, or even decline to respond, but Mr K applied himself diligently to good effect. Feigning of impairment was never a plausible consideration: he denied cognitive change, and there were no conceivable motives for embellishment of difficulty. Again, incidental recall of the Rey Figure would have provided ample opportunity to "fake bad" as would recognition memory testing with the Faces subtest, but his performance did not fall below chance. In the end, poor effort due to lowered mood is difficult to partition from the slowed mentation which is a fundamental feature of cognition in cases with depression.

Despite the difficulties encountered in assessing Mr K's cognition, a limited psychometric profile of performance was captured which established a number of important intact features. This profile could provide a useful reference point if a future review were to be suggested by an impression that Mr K's cognition was continuing to worsen.

Reflection

The key element in the neuropsychological formulation of Mr K's case involved understanding of the potential underpinning of a variety of cognitive failures on testing—and by extension, in daily life—by slowed processing speed. Consideration of this hypothesis *made neuropsychological sense* and allowed for his intact orientation and episodic memory performance. It also suggested other hypotheses about aetiology, prompting consideration of broader consequences of cerebrovascular disease beyond the known stroke, and of his deafness and possible mood disturbance. The cognitive terminology of the formulation also allowed for understanding by carers and may offer potential in terms of day-to-day management.

The Case of Mr J: A Formulation About Dementia in a High-Functioning Patient

Referral Details and Background

Mr J was a 72-year-old right-handed former chief executive officer of a multinational corporation who was referred to a cognitive neurologist with a 4-year history of word-finding difficulty, spatial disorientation and unreliable memory. The neurological examination was unremarkable but cognitive screening revealed mild constructional difficulty and rapid forgetting. The neurologist was concerned that Mr J might have Alzheimer's disease and requested a neuropsychological assessment as a contribution towards the diagnostic process.

Clinical Interview

Mr J was interviewed together with his wife. He was a good historian, although Mrs J usually conveyed a more compelling perspective on his difficulties. They said the first sign was a husky voice, followed soon afterwards by difficulty retrieving words in conversation; this was soon noticed by friends and colleagues. He used to possess an excellent memory, but forgetfulness became evident. He tended to get by using prompts and reminder notes and would forget most tasks without this kind of support. There was occasional repetitive questioning but this was not a prominent feature. He could focus attention on tasks which were engaging but tended to lose track of what he was doing around the house. Reading was intact but spoken language comprehension faltered if someone was talking too quickly. He had lost some quasi-personal semantic information: they remarked that he could not recall his father's birthday. Driving on familiar routes posed no problem, but new routes were proving tricky to negotiate. There was some personality change: he had "slowed down" a little and was less absorbed in his work. Mrs J tended to take care of the household finances but recently this had necessarily become the case. Decline had been gradual, and problems had become more prominent in the preceding year while they had been staying with family while their new house was being built. He was working 3 days a week in a senior executive role, and had few interests other than his work.

Mr J had worked in the financial sector all his adult life, and had completed a Master of Business Administration following initial degrees in commerce and law. His part-time role involved responsibility for a new area of expansion of his company.

He had sleep apnoea for which he wore a continuous positive airway pressure (CPAP) mask, and also described features of REM sleep disorder (punching and shouting out in his sleep). His sense of smell had deteriorated and his walking was slightly slowed, but he had not experienced tremor, loss of dexterity, or difficulty turning over in bed or standing on awakening. He denied hallucinations, delusions and illusions of sense of presence, and he did not experience fluctuations in consciousness. He described past episodes of atrial fibrillation and also an event around 6 months ago whereby he lost vision in one eye: this changed depending on his posture, but fully recovered after a few days. He had experienced two significant bleeds from stomach ulcers. He was a smoker in his 20s, and he typically drank a few glasses of wine a night. He experienced a few episodes of loss of consciousness playing rugby in his youth. His father died of a haemorrhagic stroke in his late 60s, following warfarin treatment of atrial fibrillation; his mother died in her 80s of "old age". Mr J had lost around 10 kg recently and he described his current mood as low. He said he had always tended to see the negative side of things, and now tended to become teary at times.

Mr J applied himself diligently throughout testing and coped well even when he was doing badly. His voice was slightly husky. Word-finding difficulties were frequent and he stumbled over a few polysyllabic words. Mood was perhaps a little lowered but affect was broad in range and congruent, and occasionally labile: he became teary when recounting a stressful period at work. He nonetheless demonstrated a wry sense of humour. On an inventory requiring reflection on experiences over the preceding week he endorsed items consistent with extremely severe depression, mild anxiety and moderate stress. Form of thought was intact and content of thought was unremarkable. He was well oriented (though the day of the week was out by one) and could provide a reasonably detailed account of recent news items. His writing was well formed, but he had difficulty drawing a clock, placing the numbers outside the circle and making a few self-corrected errors. He set the hands to a different time than specified and could not correct his error when it was pointed out.

Assessment

Summary test findings are presented in Table 13.2. Formal estimation of Mr J's premorbid intellectual level using the Wechsler Test of Adult Reading (WTAR; The Psychological Corporation 2001) suffered from a ceiling effect, suggesting the high average range (indeed a maximum score of 50/50 predicts a Full Scale IQ (FSIQ) near the upper bound of the high average range). His vocational and educational achievements, however, attested to a superior level of intellect. Against this background, intact abilities only included basic visuoperceptual functioning on the Visual Object and Space Perception Battery (VOSP; Warrington and James 1991), and focused simple attention while repeating digits verbatim (in Digit Span from the Wechsler Adult Intelligence Scale-Third edition;[1] Wechsler 1997a) with a capacity of eight (seven reliably). Remarkably, recognition memory for photographs of faces after a delay of 30 min was also intact (on WMS-III Faces II; he had seen the target faces three times by then, and told me he managed the task by focusing on prominent features such as bushy eyebrows). All other test outcomes were judged to be abnormal to some degree, and many were dramatically abnormal.

A cluster of test outcomes was placed squarely in the average range, including mental manipulation of routine and nonroutine information. He laboured when reciting months in reverse order (WMS-III Mental Control) and excused his performance by saying he does not think about the months much. Performance in repeating digits in reverse order was estimated to lie one standard deviation below levels

[1] WAIS-IV process score norms were consulted for forward and backward Digit Span (adding two points to equate the backward score), as they reflect the total achieved rather than longest span (with longest span being blind to errors committed throughout the trials).

Table 13.2 Raw and metric test scores for Mr J

Test name	Raw score	Metric score	Interpretation
Wechsler Test of Adult Reading	48	117 (FSIQ)	At least High Average
Digit Span[a]	Total: 20	90 %ile (SS = 14)	Preserved
	Forward: 13	90 %ile (SS = 14)	
Visual Object and Space Perception Battery	Dot counting: 9/10	(Pass)	
	Number location: 10/10	(Pass)	
	Cube analysis: 10/10	(Pass)	
Faces[b]	Delayed: 39	95 %ile (SS = 15)	
Mental Control[b]	24	63 %ile (SS = 11)	Mildly impaired
Similarities[a]	23	63 %ile (SS = 11)	
Digit Span[a]	Backward: 7	63 %ile (SS = 11)	
Letter Fluency[c]	34 (F: 12; A: 10; S: 12)	50 %ile (SS = 10)	
Boston Naming Test	49/60 (spontaneous)	< 25 %ile	
	58 (including cueing)	25 %ile	
Symbol Copy[a]	67	10 < %ile < 25	
Category Fluency[c]	15 (Animals: 10 Boys' names: 5)	1 %ile (SS = 3)	Markedly impaired
Category Switching[c]	5 (total correct)	< 1 %ile (SS = 2)	
	3 (switching accuracy)	< 1 %ile (SS = 2)	
Faces[b]	Immediate: 22	9 %ile (SS = 6)	
Brixton Spatial Anticipation Test	Errors: 36	< 5 %ile	
Picture Completion[a]	10	9 %ile (SS = 6)	
Digit Symbol-Coding[a]	27	5 %ile (SS = 5)	
Rey-Osterrieth Complex Figure	Copy: 21.5/36	< 1 %ile	
	3′ delay: 7.5/36	9 %ile (T = 37)	
California Verbal Learning Test-Second edition	19 (total Trials 1–5)	1 %ile (T = 28)	
	1 (SDFR)	< 1 %ile ($z = -2.5$)	
	1 (SDCR)	< 1 %ile ($z = -3.0$)	
	1 (LDFR)	< 1 %ile ($z = -2.5$)	
	1 (LDCR)	< 1 %ile ($z = -3.0$)	
	0.4 (d')	< 1 %ile ($z = -2.5$)	
	11 (hits)	2 %ile ($z = -2.0$)	
	17 (false positives)	< 1 %ile ($z = 3.5$)	

[a] Denotes subtest of the Wechsler Adult Intelligence Scale-Third edition *(WAIS-III)*
[b] Denotes subtest of the Wechsler Memory Scale-Third edition *(WMS-III)*
[c] Denotes subtest of the Delis–Kaplan Executive Function System *(D–KEFS)*

for verbatim repetition, with a capacity of five digits (four reliably). Consistent with his conversational word-finding difficulty, he had some trouble naming pictures on the Boston Naming Test, and while phonemic cues helped, they did not ameliorate the problem completely. Generation of words given initial letter cues (D–KEFS

Letter Fluency), and reasoning based on verbal material (WAIS-IV Similarities), were also performed at merely average levels, and he had trouble in the latter task expressing concepts due to word-finding difficulties. Simple copying of a set of symbols was placed around the lower bound of the average range.

The majority of test findings were unequivocally impaired. He demonstrated striking deficits in reasoning about pictorial materials (identifying missing elements in Picture Completion) and in generating flexible strategies on the Brixton Spatial Anticipation Test (Burgess and Shallice 1997). Generation of words based on a semantic theme (D–KEFS Category Fluency) was dramatically worse (by over 2 standard deviations) than when given an initial-letter cue; performance was equally impaired when required to switch between two categories (D–KEFS Category Switching). Speeded transcription of a set of symbols according to a numbered key (WAIS-III Digit Symbol-Coding) was very slow, and he verbalised his task to keep on track.

Analysis and action relating to complex visual stimuli was profoundly impaired. His copy of the Rey-Osterrieth Complex Figure was extremely disorganised in the approach taken and the end result was disfigured (see Fig. 13.1); he lost his place a number of times, resulting in translational shifts of clusters of elements into inappropriate locations.

He could learn no more than 5 words from a structured list of 16 repeated over 5 trials (CVLT-II), he remembered only one after a delay, and he was at chance picking the list words among distractors. In the nonverbal domain his memory for the figure he had copied 5 min previously was impoverished, and his immediate recognition memory for a series of photographs of faces was very poor (WMS-III Faces I).

Formulation

Mr J is a previously high-functioning executive with a 4-year history of word-finding difficulty, spatial disorientation and memory decline. There is a personal and family history of cardiovascular problems, with Mr J having atrial fibrillation and his father dying of a stroke following treatment for the same condition; he also has sleep apnoea and lowered mood.

Neuropsychological testing revealed severe deficits in a variety of cognitive domains, with profound deficits seen in learning and memory, and visuoconstruction. Flexible access to semantic memory was impaired, evident in a reversal of the usual pattern of better performance for category fluency compared with letter fluency. The "cortical" pattern of deficits was not consistent with an account in terms of depression or one implicating diffuse cerebrovascular changes (and an MRI of the brain showed no deep white matter ischaemia). Moreover, there had been no stepwise changes which might suggest a cumulative impact of multiple minor strokes (and there was no MRI evidence of strokes). The pattern could not be attributed to cerebral hypoxia due to sleep apnoea, which was mild and well treated, and while there was possible REM sleep behavioural disorder, there was no parkinsonism,

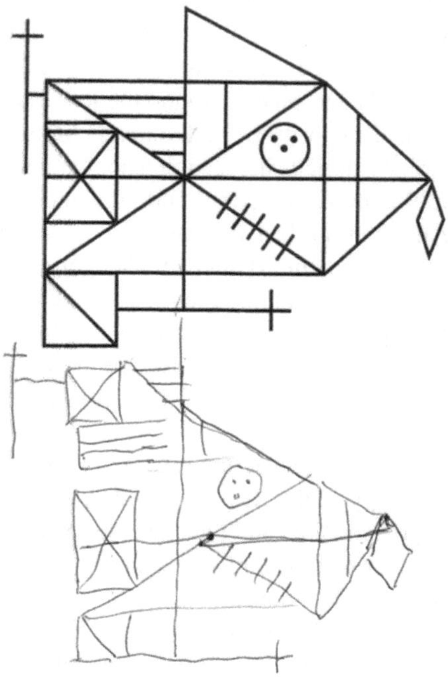

Fig. 13.1 Mr J's copy of the Rey-Osterrieth Complex Figure

fluctuations in consciousness or history of falls to implicate a diagnosis of dementia with Lewy bodies. Rather, the pattern was considered typical of Alzheimer's disease, and a subsequent FDG-PET scan revealed striking changes consistent with this diagnosis. A suggestion of atrophy from the MRI scan had initially been reported as being age-appropriate, but the referring neurologist interpreted the images as showing parietal atrophy and Scheltens Grade 3 hippocampal atrophy.

Even though neuropsychological testing revealed many signs of severe cognitive impairment, a question regarding Mr J's overall stage of decline is posed by the sizeable number of test findings placed around the average range or above. In addition, as with the case of Mr K, orientation and knowledge of recent news events were largely intact. The distribution of test outcomes relative to a threshold of impairment defined as 1.5 standard deviations below a normatively defined average level is shown in Fig. 13.2a. It is instructive to show how many of his *merely average* outcomes would be considered clearly abnormal if a threshold were to be anchored to his WTAR-predicted premorbid Full Scale IQ of 117 (bearing in mind this is likely an underestimate due to a ceiling effect on the WTAR). Figure 13.2b shows how few of his scores could be considered unimpaired when considered in light of what should be expected from Mr J normally.

The handful of relatively preserved thinking skills probably reflects his high level of *cognitive reserve* (Stern 2009), whereby a high intellectual level affords potential for flexible implementation of mental tactics leading to largely effective

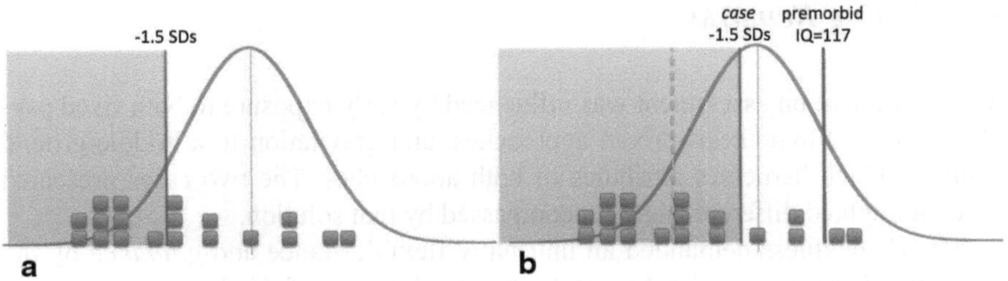

Fig. 13.2 Graphic depiction of Mr J's standard scores considered relative to **(a)** normatively defined abnormality, and **(b)** intra-individually defined abnormality

cognition (e.g. noticing idiosyncratic features such as bushy eyebrows in the face memory test). High cognitive reserve plausibly explains why Mr J was still able to function adequately at work, but reserve is thought to provide only short-term respite from the impact of brain disease, with rapid decline often becoming apparent once the pillars of reserve are eroded. Considering this potential for rapid decline, Mr J was counselled about retiring from work, and also ceasing driving, to avoid potentially grave consequences of cognitive errors which could be made in the business arena, and also on the road.

Reflection

The focus of formulation in Mr J's case centred on his high premorbid intellectual ability and likely associated cognitive reserve, which probably provided scaffolding for gradually failing thinking skills. These kinds of considerations are routine for most clinical neuropsychologists, but an explicit and reliable framework for making such considerations is not readily available.

In the context of a psychometric approach to assessment, a "numerical formulation" can be made by appeal to formal estimates of premorbid function such as the WTAR-predicted FSIQ. This method was used in Mr J's case primarily as a heuristic device, with explicit acknowledgment that it probably underestimated his expected abilities due to a ceiling effect. It also assumes that all cognitive abilities are equipotential in the first place, and that they decline together in synchrony; both of these assumptions cannot be upheld in any given case, and in particular, in cases representing the upper and lower tails of intellectual ability. A further limitation relates to the tests in use. The WTAR, for example, references verbally based expectations for other tests from the Wechsler batteries, but cannot speak for many other tests used by neuropsychologists. Furthermore, most tests are intrinsically unreliable when used with at the extremes of normally distributed cognitive abilities. Other adjustment methods appeal to demographic predictive equations, but the precision promised by these techniques falls short when the demographic conditions of the case in question do not match with those of the source data.

Concluding Remarks

My perspective on assessment was influenced by early exposure to both fixed psychometric and hypothesis-driven approaches, and gravitation to a middle-ground solution which harnesses attributes of both approaches. The two cases presented here highlighted different angles encompassed by that solution.

Mr K's deafness demanded an unusually flexible stance and *guidance* by the test data; formulation clearly involved consideration of predisposing vascular risks, and deafness as a precipitating and maintaining factor. The cognitive aspect of formulation proposed processing speed as an underpinning feature, which opened opportunities for considering other differentials such as cerebrovascular disease and depression. It also emphasised qualitative features such as intact orientation and what Mr K *could* achieve on testing, advocating against a diagnosis of Alzheimer's disease.

In contrast, formulation of Mr J's case leaned heavily on the data, but appealed to an overarching reference point of a WTAR-predicted FSIQ for their interpretation. The flexible battery precluded "by the book" comparisons of this premorbid estimate with WAIS-III index- or IQ-level summary scores—but these kinds of comparisons were not on the hypothesis-testing agenda in any case. Rather, individual test scores were interpreted against a general expectation that performances should have been distributed more or less around a level corresponding to a normative z-score of greater than 1. High premorbid intellect could be considered a predisposing factor in terms of masking a diagnosis, rather than suggesting one. On this account, cognitive reserve was scaffolding his functioning (he was well oriented and could discuss recent news events, and concerns had not been voiced about his performance at work), and a diagnosis might not have been reached if explicit consideration of decline relative to premorbid levels had not been given.

Adopting the perspective of *cognitive neuropsychological assessment*, I would suggest that clinicians using a typical flexible battery of tests can use the best psychometric tools available to *test* a specific patient, and then formulate an opinion drawing on multiple sources of data. These will necessarily include demographic aspects such as educational and vocational achievements (which in some cases may be difficult to quantify), qualitative features of the history and quasi-cognitive features of the case which may be difficult to quantify with customary rigor (e.g. aspects of mood state or personality captured by subjective questionnaires). The unique contribution a neuropsychologist can make, however, will be to answer a question about cognitive impairment with a formulation framed in cognitive terms.

References

Baddeley, A., Emslie, H., & Nimmo-Smith, I. (1994). *Doors and People*. Bury St Edmunds: Thames Valley Test Company.

Bowden, S. C. (1995). Hypothesis-testing in Australian neuropsychology. *Australian Psychologist, 30*(1), 35–38.

Burgess, P. W., & Shallice, T. (1997). *The Hayling and Brixton tests*. Thurston: Thames Valley Test Company.
Caine, D. (1995). Some determinants of method in neuropsychology. *Australian Psychologist, 30*(1), 39–41.
Crowe, S. F. (2010). *Evidence of absence: A guide to cognitive assessment in Australia*. Bowen Hills: Australian Academic.
Delis, D. C., Kramer, J. H., Kaplan, E., & Ober, B. A. (2000). *California Verbal Learning Test* (2nd ed.). (Adult Version). San Antonio: The Psychological Corporation.
Delis, D. C., Kaplan, E., & Kramer, J. H. (2001). *The Delis-Kaplan Executive Function System (D-KEFS)*. San Antonio: The Psychological Corporation.
Kaplan, E. F., Goodglass, H., & Weintraub, S. (2001). *The Boston Naming Test* (2nd ed.). Philadelphia: Lippincott Williams & Wilkins.
Kaufman, A. S. (1990). *Assessing adolescent and adult intelligence*. Needham: Allyn and Bacon.
Lin, F. R., Metter, E. J., O'Brien, R. J., Resnick, S. M., Zonderman, A. B., & Ferrucci, L. (2011). Hearing loss and incident dementia. *Archives of Neurology, 68*(2), 214–220.
Mapou, R. L. (1995a). A cognitive framework for neuropsychological assessment. In R. L. Mapou & J. Spector (Eds.), *Clinical neuropsychological assessment: A cognitive approach* (pp. 295–337). New York: Plenum Press.
Mapou, R. L. (1995b). Introduction. In R. L. Mapou & J. Spector (Eds.), *Clinical neuropsychological assessment: A cognitive approach* (pp. 1–13). New York: Plenum Press.
Meyers, J. E., & Meyers, K. R. (1995). *Rey complex figure test and recognition trial*. Odessa: Psychological Assessment Resources.
Pearson. (2009). *Advanced clinical solutions for the WAIS-IV and WMS-IV: Administration and scoring manual*. San Antonio: Author.
Rey, A. (1958). *L'examen clinique en psychologie*. Paris: Presse Universitaire de France.
Riddoch, M. J., & Humphreys, G. W. (Eds.). (1994). *Cognitive neuropsychology and cognitive rehabilitation*. Hove: Lawrence Erlbaum.
Robertson, I. H., Ward, T., Ridgeway, V., & Nimmo-Smith, I. (1994). *The Test of Everyday Attention*. Bury St Edmunds: Thames Valley Test Company.
Saling, M. M. (1995). Neuropsychology in the clinic: A comment on Caine (1995) and Bowden (1995). *Australian Psychologist, 30*(1), 42–44.
Stern, Y. (2009). Cognitive reserve. *Neuropsychologia, 47*(10), 2015–2028.
The Psychological Corporation. (2001). *Wechsler Test of Adult Reading*. New York: Author.
Walsh, K. W. (1991). *Understanding brain damage: A primer of neuropsychological evaluation* (2nd ed.). Edinburgh: Churchill Livingstone.
Walsh, K. (1992). Some gnomes worth knowing. *Clinical Neuropsychologist, 6*(2), 119–133.
Walsh, K. (2001). ASSBI's founding president reminisces. *Brain Impairment, 2*(1), 39–47.
Warrington, E. K., & James, M. (1991). *Visual Object and Space Perception Battery*. Bury St Edmunds: Thames Valley Test Company.
Wechsler, D. (1997a). *Wechsler Adult Intelligence Scale* (3rd ed.). San Antonio: The Psychological Corporation.
Wechsler, D. (1997b). *Wechsler Memory Scale* (3rd ed.). San Antonio: The Psychological Corporation.
Wechsler, D. (2008). *Wechsler Adult Intelligence Scale* (4th ed.). San Antonio: Pearson.
Wechsler, D. (2009). *Wechsler Memory Scale* (4th ed.). San Antonio: Pearson.

Index

J. A. B. Macniven (ed.), *Neuropsychological Formulation*,
DOI 10.1007/978-3-319-18338-1

MIX
Papier aus verantwortungsvollen Quellen
Paper from responsible sources
FSC® C105338

If you have any concerns about our products,
you can contact us on
ProductSafety@springernature.com

In case Publisher is established outside the EU,
the EU authorized representative is:
Springer Nature Customer Service Center GmbH
Europaplatz 3, 69115 Heidelberg, Germany

Printed by Libri Plureos GmbH
in Hamburg, Germany